Cancer Clinical Trials

Current and Controversial Issues in Design and Analysis

Chapman & Hall/CRC Biostatistics Series

Published Titles

Adaptive Design Methods in Clinical Trials, Second Edition
Shein-Chung Chow and Mark Chang

Adaptive Designs for Sequential Treatment Allocation
Alessandro Baldi Antognini and Alessandra Giovagnoli

Adaptive Design Theory and Implementation Using SAS and R, Second Edition
Mark Chang

Advanced Bayesian Methods for Medical Test Accuracy
Lyle D. Broemeling

Advances in Clinical Trial Biostatistics
Nancy L. Geller

Applied Meta-Analysis with R
Ding-Geng (Din) Chen and Karl E. Peace

Basic Statistics and Pharmaceutical Statistical Applications, Second Edition
James E. De Muth

Bayesian Adaptive Methods for Clinical Trials
Scott M. Berry, Bradley P. Carlin, J. Jack Lee, and Peter Muller

Bayesian Analysis Made Simple: An Excel GUI for WinBUGS
Phil Woodward

Bayesian Methods for Measures of Agreement
Lyle D. Broemeling

Bayesian Methods for Repeated Measures
Lyle D. Broemeling

Bayesian Methods in Epidemiology
Lyle D. Broemeling

Bayesian Methods in Health Economics
Gianluca Baio

Bayesian Missing Data Problems: EM, Data Augmentation and Noniterative Computation
Ming T. Tan, Guo-Liang Tian, and Kai Wang Ng

Bayesian Modeling in Bioinformatics
Dipak K. Dey, Samiran Ghosh, and Bani K. Mallick

Benefit-Risk Assessment in Pharmaceutical Research and Development
Andreas Sashegyi, James Felli, and Rebecca Noel

Benefit-Risk Assessment Methods in Medical Product Development: Bridging Qualitative and Quantitative Assessments
Qi Jiang and Weili He

Biosimilars: Design and Analysis of Follow-on Biologics
Shein-Chung Chow

Chapman & Hall/CRC Biostatistics Series

Cancer Clinical Trials

Current and Controversial Issues in Design and Analysis

Edited by

Stephen L. George

Duke University School of Medicine

Durham, North Carolina, USA

Xiaofei Wang

Duke University School of Medicine

Durham, North Carolina, USA

Herbert Pang

The University of Hong Kong

Hong Kong, China

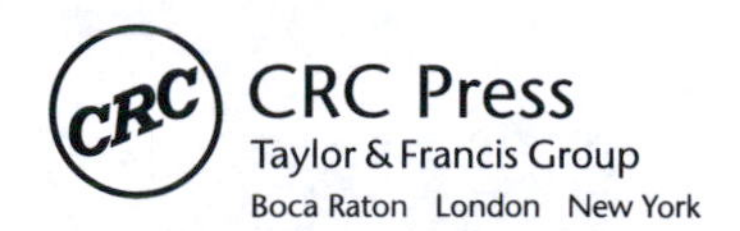

CRC Press is an imprint of the
Taylor & Francis Group, an **informa** business
A CHAPMAN & HALL BOOK

CRC Press
Taylor & Francis Group
6000 Broken Sound Parkway NW, Suite 300
Boca Raton, FL 33487-2742

Printed on acid-free paper
Version Date: 20160414

International Standard Book Number-13: 978-1-4987-0688-9 (Hardback)

Visit the Taylor & Francis Web site at
http://www.taylorandfrancis.com

and the CRC Press Web site at
http://www.crcpress.com

Printed and bound in the United States of America by Publishers Graphics,
LLC on sustainably sourced paper.

To Ed Gehan and Marvin Zelen, who early in my career taught me much about the art and science of cancer biostatistics and served as role models while doing so.
– Stephen L. George

To my beloved family and in memory of my father.
– Xiaofei Wang

To my parents and mentors at Duke, the CALGB, and the Alliance for their support and guidance in my quest for knowledge in the field of cancer clinical trials.
– Herbert Pang

Contents

Preface

There are many important and controversial topics in the design and analysis of cancer clinical trials, including adaptive approaches, biomarker-based trials, and dynamic treatment regime trials. This book provides readers with a current understanding of the critical issues in these and other topics with state-of-the-art approaches. Each chapter is written by well-known statisticians from academic institutions, regulatory agencies (FDA), the National Cancer Institute, or the pharmaceutical industry, all with extensive experience in cancer clinical trials. Examples are taken from actual cancer clinical trials. The topics covered are:

- Endpoints for cancer clinical trials (Chapter 1)
- Use of historical data (Chapter 2)
- Multiplicity (Chapter 3)
- Analysis of safety data (Chapter 4)
- Development and validation of predictive signatures (Chapter 5)
- Phase I trials and dose-finding (Chapter 6)
- Design and analysis of phase II cancer clinical trials (Chapter 7)
- Sample size for survival trials in cancer (Chapter 8)
- Non-inferiority trials (Chapter 9)
- Quality of life (Chapter 10)
- Biomarker-based clinical trials (Chapter 11)
- Adaptive clinical trial designs in oncology (Chapter 12)
- Dynamic treatment regimes (Chapter 13)

Our focus is on cancer clinical trials and the topics covered are important in cancer trials. Many of these topics have less understood or controversial aspects. In addition, most of the issues addressed in this book are important for clinical trials in other settings. The primary audience for readers of this book will be statisticians with university postgraduate training working in cancer clinical trials in industry, government, and academia. Although it is not intended as a textbook, teachers of clinical trials classes may find this book useful as a supplementary text in their classes.

We would like to acknowledge the partial support from the National Cancer Institute of the National Institutes of Health under award number CA142538.

Stephen L. George
Xiaofei Wang
Herbert Pang

Editors

Stephen L. George, Ph.D., is Professor Emeritus of Biostatistics in the Department of Biostatistics and Bioinformatics in the Duke University School of Medicine. He served for over 20 years as Director of Biostatistics in the Duke Comprehensive Cancer Center and Director of the Statistical Center of the Cancer and Leukemia Group B (CALGB). He has been closely involved in the design, conduct, and analysis of cancer clinical trials and other research projects in cancer throughout his career. He has served on and chaired data monitoring committees for treatment and prevention trials in cancer and other diseases. Dr. George is a Fellow of the American Statistical Association and of the Society for Clinical Trials; served as Treasurer and a member of the Executive Committee of the International Biometric Society for eight years; is a past President for the Society for Clinical Trials; and served for four years as the biostatistician for the Oncologic Drugs Advisory Committee for the Food and Drug Administration.

Xiaofei Wang, Ph.D., obtained his Ph.D. in Biostatistics from the University of North Carolina at Chapel Hill. He is currently an Associate Professor of Biostatistics and Bioinformatics at Duke University School of Medicine, a member of Duke Cancer Institute (DCI), and the Director of Statistics of the Alliance Statistics and Data Center. The Alliance for Clinical Trials in Oncology is part of the NCI's Clinical Trials Network (NCTN). He has been involved in design and analysis of cancer clinical trials and translational studies in the past twelve years at Alliance, CALGB, and DCI. He is an associate editor for Statistics in Biopharmaceutical Research and has served on special emphasis panels for NIH and FDA grants. His methodology research is focused on the development of novel designs and methods for biomarker-integrated clinical studies, and methods for analyzing patient data from multiple sources.

Herbert Pang, Ph.D., obtained his Ph.D. in Biostatistics from Yale University and B.A. in Mathematics and Computer Science from the University of Oxford. He is an assistant professor at the School of Public Health, Li Ka Shing Faculty of Medicine (LKSFM), the University of Hong Kong. Dr. Pang now holds an adjunct faculty position in the Department of Biostatistics and Bioinformatics at Duke University. He has been involved in the design, monitoring, and analysis of cancer clinical trials, translational, and big data-omics research in cancer for the CALGB, Alliance, Duke Cancer Institute, and LKSFM. He served on the editorial board of the Journal of Clinical Oncology. Dr. Pang received the Yale Graduate Fellowship, travel award/grant from the NIH, American Association for Cancer Research, Burroughs Wellcome Fund, and American Statistical Association, as well as the US Chinese Anti-Cancer Association-Asian Fund for Cancer Research Scholar Award.

Contributors

Frank Bretz
Norvatis
Basel, Switzerland

Mark R. Conaway
Department of Public Health Sciences
University of Virginia
Charlottesville, Virginia

Marie Davidian
Department of Statistics
North Carolina State University
Raleigh, North Carolina

Diane Fairclough
Department of Biostatistics & Informatics
University of Colorado
Aurora, Colorado

Boris Freidlin
Biometric Research Branch
Division of Cancer Treatment and Diagnosis
National Cancer Institute
Bethesda, Maryland

Stephen L. George
Department of Biostatistics & Bioinformatics
Duke University
Durham, North Carolina

Ekkehard Glimm
Norvatis
Basel, Switzerland

Thomas Gwise
Office of Biostatistics
Center for Drug Evaluation and Research
US Food and Drug Administration
Silver Spring, Maryland

Qi Jiang
Global Biostatistical Science
Amgen
Thousand Oaks, California

Sin-Ho Jung
Department of Biostatistics & Bioinformatics
Duke University
Durham, North Carolina

Edward L. Korn
Biometric Research Branch
Division of Cancer Treatment and Diagnosis
National Cancer Institute
Bethesda, Maryland

Eric Laber
Department of Statistics
North Carolina State University
Raleigh, North Carolina

Edward Lakatos
BiostatHaven Inc
Croton on Hudson, New York

J. Jack Lee
Department of Biostatistics
The University of Texas MD Anderson Cancer Center
Houston, Texas

Lisa M. McShane
Biometric Research Branch
National Cancer Institute
Bethesda, Maryland

Beat Neuenschwander
Oncology Biometrics and Data Management
Novartis Pharma AG
Basel, Switzerland

Herbert Pang
School of Public Health
Li Ka Shing Faculty of Medicine
The University of Hong Kong
Hong Kong SAR, China

Michael C. Sachs
Biometric Research Branch
National Cancer Institute
Bethesda, Maryland

Heinz Schmidli
Statistical Methodology
Novartis Pharma AG
Basel, Switzerland

Steven Snapinn
Global Biostatistical Science
Amgen
Thousand Oaks, California

Rajeshwari Sridhara
Office of Biostatistics
Center for Drug Evaluation and Research
US Food and Drug Administration
Silver Spring, Maryland

Lorenzo Trippa
Department of Biostatistics
Harvard T. H. Chan School of Public Health
Dana-Farber Cancer Institute
Boston, Massachusetts

Anastasios (Butch) Tsiatis
Department of Statistics
North Carolina State University
Raleigh, North Carolina

Nolan A. Wages
Department of Public Health Sciences
University of Virginia
Charlottesville, Virginia

Simon Wandel
Oncology Biometrics and Data Management
Novartis Pharma AG
Basel, Switzerland

Xiaofei Wang
Department of Biostatistics & Bioinformatics
Duke University
Durham, North Carolina

Dong Xi
Norvatis
East Hanover, New Jersey

Part I

General Issues

1

Endpoints for Cancer Clinical Trials

Stephen L. George

Xiaofei Wang

Herbert Pang

CONTENTS

1.1 Introduction

The selection of appropriate endpoints for a clinical trial is an extremely important step in determining the appropriate design and analysis for the trial [106, 107]. An endpoint is ordinarily taken to mean an efficacy endpoint, a measure of the clinical efficacy of the treatments under consideration, although safety endpoints are also important. In this chapter we focus primarily on the key efficacy endpoints commonly used in cancer clinical trials, describing their strengths and weaknesses and, where appropriate, controversies surrounding their use.

In cancer trials, the most common practice is to specify a single primary endpoint and a primary trial objective based on this endpoint, used for setting the key design and analysis specifications. Other endpoints and objectives are usually relegated to secondary or exploratory roles. However, an increasingly common practice is to define co-primary endpoints and objectives, necessitating appropriate statistical adjustments for the resultant multiplicity [96].

Examples of endpoints commonly used in cancer clinical trials include overall survival, generally agreed to be the gold standard efficacy endpoint; tumor response rate or other endpoints based on tumor measurements; composite endpoints such as progression-free survival and similar endpoints combining individual endpoints that may serve as surrogate endpoints for overall survival; patient-reported endpoints such as quality of life; and promising new approaches for defining endpoints including pharmacokinetic and pharmacodynamics responses, imaging techniques, and biomarker-based endpoints. These endpoints are summarized in Table 1.1 and are all discussed in more detail in the following sections of this chapter.

The particular endpoints chosen for a clinical trial will depend on many factors including the phase of the trial, the cost and feasibility of assessing the endpoint, the follow-up studies planned, and other factors. A simple statement of an endpoint to be used is not sufficient to define the specific aspect of the endpoint and the specific objectives that will be addressed in the trial. For example, comparing treatments via an endpoint such as overall survival or other time-to-event endpoints can be assessed in terms of the entire survival distribution, hazard ratios, median survival time differences, survival probabilities at some prespecified time point (e.g., 5 years), or other measures. The exact specification of the endpoint is an important detail and will determine key aspects of both design and analysis of the trial.

TABLE 1.1: Endpoints in Cancer Clinical Trials

Endpoint	Advantages	Disadvantages
OS	Clinically relevant outcome Easily measured	Affected by crossover designs and subsequent therapies Longer follow-up time required Includes deaths from other causes
PFS, TTP	Not confounded by post-progression survival Smaller sample size than for OS	Subject to assessment and investigator bias Interval-censored data Only partially validated as a surrogate in most diseases Missing data issues
Tumor RR	Standardized, easily applicable to multicenter trials Early outcome Useful in early phase trials	Measurement imprecision Difficult to assess some tumor types (e.g., mesothelioma) Correlation with patient benefit variable
Quality of life	Indicative of direct patient benefit Patient-reported outcome	Multiple comparisons problems Requires validated instruments Time-intensive evaluation Missing data issues
Pharmacokinetics/ Pharmacodynamics	Very early assessment of drug activity Possibly allows for dose adjustment	Costly and time-consuming Not a direct measure of clinical benefit
Imaging	May allow early assessment of antitumor effect	May add little to response assessment Costly and time-consuming Difficult to combine results across institutions
Molecular biomarkers	May be predictive and allow patient enrichment May provide additional insight into resistance mechanisms	Usually not validated as a surrogate of efficacy

There have been recent efforts by regulatory authorities and others to define the appropriate endpoints for trials of cancer treatment, both in general and for specific diseases. For example, the US Food and Drug Administration (FDA) has issued general guidelines for industry on endpoints appropriate for use when seeking regulatory approval for marketing of cancer drugs and biologics [98]. Specific FDA guidance documents for non-small cell lung cancer (NSCLC) and for imaging endpoints have also been published [100, 101]. Similarly, a European project entitled Definition for the Assessment of Time-to-event Endpoints in CANcer trials (DATECAN) aims to provide recommendations for time-to-event endpoints used in cancer clinical trials [10]. DATECAN guidelines for GIST tumors and pancreatic cancer have been recently published [9, 13]. Recommendations for hepatocellular carcinoma [63] and others have been published.

1.2 Overall Survival

Overall survival (OS), the time from randomization (for randomized trials) or from trial registration (for non-randomized trials) to death from any cause, is generally acknowledged as the gold standard endpoint for cancer clinical trials [76]. It reflects an obviously important clinical outcome, is easy to measure, and does not suffer from potential ascertainment or other biases existing for other endpoints. However, trials with objectives related to OS are generally quite large and may require a lengthy follow-up period. Surrogate endpoints for overall survival, discussed in detail below, are often used to reduce the size and duration of a planned trial.

In addition, there are other limitations and drawbacks in analysis and interpretation when using OS as a primary endpoint in cancer trials. For example, Phase I and II clinical trials are relatively small trials designed to determine an appropriate dose or schedule for an agent or to detect some minimal activity and, with rare exceptions, OS would in general not be an appropriate primary endpoint for such trials. Even for phase III cancer trials, in which OS is nearly always an important endpoint, there are difficulties. Most cancer therapies are given over a prolonged period of time, thereby increasing the probability of non-adherence to the assigned treatment. Even with excellent adherence to the originally assigned treatment regimen, cancer patients typically move through various disease states prior to death (e.g., patients may experience a disease recurrence or disease progression), often requiring additional treatments at each change in state. These treatments are often difficult or impossible to specify fully in advance and in many settings (e.g., breast cancer) there are effective post-trial therapies that complicate the interpretation of OS [86]. Thus, a clinical trial designed to compare the OS of two initial treatments becomes increasingly difficult to interpret if there are intervening additional treatments given prior to death. An extreme example occurs when crossover or switch to the alternative treatment is allowed at progression or relapse [110].

1.3 Endpoints Based on Tumor Measurements

1.3.1 RECIST Criteria

In solid tumors, tumor response is measured in terms of tumor growth or shrinkage. Although it is still subject to criticism, response evaluation criteria in solid tumor (RECIST) has become widely accepted as the preferred method to assess tumor changes. RECIST was first published in 2000 as version 1.0 [97] and revised in 2009 as version 1.1 [34]. The establishment of RECIST was based on the WHO criteria [109], the first internationally recognized criteria for assessment of solid tumor response. Unlike the WHO criteria, which measures tumor responses based on 2D imaging, RECIST uses 1D imaging assessment to define response. To evaluate tumor changes per RECIST, tumor lesions are classified as being target or non-target prior to study entry, and lesions characteristics (e.g., location), measures and the method used to assess the lesions are recorded. At prespecified time intervals, pre-identified lesions are repeatedly measured and any new identified lesions are also evaluated. The overall tumor response at each time point is defined as follow:

- Complete Response (CR)

  Disappearance of all lesions (target and non-target)

  No new lesions diagnosed

  Sustained at least four weeks, when confirmation is required

- Partial Response (PR)

  Greater than 30% decrease in the sum of the longest diameters (SLD) of target lesions taking the baseline SLD as reference

  No evidence of progression in any of the non-target lesions diagnosed at baseline

  No new lesions diagnosed

- Progressive Disease (PD)

  Greater than 20% increase in the SLD of target lesions taking the smallest SLD as reference, where the smallest SLD should be more than $5mm$

  The progression of a non-target lesion

  The appearance of a new lesion

- Stable (SD)

  Neither sufficient shrinkage to qualify for PR nor sufficient increase to qualify for PD, taking as reference the smallest SLD since the treatment started

Table 1.2 summarizes how overall response is determined based on tumor changes in target, non-target, and new lesions at the patient level. Best overall response (BOR) for a patient is defined as the best response evaluated from the start of the treatment until disease progression/recurrence. BOR represents the best response level achieved among all overall responses with the rule that CR is better than PR and PR is better than SD. Study endpoints to measure drug activities can be defined on the occurrence and the durance of certain response types. Objective response rate (ORR) denotes the proportion of patients with at least one CR/PR. Disease control rate (DCR) is the proportion of patients with at least one CR/PR/SD. Response duration (DR) is the time from first assessment of CR/PR until date of progression or last tumor assessment. Per RECIST 1.1, when response rate and its confidence interval are reported for a clinical trial, all patients included in a clinical trial should be assigned one of the following categories: 1) CR, 2) PR, 3) SD, 4) PD, 5) early death from malignant disease or toxicity or other cause, and 6) unknown (not assessable, insufficient data). All of the patients who met eligibility criteria should be included in the denominator when calculating the response rate. Patients in response categories 4–6 should be considered as disease progression. Supplementary analyses may be performed on various subsets of patients, e.g., excluding those with protocol deviations or early death. For most solid tumors, endpoints, such as progression-free survival (PFS) or time to progression (TTP), are also based on assessments of tumor changes per RECIST. For example, TTP is the time from the start of the treatment until tumor progression (PD) with other events, including death, treated as "censored."

TABLE 1.2: Evaluation of Best Overall Response (BOR)

Target Lesions	**Non-target Lesions**	**New Lesions**	**Overall Response**
CR	CR	No	CR
CR	Incomplete response/SD	No	PR
PR	Non-PD	No	PR
SD	Non-PD	No	SD
PD	Any	Yes or No	PD
Any	PD	Yes or No	PD
Any	Any	Yes	PD

1.3.2 Response Rate as Primary Endpoints

In many diseases and treatment settings, there exists a strong association between tumor response and progression (or survival). It is also commonly believed that drugs that induce tumor response are biologically active and may lead to improved survival or decreased symptoms. Response rate can be assessed using smaller trials in less time because of a bigger effect size and shorter required follow-up as compared to PFS and OS. For these reasons, response rate is frequently used as the primary endpoint for phase II trials with both single-arm and randomized designs. The hope is that the trials with response rate as the primary endpoint will lead to an early decision of whether a drug is promising enough to warrant further investigation in phase III trials.

The RECIST criteria for tumor response were designed primarily to assess cytotoxic agents and the appropriateness of evaluating tumor response to target agents and immunotherapy via RECIST has been challenged. In many recent clinical trials that involve molecularly targeted agents, tumor shrinkage has failed to translate into clear clinical benefit of patient symptom and survival. One possible reason is that the early activity of target agents, such as the EGFR-inhibitors and the VEGF-inhibitors, that occurs before tumor shrinkage might not be measured appropriately with conventional criteria such as RECIST [68]. There are also cases of cytostatic agents that significantly prolong PFS and OS but don't significantly change the size of the tumor. In evaluating immunotherapeutic agents, such as ipilimumab, there is evidence that durable modest regressions or prolonged disease stability may be signalling a sustained improvement of survival, but tumor response per RECIST does not consider these aspects of tumor response. As a result, modified immune-response-related criteria were proposed to optimize the assessment of tumor response or progression to immunotherapy [71, 108]. For these and other reasons, the use of response rate to measure tumor response in phase II trials is becoming drug- and/or disease-specific. Meanwhile, more randomized phase II trials are now conducted with PFS or OS as primary endpoints with inflated type I error [85] to control the size of the trial. Alternative strategies, such as designs utilizing RR as a co-primary endpoint with PFS [84] and randomized discontinuation designs [79], have also been proposed to address the problem of a weak connection between response rate and gold standard endpoints such as PFS and OS.

Response rate is rarely chosen as the primary endpoint in phase III trials. The current stance of FDA is that cancer drug approval should be based on more direct evidence of clinical benefit, such as improvements in overall survival (OS), health-related quality of life, tumor-related symptoms, and/or physical functioning [76]. However, exceptions do exist. For example, response rate has been used as the primary endpoint for FDA accelerated approval trials, where limited accrual is anticipated for rare diseases. Complete response (CR) has also led to regular approval of drugs for treating acute leukemia [25], because response of significant magnitude and duration has been shown to be associated with longer OS in this disease.

1.3.3 Tumor Response as Continuous Variable

Concerns over the high failure rate in phase III trials has led to pursuing alternatives to RECIST response as a phase II endpoint. One criticism of using response rate per RECIST as the phase II primary endpoint is the arbitrariness of classifying patients into four categories: CR, PR, SD, and PD. For example, when a patient experiences a 19% versus 21% increase in disease, this indicates a difference between SD and PD per RECIST. Similarly, 29% versus 31% decrease in disease signals a difference between SD and PR. In reality, such small changes in SLD do not constitute a substantial change in the patient's disease state. The arbitrariness of response classification underscores the inherent difficulty in using categorical measures to summarize tumor changes for drug effect evaluation in clinical trials.

Important information is potentially ignored when the continuum of tumor change is categorized into groups [61]. The use of tumor response as a continuous variable has been hypothesized to be more informative than categorical variables [3, 4]. Waterfall and spider plots are data visualization techniques that display tumor shrinkage as observed % change of SLD from baseline. This continuous 'measure' provides a visual indication of the treatment effect in reducing the tumor burden [32]. As an example, CALGB 30704 is a randomized phase II trial comparing pemetrexed, sunitinib, or their combination as second-line chemotherapy for advanced non-small cell lung cancer (NSCLC) [49]. Tumor burden, measured as the SLD of target lesions, was collected for all randomized patients within 30 days of registration and then every 2 cycles during protocol treatments and every 6 weeks until progression. Waterfall plot and spider plot are used to display the percent change of tumor burden during treatment relative to baseline for 39 patients on pemetrexed and 37 patients on sunitinib. As illustrated in Figure 1.1, each vertical line of a water plot represents the tumor shrinkage of each patient receiving the treatment. One advantage of waterfall plot is its capability of showing tumor measures for patients within the RECIST categories. In Figure 1.2, a spider plot represents tumor percent growth of these patients relative to baseline. Waterfall plot and spider plot have become important tools to display graphically the continuous percent change of tumor measurements. The continuous measures can be analyzed quantitatively by summarizing the mean (SD) and compared between groups using a t or Wilcoxon test. Waterfall plots and spider plots have been used effectively to show the benefit of some treatments, such as sorafenib in renal cell carcinoma [81] and erlotinib in NSCLC [90].

Treating tumor changes as a continuous variable is also considered to correlate better with patient survival. Unfortunately, studies so far have shown no improvement in the usefulness of assessing tumor response as a continuous variable as compared with RECIST measures [3, 4, 32, 64, 89]. In renal

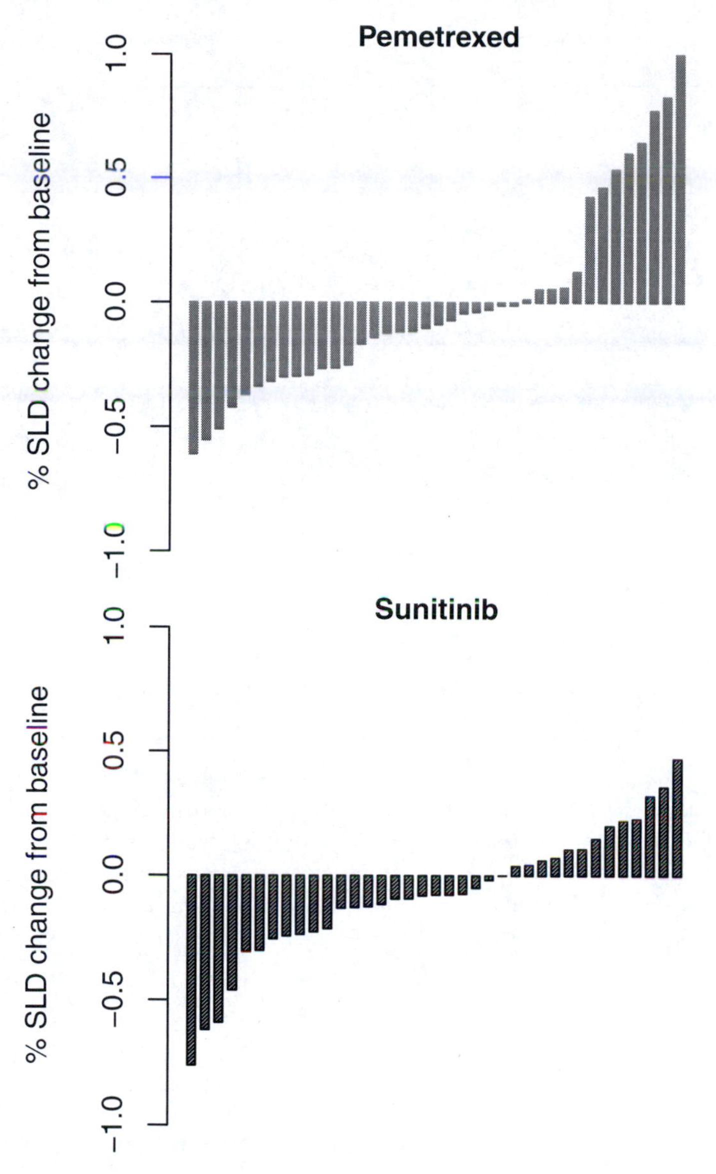

FIGURE 1.1: Waterfall plot for tumor shrinkage as continuous measurement.

cell cancer, Stein et al. [94] used mathematical models to calculate constants that describe the exponential decrease and growth of the tumor burden for each patient treated on a phase III trial comparing sunitinib vs. interferon-α. They found that the median tumor growth constant of patients receiving sunitinib was significantly lower than for those receiving interferon-α, which is consistent with survival benefit of sunitinib over interferon found in the phase

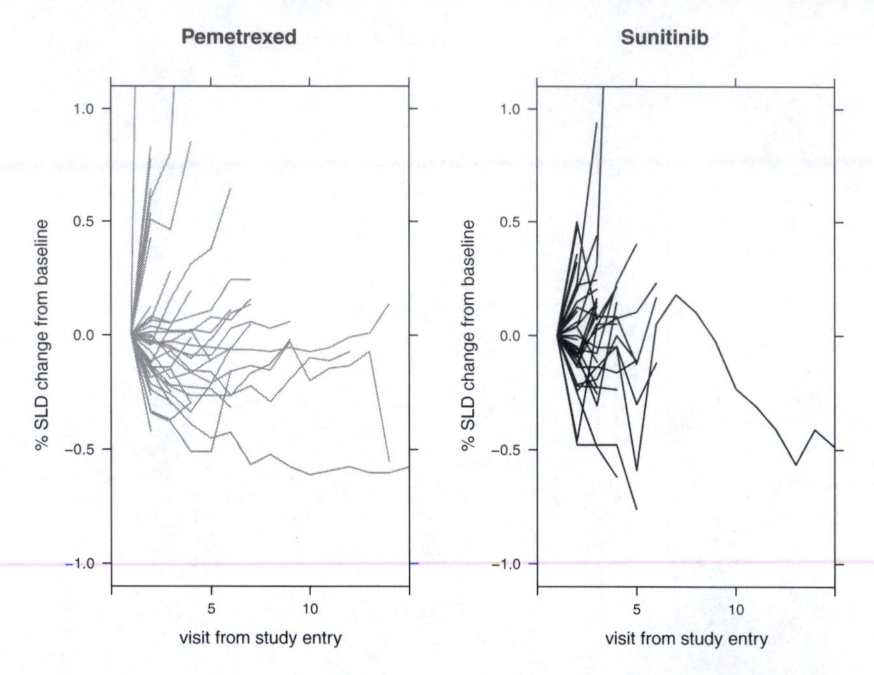

FIGURE 1.2: Spider plot for tumor shrinkage as continuous measurement.

III trial [70]. The investigators suggested that calculation of a tumor growth constant could be an effective surrogate endpoint for overall survival. Tumor growth modeling has also been studied in lung cancer [103] and has led to the proposal of a randomized trial that uses early tumor growth, rather than PFS, as a primary endpoint [55]. The utility of analyzing tumor growth as a continuous variable or the estimation of parameters of tumor growth model has yet to prove its value.

1.4 Progression-free Survival and Other Composite Endpoints

A composite endpoint is one in which there are several components. In cancer, the most common examples are progression-free survival (PFS) for advanced cancer, defined as the time to progression or death, whichever comes first, and, for early stage cancer, disease-free survival (DFS) or recurrence-free survival (RFS), defined as the time to disease recurrence or death, whichever comes first [15]. These are the composite analogues of the endpoints time to progression (TTP) and time to recurrence (TTR), respectively, which do not count death without progression or recurrence as an event. Other composite endpoints such as duration of disease control (DDC) and time to failure of strategy (TFS) have also been proposed in specific settings such as advanced colorectal cancer [22], but have been rarely used to date.

There are many important statistical issues to consider when using time-to-event composite endpoints [11, 20, 31, 40, 50, 59, 73]. One complication is that the contribution of the individual components may be lost and, for the most commonly used composite endpoints in cancer described above (PFS, DFS), there is a "competing risks" problem [67]. In addition, the treatment effects on one component (e.g., deaths from other causes) may be very different from the effect on other components (e.g., disease progression), complicating the interpretation of the results. And if it is thought that the composite endpoint can serve in some sense as a "surrogate" for overall survival, one is faced with the task of validating that this is true in the particular setting under study, a difficult task discussed in a later section of this chapter. Careful analyses of additional outcomes after progression or recurrence, such as time to subsequent progression and post-progression survival, may provide additional insights in addition to PFS and OS [29, 65]. In general, the correlation between PFS and OS has been found to be inversely related to the duration of post-progression survival [2].

Nevertheless, composite endpoints have become increasingly used in cancer clinical trials and PFS and DFS in particular have been commonly used to approve new therapies for specific indications in the U.S. and Europe [35], either as the basis for accelerated approval when PFS or DFS can be considered as "surrogates" for overall survival or for full approval when they can be considered as measures of direct clinical benefit themselves [98]. Indeed, improvement in PFS is now the most common endpoint used as the basis for FDA approval of an indication in the advanced or metastatic disease setting [82]. And these endpoints are becoming more common in all clinical trials. In trials involving breast, colorectal, and non-small cell lung cancer patients reported in the *Journal of Clinical Oncology* from 1975 through 2009 the percentage of trials using PFS or TTP was only 4% (13 of 321) prior to 2005 but 26% (35 of 137) from 2005 through 2009 [14, 56]. The increasing popularity of PFS is due in part because the endpoint is reached early and in part because in many diseases, whether or not the endpoint is a surrogate for overall survival, improvement in the composite endpoint itself reflects treatment benefit. For example delay in progression may delay symptoms and additional treatment complications even if overall survival is not affected, so an improvement in PFS may be a clinical benefit even with no improvement in overall survival. In addition, for composite endpoints such as PFS or DFS, post-progression (or post-recurrence) treatment and survival do not complicate the assessment and interpretation of the results.

Any time-to-event endpoint requires a clear definition of an "event" and clear rules for censoring. In the case of overall survival the conventions are straightforward. A death (any cause) represents an event and censoring occurs at the last time the patient is known to be alive. For composite endpoints such as PFS or DFS, the definitions and conventions are not so obvious and studies in the same disease may use different definitions and conventions [38]. In addition, the definition of progression, generally based on the Response Evaluation Criteria In Solid Tumors (RECIST) [34], is not without difficulties [72]. Guidance for the appropriate definitions and conventions for PFS and DFS have been provided by regulatory agencies [36, 100, 101] and others [28, 95].

1.5 Surrogate Endpoints

1.5.1 Definition

Because of the complexity and the high cost of developing and demonstrating clinically meaningful efficacy and tolerable toxicity, the approval for effective and safe cancer drugs has been slow. On the other hand, there are increasingly more cancer drugs available to test in clinical trials. This has created a call for alternative and potentially faster approval processes based on surrogate endpoints. Overall survival (OS) is the gold standard endpoint for evaluating the effect of new therapy in cancer. However, compared to progression-free survival (PFS), it requires large number of patients and long follow-up to accumulate sufficient number of events to achieve adequate statistical power. There is a great need in cancer research to find and validate surrogate endpoints, that are able to accurately capture the treatment effect, that are cheap to measure, and that achieve the required number of events earlier than OS. Meanwhile, the rapid advances in molecular biology, in particular the -omics revolution and the advent of new drugs with molecular mechanisms, dramatically increase the number of biomarkers that can potentially be used as surrogate endpoints [62].

The definition of a surrogate endpoint is complex and controversial. According to the NIH Biomarkers Definitions Working Group [26], a clinical endpoint is a characteristic or variable that reflects how a patient feels, functions or survives, and a surrogate endpoint is defined as a biomarker intended to act as a clinical endpoint. The property of a surrogate is that the "effect of the intervention on the clinical endpoint is reliably predicted by the effect of the intervention on the surrogate endpoint" [39]. Consider a simple setting, where Z is a binary indicator for treatment group, S is the surrogate endpoint to be validated, T is true endpoint. For example, Z may be a new target agent for treating metastatic non-small cell lung cancer, S is progression-free survival and T is overall survival time. A good candidate for a surrogate endpoint S is measured earlier than the true endpoint (T), is an intermediate biological indicator in a disease progression process, but ultimately, surrogate endpoint should serve as a substitute for the true endpoint and make a trial cheaper and faster to conduct.

A surrogate endpoint is an alternative endpoint (e.g., biological markers, physical sign, etc.) that if validated allows conclusions to be made about the effect of a treatment on a true endpoint (e.g., a clinical meaningful endpoint), often requiring a shorter "observation" period. An example is the use of objective response rate (ORR) and progression-free survival (PFS) in phase II/III trials. It is important to note that a surrogate endpoint may be valid for a particular indication (e.g., a particular drug for colon cancer) and not for other indications (e.g., the same drug for non-small cell lung cancer).

1.5.2 Surrogate Endpoint Validation

The evaluation and validation of putative surrogate endpoints in clinical trials is a controversial topic in methodological and applied statistics. Prentice [78] proposed a definition of a surrogate endpoint as "a response variable for which a test of the null hypothesis of no relationship to the treatment groups under comparison is also a valid test of the corresponding null hypothesis based on the true endpoint." A validation of perfect surrogacy ($Z \rightarrow S \rightarrow T$) in particular involves validation of the following four conditions:

- Treatment has a significant impact on the surrogate endpoint: $f(T|Z) \neq f(T)$
- Treatment has a significant impact on the true endpoint: $f(T|Z) \neq f(T)$
- The surrogate endpoint has a significant impact on the true endpoint: $f(T|S) \neq f(T)$
- The full effect of treatment upon the true endpoint is captured by the surrogate: $f(T|S, Z) = f(T|S)$

Under these conditions, it can be shown that a test of null hypothesis $E(S|Z = 0) = E(S|Z = 1)$ is a valid test of $E(T|Z = 0) = E(T|Z = 1)$, or S is a perfect surrogate endpoint for T.

Freedman et al. [42] argued that Prentice's fourth criterion raises a conceptual difficulty since it requires the statistical test for treatment effect on the true endpoint to be nonsignificant after adjustment for the surrogate. These authors argued that the nonsignificance of this test does not prove that the effect of treatment upon the true endpoint is fully captured by the surrogate. In particular, they proposed a proportion of treatment effect explained (F) for less than perfect surrogacy. Consider $Z \rightarrow S \rightarrow T$ and $Z \rightarrow T$. For example, $E(T|Z) = \alpha_0 + \alpha_1 Z$ and $E(T|Z, S) = \beta_0 + \beta_1 Z + \beta_2 S$. The proportion of treatment effect explained by S is defined as

$$F = \frac{\text{the treatment effect on } T \text{ explained by } S}{\text{the treatment effect on } T} = \frac{\alpha_1 - \beta_1}{\alpha_1}$$

It has been argued that what is required to replace the clinical endpoint by the surrogate is that the effect of the treatment on the surrogate endpoint reliably predicts the effect on the clinical endpoint [19].

For these and other reasons, Prentice's criteria have been criticized as too restrictive and a validation of perfect surrogacy is unrealistic and unnecessary. Since then, more than a dozen different statistical surrogacy evaluation methods have been proposed [60, 105]. In recent years, surrogacy evaluation based on multiple trials, as initiated with a Bayesian random effect meta-analysis proposed by Daniels and Hughes [30] and fully developed by Buyse et al. [18], has increasingly become the preferred method. Under this framework, assessment of surrogacy should take place at both the patient level and the trial level [69]. For illustration, we consider a simple setting with continuous surrogate and true endpoints. Consider the simple meta-analysis framework proposed by Daniels and Hughes [30] and Buyse et al. [18], where data are observed on Z, S and T in $n-1$ similar trials. The goal is to estimate the treatment effect of Z on T in nth trial. At the nth trial, the data are observed on Z, S and partially on T. Methods based on hierarchical models are used to estimate within-trial and between-trial measures of association have been suggested.

Suppose we have n randomized trials, $i = 1, \cdots, n$ with m patients per trial. For individual j in the ith trial, let T_{ij} and S_{ij} be the random variables denoting the true and surrogate endpoints, respectively, and let Z_{ij} be the indicator variable for treatment. A classical hierarchical, random-effects modeling strategy can be defined as

$$\begin{aligned} S_{ij} &= \mu_S + m_{Si} + \alpha Z_{ij} + a_i Z_{ij} + \epsilon_{Sij} \\ T_{ij} &= \mu_T + m_{Ti} + \beta Z_{ij} + b_i Z_{ij} + \epsilon_{Tij} \end{aligned}$$

where μ_S and μ_T are fixed intercepts, α and β are fixed treatment effects, m_{Si} and m_{Ti} are random intercepts and a_i and b_i are random treatment effects in trial i for the surrogate and true endpoints, respectively. ϵ_{Sij} and ϵ_{Tij} are correlated error terms, assumed to be zero-mean normally distributed, as the vector of random effects $(m_{Si}, m_{Ti}, a_i, b_i)$ is assumed to be mean-zero normally distributed.

After fitting the above models, surrogacy is captured by means of two quantities: the "individual level" and "trial level" coefficients of determination, denoted, respectively, R^2_{indiv} and R^2_{trial}. R^2_{indiv} measures the association between S and T at the level of the individual patient, after adjustment for Z, while R^2_{trial} quantifies the association between the treatment effects on S and T at the trial level. R^2_{indiv} is based on the component of variance-covariance matrix of ϵ_{Sij} and ϵ_{Tij} and takes the following form:

$$R^2_{indiv} = R^2_{\epsilon_{Tij}|\epsilon_{Sij}} = \frac{\sigma^2_{ST}}{\sigma_{SS}\sigma_{TT}}$$

R^2_{trial} is given by

$$R^2_{trial} = R^2_{b_i|m_{Si},a_i} = \frac{\begin{pmatrix} d_{Sb} \\ d_{ab} \end{pmatrix}^T \begin{pmatrix} d_{SS} & d_{Sa} \\ d_{Sa} & d_{aa} \end{pmatrix}^{-1} \begin{pmatrix} d_{Sb} \\ d_{ab} \end{pmatrix}}{d_{bb}}$$

A surrogate could be adopted when R^2_{indiv} and R^2_{trial} are both sufficiently close to one. The standard error of R^2_{trial} can be calculated using the delta method [16]. Such two-level surrogacy measures based on meta-analytic procedures have been investigated for various types of endpoints [16]. The Copula R^2 trial proposed by Burzykowski et al. [17] is the most popular trial-level surrogacy measure in cancer clinical trials when both endpoints are survival outcomes.

In one sense, the correlation between trials is more important than the correlation at individual level. For trial-level correlation, under the meta-analytic framework, estimates of the treatment effects on both endpoints within each trial are obtained, and conventional measure of R^2 using weighted least square regression can be used. These conventional measures assume the estimated treatment effects on S and T are fixed and ignore the correlation between endpoints within a same patient and therefore are considered less statistically sophisticated. However, both the conventional and the model-based trial-level surrogacy measures quantify the ability to predict the treatment effect on a true endpoint based on observed treatment effect on the surrogate endpoint. In practice, these correlations and the coefficient-of-determination-type surrogacy measures have been utilized by the Adjuvant Colon Cancer Endpoints (ACCENT) Group and other individual investigators (e.g., [87, 91]). This research led to the acceptance of disease-free survival (DFS) as a surrogate endpoint for overall survival (OS) in adjuvant colon cancer studies by FDA.

1.5.3 Remaining Issues

By contrast with traditional endpoints used in trials, surrogate endpoints, such as progression-free survival, remain controversial but suggest a potential for earlier assessment of treatment effect of interest. Trial designs need to integrate new endpoints with traditional endpoints to ensure they are better predictors of the primary outcome. It remains to see if stringent validation and assessment in accordance with the Prentice criteria [78] is necessary. There are many examples in which positive results were found in PFS but for which the treatment effect ultimately failed to translate into meaningful improvement in OS. In addition, the current validation of surrogate endpoints offers essentially a number of statistics that characterize in various ways the concordance of PFS and OS results, in addition to R^2 [8]. These measures are all largely descriptive and do not lend themselves to a definitive criterion for determining whether the use of the surrogate endpoint is justified. The strength of surrogacy is inherently dependent on the size of treatment effect on OS, the heterogeneity of underlying patient population, treatment setting (adjuvant or metastatic) and type of treatments (cytotoxic or cytostatic agents). Before new statistical methods are used to evaluate the impact of these factors on PFS and other endpoints as surrogate endpoints for OS, one should be cautious in interpreting the findings of surrogacy endpoint validation for different indications of different diseases.

1.6 Patient-reported Outcomes

1.6.1 Patient-reported Outcomes

Patient-reported outcomes (PRO) provide patients' perspective in the interpretation of clinical benefit from treatments. It is an important measure that can enhance our clinical decision making ability. In trials of cancer therapies for incurable disease, symptoms and quality of life of the patient is as important as the gains in survival. With the growing interest in the research community, the Patient-Centered Outcomes Research Institute (PCORI), a nonprofit nongovernmental organization, was established in 2010 to facilitate the advancement of patient focused comparative effectiveness research. In November 2013, the Methodology Committee of the PCORI released their Methodology Report to provide guidance for the achievement of that goal.

1.6.2 Types of PRO for Treatment Comparisons

PRO has become more commonly used as a primary endpoint or remained as a key secondary endpoint in cancer trials. Examples of indications for which PROs consistently serve as primary endpoints include painful conditions, such as neuropathic pain [93]. For regulatory approvals, FDA also provides guidance on setting up endpoint models. Endpoint models depict the role of PROs (i.e., a primary, key secondary or exploratory endpoint) and its relationship with other clinical trial endpoints. Below we describe two basic types of PRO for treatment comparisons.

1.6.3 Health Status, Functional and Symptoms Outcomes

The Functional Assessment of Cancer Therapy (FACT) [21] is an example of a widely used PRO instrument in cancer research. The several questionnaires and related subscales mainly measure physical functions, cognitive functioning, emotional function and social well-being of cancer patients. Other functional dimensions that one may consider in their PRO instruments include neuropsychological, psychological, and sexual functioning. For symptoms outcomes focusing on the sensation or perception of change related to health function, the same author Cleeland developed the two popular tools, MD Anderson Symptom Assessment Inventory [24], for symptoms in general, and the Brief Pain Inventory [23], for pain specifically.

1.6.4 General and Cancer-specific Quality of Life Outcomes

PROs that assess quality of life outcomes fall into two categories, generic and cancer-specific quality of life outcomes. The 36-item Short Form Health Survey (SF-36) is a set of generic quality of life measures developed from the Medical Outcomes Study [104]. Another popular PRO is the Patient-reported Outcomes Measurement Information System (PROMIS), which began in 2004 and was further expanded by the NIH, currently has two active studies on cancer including Georgetown's Validation of PROMIS in Diverse Cancer Populations and Supplement study and Duke's Validating and Extending the PROMIS Sexual Function Measure for Clinical Research. In contrast to general PROs, cancer-specific PRO is specific for oncology research. The European Organization for Research and Treatment of Cancer Quality of Life Questionnaire (EORTC-QLQ) is a great example of a widely used cancer-specific PRO instrument [1].

1.6.5 Criteria Used for PRO Instruments Selection

In most instances, researchers often choose well-validated and reliable self-reported instruments to measure PRO in clinical trials. Newly developed PRO tailored to measure the relevant endpoint may be better at detecting differences and changes. However, it is still important for researchers to understand metrics that are used to evaluate PROs. Below we briefly outline these metrics: reliability, validity, and the responsiveness to changes.

1.6.6 Reliability

Reliability measures the ability of PRO to yield consistent and reproducible estimates. PRO instruments are subject to measurement error. Reliability can be used to estimate the variation in PRO scores due to measurement error. Reliability is mainly divided into three methods: 1) test-retest intra-interviewer reliability, 2) inter-interviewer reliability, and 3) internal consistency. Test-retest intra-interviewer reliability is used to measure how consistent the PRO is by assessing the stability of the PRO scores for a single patient at two consecutive time points. Inter-interviewer reliability is used to measure the agreement of PRO scores when the instrument is administered by two or more different interviewers. These two types of reliability can be examined by the use of intraclass correlation coefficient and interclass correlation coefficient (Pearson's r), respectively. Internal consistency is used to assess the degree in which the items comprising the PRO instrument measure the same underlying concept. Internal consistency is commonly assessed by Cronbach's alpha. It is defined as

$$\alpha = \frac{K}{K-1}\left(1 - \frac{\sum_i^K \sigma_{Y_i}^2}{\sigma_X^2}\right)$$

where K = number of questions, $\sigma_{Y_i}^2$ = variance of component i for the current sample of patients, σ_X^2 = variance of the observed total test scores.

1.6.7 Validity

Validity is another important aspect of a good PRO instrument. To aid interpretation, validity provides an assessment of checking whether the PRO instrument measures what it is intended to.

Content validity

Content validity is the extent to which the instrument measures the concept of interest [99]. It is specific to the condition and cancer treatment under study. Content validity can be assessed both qualitatively and quantitatively. In 2011, the International Society for Pharmacoeconomics and Outcomes Research (ISPOR) task force published good research practices for establishing and reporting the evidence of content validity [75]. These qualitative steps are: 1) determination of the context of use, 2) development of the research protocol for the qualitative concept elicitation, 3) concept elicitation interviews and data collection among the cancer patients of interest, 4) analysis of the qualitative data, and 5) documentation of concept development and elicitation methods and results. Quantitative assessment for content validity, including item response theory and Rasch model, is also commonly conducted. Shortcomings in classical test theory has led statisticians to develop an alternative theory, item response theory (IRT). IRT model falls under the class of latent variable model. IRT is based on three assumptions, which are often desirable during the validation steps of PRO instruments: 1) unidimensionality, stating that the responses of patients on a questionnaire can be explained by one latent trait that the instrument aims to measure, 2) local independence, meaning that the observed items are conditionally independent of each other given an individual score on the latent trait, and 3) monotonicity, stating that the probability to have a positive response to a given item does not decrease with the latent variable [6, 48]. Commonly used IRT models are the Rasch models. Consider the response scale for a PRO instrument goes from k=1 to m, for example, m = 5 for the 5-point Likert scale. The probability that a subject $i(i = 1, \ldots, n)$ scoring at or above category k on question j with latent trait θ_i is as follows:

$$P(X_j \geq k|\theta) = \frac{exp(\gamma_j(\theta_i - \beta_{j(k-1)})}{1 + exp(\gamma_j(\theta_i - \beta_{j(k-1)}))}$$

where $k = 1, \ldots, m, X_j$ is the participant's response to question j, γ_j is the discrimination parameter, and the β_{jk}s are the threshold parameter. For $m = 5$, β_{j1} to β_{j4} will be estimated. IRT and Rasch model remain a popular research topic [6, 27, 48]. The EORTC Quality of Life Group has mentioned in their scoring manual that they are exploring alternative scoring procedures, such as the use of IRT and Rasch models.

Construct validity
Construct validity is defined as evidence that relationships among domains and concepts conform to a priori hypotheses concerning logical relationships that should exist with measures of related concepts or scores [99]. An underlying construct such as pain can be expected to have a set of quantitative relationships with other constructs like analgesics use. For example, those with less pain may have lower analgesic use. Confirmatory factor analyses are statistical techniques commonly used to identify separate domains within a PRO instrument.

1.6.8 Responsiveness of Instruments to Change

Responsiveness of instruments to change is concerned with the ability to identify differences in scores over time in patients whose health is known to have changed. FDA review considers within person change over time and effect size statistic. The latter is equal to the mean change in instrument scores divided by the baseline standard deviation [57].

1.7 Promising New Approaches

1.7.1 Limitations of Traditional Endpoints

Overall survival has long been the gold standard as an endpoint for cancer clinical trials. However, it is not without its limitations. Not only does overall survival require longer follow-up, but it may also be confounded by factors such as non-cancer related deaths and crossover to experimental therapy after progression. Moreover, as numerous life prolonging therapies for cancer become available, it makes the interpretation of overall survival more difficult as the primary endpoint. This has made it increasingly difficult to demonstrate survival gains for new and promising therapeutic options in cancer research. For example, statistically significant findings are infrequently established in non-small cell lung cancer. In chronic myeloid leukemia, survival can underestimate the probability of being alive and in remission after the achievement of the first remission while receiving therapy [47]. Other traditional endpoints such as response rate are also problematic in the context of immunotherapy as response patterns of patients are less predictable.

1.7.2 Pharmacokinetic and Pharmacodynamics Responses

The manufacturing process of biologic drugs is complex and can be difficult to be replicated exactly. The term biosimilar was introduced to describe medicines that are highly similar and can serve as a generic drug for a reference biologic drug. However, use of standard endpoints such as OS and PFS may require thousands of patients treated for several years, which may be unrealistic for some biosimilar cancer clinical trials. The FDA encourages the use of endpoints that enable more precise comparisons of relevant therapeutic effects even if it deviates from those in the reference drug's clinical trials [102]. The area under the concentration-time curve (AUC) is commonly used as a primary endpoint in early phase bioequivalence studies. Various forms of non-compartmental pharmacokinetic AUC parameters are available. AUC_{0-t} or AUC_{last} is AUC from time zero up to the last measurable concentration. $AUC_{0-\infty}$ is AUC from time zero to infinite time. $AUC_{0-\tau}$ is AUC from time zero to the end of dosing interval. Another endpoint mostly used as a secondary outcome is C_{max}, defined as the maximum concentration observed. It is commonly used as a secondary endpoint. Other similar measurements are used as secondary endpoints for biosimilar trials. These pharmacokinetic and pharmacodynamics endpoints are often analyzed by ANOVA. Some of these endpoints have also been used in phase IV studies such as the bioequivalence study of Temozolomide in patients with central nervous system tumors.

1.7.3 Imaging Techniques

Imaging has gained popularity in cancer clinical trials in the past decade due to its non-invasive nature. It has evolved into the primary endpoint of response in most phase 2 studies [80]. Given the shortcomings of RECIST, the RECIST 1.1 has incorporated fluorodexyglucose positron emission tomography (FDG-PET) on a limited basis as an indicator of disease progression [34]. Dynamic contrast-enhanced magnetic resonance imaging (DCE-MRI) which characterizes tumor neovasculature was first published by Dowlati et al. [33] and Galbraith et al. [45]. DCE-MRI has now become one of the most widely used imaging techniques. Volume transfer constant K^{trans} and initial area under the gadolinium curve (IAUGC) are two preferred endpoints for DCE-MRI. K^{trans} requires a two-compartment model that reflects contrast delivery and transport across the vascular endothelium [92]. IAUGC does not require a model which makes it relatively robust and comparable across sites [37]. Other emerging imaging endpoints include: diffusion-weighted magnetic resonance imaging and fluorodeoxythymidine-PET for probing tissue cellularity, and magnetic resonance spectroscopy imaging for providing spatial data of metabolites.

1.7.4 Immune Biomarkers-based Endpoints

Immunotherapy has played an ever-increasing role in cancer research. In the past few months from September 2014 to March 2015, FDA has approved three immunotherapy treatments: Pembrolizumab for metastatic melanoma, Blinatumomab for acute lymphoblastic leukemia, and Nivolumab for advanced melanoma and squamous non-small cell lung cancer. The number of cancer immunotherapy trials is also rapidly expanding. However, traditional clinical trial endpoints, like overall survival, are not immunotherapy focused and take longer follow-up. The measurement of the T-cell immune response is an attractive primary endpoint that could be assessed when conducting phase 2 trials. A commonly used T-cell immune response assay is the enzyme-linked immunospot assay, or ELISPOT. ELISPOT assay measures antigen-specific T cells and their function usually in the form of interferon-gamma [12]. Other cytokines and granzymes can be also be detected. The ELISPOT endpoint is usually defined as the change from baseline to a specific timepoint, for example, at end of first-line chemotherapy or radiation. From 2011, a number of randomized phase II immunotherapies trials using ELISPOT as a major primary endpoint are being evaluated (see Clinicaltrials.gov: NCT02159950, NCT01616303, NCT01496131, NCT01507103, NCT01431391, NCT01504542, NCT01307618). ELISPOT like other T-cell immune response assays is known to have high variability from laboratory to laboratory. There are efforts made to setup guidelines for assay harmonization, such as the preliminary guidelines published in 2008 [53]. In 2013, immune-related response criteria (irRC) based on the RECIST one-dimension measurements were proposed to better capture two potential patterns of response not considered by standard RECIST [71]. In phase III trials, due to delayed treatment effect, milestone survival as the clinical endpoint for survival has been recommended [51]. As proportional hazards may not be appropriate for time-to-event endpoints in the setting of delayed treatment effects, the weighted Cox regression or restricted mean survival time are good alternatives [83, 88].

1.7.5 Criteria for Evaluating Biomarker-based Endpoints

This section briefly outlines the evaluation of biomarkers as a clinical endpoint. The National Academy of Medicine, previously known as the Institute of Medicine (IOM), outlines a biomarker evaluation framework consisting of three steps: analytical validation, qualification, and utilization [52]. Analytical validation — the biomarker endpoint should be reliable and reproducible across laboratories and clinical centers. It also needs to have good performance characteristics such as sensitivity and specificity. Qualification — the biomarker should be evaluated for its association with the disease. There should also be cumulative evidence to demonstrate that the biomarker endpoint establishes surrogacy for the clinical endpoint of interest. To make this assessment usually a meta-analytic approach is needed [66]. Utilization — the decision to use a biomarker endpoint for a trial should be based on the particular context. Strong and compelling quantitative evidence should be coupled with clinical relevance and biological plausibility [46]. Gene signatures have been developed to correlate with survival, for example Th1 in colorectal cancer [43]. In the future, there will be a growing demand for the design of biomedical studies involving high-dimensional data and survival outcomes; this was considered in a recent study [74]. The development of new measures for surrogacy assessments remains as a current research topic [58].

1.8 Summary

Although overall survival is undisputed as the gold standard endpoint in cancer clinical trials, there are many other endpoints that have proven useful in developing and testing new treatments. Progression-free survival rivals the importance of overall survival in many advanced disease settings and has been shown to be a useful surrogate for overall survival in many, but not all, cases. These and other traditional endpoints based on some combination of tumor measurements and survival will continue to serve as key outcome measures in future clinical trials. Further work on the appropriate use of specific endpoints in specific settings should lead to more efficient studies. In addition, increased use of patient-reported outcomes and more novel endpoints will supplement traditional endpoints to provide a more complete and nuanced understanding of the effects of treatments evaluated in clinical trials.

The use of patient reported outcomes as primary and key secondary endpoints in clinical trials has increased over the past decade and will remain important in the future [7, 41, 44]. The data collection landscape has also started to change with real-time data capture using electronic PROs. Utility measure as an endpoint in cost effectiveness is expected to play a key role in future PRO studies [54, 77].

The advancement of imaging technologies and the growth of biosimilar and immunotherapy cancer trials have aided the development of new promising endpoints. Some of these less established endpoints are still in their infancy and will continue to evolve and to be refined. Validation of biomarker endpoints requires time and resources. However, it is certainly worth the effort if use of a novel biomarker endpoint can gain efficiency over trials using a traditional endpoint. As an interesting recent example, the use of video game training has been investigated as a biomarker or cognitive endpoint for individuals at risk of developing Alzheimer's disease [5]. There is little doubt that in the future that there will be similar innovative endpoints developed and selected for use in cancer clinical trials.

Acknowledgments

Research reported in this paper was supported in part by the National Cancer Institute of the National Institutes of Health under award number CA142538.

Bibliography

[1] N. K. Aaronson, S. Ahmedzai, B. Bergman, M. Bullinger, A. Cull, N. J. Duez, A. Filiberti, H. Flechtner, S. B. Fleishman, et al. The European Organization for Research and Treatment of Cancer QLQ-C30: a quality-of-life instrument for use in international clinical trials in oncology. *Journal of the National Cancer Institute*, 85(5):365–376, 1993.

[2] E. Amir, B. Seruga, R. Kwong, I. F. Tannock, and A. Ocaña. Poor correlation between progression-free and overall survival in modern clinical trials: are composite endpoints the answer? *European Journal of Cancer*, 48(3):385–388, 2012.

[3] M.-W. An, X. Dong, J. Meyers, Y. Han, A. Grothey, J. Bogaerts, D. J. Sargent, and S. J. Mandrekar. Evaluating continuous tumor measurement-based metrics as phase II endpoints for predicting overall survival. *Journal of the National Cancer Institute*, 107(11):djv239, 2015.

[4] M.-W. An, S. J. Mandrekar, M. E. Branda, S. L. Hillman, A. A. Adjei, H. C. Pitot, R. M. Goldberg, and D. J. Sargent. Comparison of continuous versus categorical tumor measurement–based metrics to predict overall survival in cancer treatment trials. *Clinical Cancer Research*, 17(20):6592–6599, 2011.

[5] J. A. Anguera, J. Boccanfuso, J. L. Rintoul, O. Al-Hashimi, F. Faraji, J. Janowich, E. Kong, Y. Larraburo, C. Rolle, E. Johnston, et al. Video game training enhances cognitive control in older adults. *Nature*, 501(7465):97–101, 2013.

[6] S. Arima. Item selection via Bayesian IRT models. *Statistics in Medicine*, 34(3):487–503, 2015.

[7] E. Basch. Toward patient-centered drug development in oncology. *New England Journal of Medicine*, 369(5):397–400, 2013.

[8] C. B. Begg. Justifying the choice of endpoints for clinical trials. *Journal of the National Cancer Institute*, 105(21):1594–1595, 2013.

[9] C. A. Bellera, N. Penel, M. Ouali, S. Bonvalot, P. G. Casali, O. S. Nielsen, M. Delannes, S. Litiere, F. Bonnetain, T. S. Dabakuyo, et al. Guidelines for time-to-event end point definitions in sarcomas and gastrointestinal stromal tumors (GIST) trials: results of the DATECAN initiative (Definition for the Assessment of Time-to-event Endpoints in CANcer trials). *Annals of Oncology*, 26(5):865–72, 2015.

[10] C. A. Bellera, M. Pulido, S. Gourgou, L. Collette, A. Doussau, A. Kramar, T. S. Dabakuyo, M. Ouali, A. Auperin, T. Filleron, C. Fortpied, et al. Protocol of the Definition for the Assessment of Time-to-event Endpoints in CANcer trials (DATECAN) project: formal consensus method for the development of guidelines for standardised time-to-event endpoints' definitions in cancer clinical trials. *European Journal of Cancer*, 49(4):769–81, 2013.

[11] S. Bhattacharya, G. Fyfe, R. J. Gray, and D. J. Sargent. Role of sensitivity analyses in assessing progression-free survival in late-stage oncology trials. *Journal of Clinical Oncology*, 27(35):5958–5964, 2009.

[12] M. Bilusic and J. L. Gulley. Endpoints, patient selection, and biomarkers in the design of clinical trials for cancer vaccines. *Cancer Immunology, Immunotherapy*, 61(1):109–17, 2012.

[13] F. Bonnetain, B. Bonsing, T. Conroy, A. Dousseau, B. Glimelius, K. Haustermans, F. Lacaine, J. L. Van Laethem, T. Aparicio, D. Aust, et al. Guidelines for time-to-event end-point definitions in trials for pancreatic cancer. Results of the DATECAN initiative (Definition for the Assessment of Time-to-event End-points in CANcer trials). *European Journal of Cancer*, 50(17):2983–2993, 2014.

[14] C. M. Booth and E. A. Eisenhauer. Progression-free survival: meaningful or simply measurable? *Journal of Clinical Oncology*, 30(10):1030–1033, 2012.

[15] T. Brody. *Clinical Trials: Study Design, Endpoints and Biomarkers, Drug Safety, and FDA and ICH Guidelines.* Academic Press, Boston, MA, 2012.

[16] T. Burzykowski, G. Molenberghs, and M. Buyse. *The Evaluation of Surrogate Endpoints.* Springer Science & Business Media, 2006.

[17] T. Burzykowski, G. Molenberghs, M. Buyse, H. Geys, and D. Renard. Validation of surrogate end points in multiple randomized clinical trials with failure time end points. *Journal of the Royal Statistical Society: Series C (Applied Statistics)*, 50(4):405–422, 2001.

[18] M. Buyse, G. Molenberghs, T. Burzykowski, D. Renard, and H. Geys. The validation of surrogate endpoints in meta-analyses of randomized experiments. *Biostatistics*, 1(1):49–67, 2000.

[19] M. Buyse, G. Molenberghs, X. Paoletti, K. Oba, A. Alonso, W. der Elst, and T. Burzykowski. Statistical evaluation of surrogate endpoints with examples from cancer clinical trials. *Biometrical Journal*, 2015.

[20] K. J. Carroll. Analysis of progression-free survival in oncology trials: some common statistical issues. *Pharmaceutical Statistics*, 6(2):99–113, 2007.

[21] D. F. Cella, D. S. Tulsky, G. Gray, B. Sarafian, E. Linn, A. Bonomi, M. Silberman, S. B. Yellen, P. Winicour, and J. Brannon. The Functional Assessment of Cancer Therapy scale: development and validation of the general measure. *Journal of Clinical Oncology*, 11(3):570–9, 1993.

[22] B. Chibaudel, F. Bonnetain, Q. Shi, M. Buyse, C. Tournigand, D. J. Sargent, C. J. Allegra, R. M. Goldberg, and A. de Gramont. Alternative end points to evaluate a therapeutic strategy in advanced colorectal cancer: Evaluation of progression-free survival, duration of disease control, and time to failure of strategy - An Aide et Recherche en Cancérologie Digestive Group Study. *Journal of Clinical Oncology*, 29(31):4199–4204, 2011.

[23] C. S. Cleeland. Measurement of pain by subjective report. In C. R. Chapman and J. D. Loeser, editors, *Advances in Pain Research and Therapy*, pages 391–403. Raven Press, New York, NY, USA, 1989.

[24] C. S. Cleeland, T. R. Mendoza, X. S. Wang, C. Chou, M. T. Harle, M. Morrissey, and M. C. Engstrom. Assessing symptom distress in cancer patients: the M.D. Anderson Symptom Inventory. *Cancer*, 89(7):1634–46, 2000.

[25] M. H. Cohen, G. Williams, J. R. Johnson, J. Duan, J. Gobburu, A. Rahman, K. Benson, J. Leighton, S. K. Kim, R. Wood, et al. Approval summary for imatinib mesylate capsules in the treatment of chronic myelogenous leukemia. *Clinical Cancer Research*, 8(5):935–942, 2002.

[26] W. Colburn, V. G. DeGruttola, D. L. DeMets, G. J. Downing, D. F. Hoth, J. A. Oates, C. C. Peck, R. T. Schooley, B. A. Spilker, J. Woodcock, et al. Biomarkers and surrogate endpoints: Preferred definitions and conceptual framework. Biomarkers Definitions Working Group. *Clinical Pharmacol & Therapeutics*, 69:89–95, 2001.

[27] M. P. Couper and F. Kreuter. Using paradata to explore item level response times in surveys. *Journal of the Royal Statistical Society: Series A*, 176(1):271–286, 2013.

[28] J. Dancey, L. Dodd, R. Ford, R. Kaplan, M. Mooney, L. Rubinstein, L. Schwartz, L. Shankar, and P. Therasse. Recommendations for the assessment of progression in randomised cancer treatment trials. *European Journal of Cancer*, 45(2):281–289, 2009.

[29] J. E. Dancey. Assessing benefit in trials: Are we making progress in assessing progression in cancer clinical trials? *Cancer*, 121(11):1728–1730, 2015.

[30] M. J. Daniels and M. D. Hughes. Meta-analysis for the evaluation of potential surrogate markers. *Statistics in Medicine*, 16(17):1965–1982, 1997.

[31] J. Denne, A. Stone, R. Bailey-Iacona, and T.-T. Chen. Missing data and censoring in the analysis of progression-free survival in oncology clinical trials. *Journal of Biopharmaceutical Statistics*, 23(5):951–970, 2013.

[32] N. Dhani, D. Tu, D. J. Sargent, L. Seymour, and M. J. Moore. Alternate endpoints for screening phase II studies. *Clinical Cancer Research*, 15(6):1873–1882, 2009.

[33] A. Dowlati, K. Robertson, M. Cooney, W. P. Petros, M. Stratford, J. Jesberger, N. Rafie, B. Overmoyer, V. Makkar, B. Stambler, A. Taylor, et al. A phase I pharmacokinetic and translational study of the novel vascular targeting agent combretastatin a-4 phosphate on a single-dose intravenous schedule in patients with advanced cancer. *Cancer Research*, 62(12):3408–16, 2002.

[34] E. A. Eisenhauer, P. Therasse, J. Bogaerts, L. H. Schwartz, D. Sargent, R. Ford, J. Dancey, S. Arbuck, S. Gwyther, M. Mooney, L. Rubinstein, et al. New response evaluation criteria in solid tumours: revised RECIST guideline (version 1.1). *European Journal of Cancer*, 45(2):228–47, 2009.

[35] European Medicines Agency. Guideline on the evaluation of anticancer medicinal products in man, 2012.
http://www.ema.europa.eu/ema/pages/includes/document/
open_document.jsp?webContentId=WC500137128.

[36] European Medicines Agency. Methodological consideration for using progression-free survival (PFS) or disease-free survival (DFS) in confirmatory trials (appendix 1 to the guideline on the evaluation of anticancer medicinal products in man), 2012.
http://www.ema.europa.eu/ema/pages/includes/document/
open_document.jsp?webContentId=WC500137126.

[37] F. M. Fennessy, R. R. McKay, C. J. Beard, M. E. Taplin, and C. M. Tempany. Dynamic contrast-enhanced magnetic resonance imaging in prostate cancer clinical trials: potential roles and possible pitfalls. *Translational Oncology*, 7(1):120–9, 2014.

[38] F. Fiteni, V. Westeel, X. Pivot, C. Borg, D. Vernerey, and F. Bonnetain. Endpoints in cancer clinical trials. *Journal of Visceral Surgery*, 151(1):17–22, 2014.

[39] T. R. Fleming and D. L. DeMets. Surrogate end points in clinical trials: are we being misled? *Annals of Internal Medicine*, 125(7):605–613, 1996.

[40] T. R. Fleming, M. D. Rothmann, and H. L. Lu. Issues in using progression-free survival when evaluating oncology products. *Journal of Clinical Oncology*, 27(17):2874–2880, 2009.

[41] L. Frank, E. Basch, and J. V. Selby. The PCORI perspective on patient-centered outcomes research. *Journal of the American Medical Association*, 312(15):1513–4, 2014.

[42] L. S. Freedman, B. I. Graubard, and A. Schatzkin. Statistical validation of intermediate endpoints for chronic diseases. *Statistics in Medicine*, 11(2):167–178, 1992.

[43] W. H. Fridman, F. Pages, C. Sautes-Fridman, and J. Galon. The immune contexture in human tumours: impact on clinical outcome. *Nature Reviews Cancer*, 12(4):298–306, 2012.

[44] S. E. Gabriel and S. L. T. Normand. Getting the methods right — the foundation of patient-centered outcomes research. *New England Journal of Medicine*, 367(9):787–790, 2012.

[45] S. M. Galbraith, G. J. Rustin, M. A. Lodge, N. J. Taylor, J. J. Stirling, M. Jameson, P. Thompson, D. Hough, L. Gumbrell, and A. R. Padhani. Effects of 5,6-dimethylxanthenone-4-acetic acid on human tumor microcirculation assessed by dynamic contrast-enhanced magnetic resonance imaging. *Journal of Clinical Oncology*, 20(18):3826–40, 2002.

[46] E. Green, G. Yothers, and D. J. Sargent. Surrogate endpoint validation: statistical elegance versus clinical relevance. *Statistical Methods in Medical Research*, 17(5):477–86, 2008.

[47] J. Guilhot, C. Preudhomme, F. X. Mahon, and F. Guilhot. Analyzing molecular response in chronic myeloid leukemia clinical trials: pitfalls and golden rules. *Cancer*, 121(4):490–7, 2015.

[48] J. B. Hardouin, S. Amri, M. L. Feddag, and V. Sebille. Towards power and sample size calculations for the comparison of two groups of patients with item response theory models. *Statistics in Medicine*, 31(11-12):1277–90, 2012.

[49] R. S. Heist, X. Wang, L. Hodgson, G. A. Otterson, T. E. Stinchcombe, L. Gandhi, M. A. Villalona-Calero, P. Watson, E. E. Vokes, and M. A. Socinski. A randomized phase II study to assess the efficacy of pemetrexed or sunitinib or pemetrexed plus sunitinib in the second-line treatment of advanced non-small cell lung cancer. *Journal of Thoracic Oncology*, 9(2):214, 2014.

[50] S. Hong, N. Schmitt, A. Stone, and J. Denne. Attenuation of treatment effect due to measurement variability in assessment of progression-free survival. *Pharmaceutical Statistics*, 11(5):394–402, 2012.

[51] A. Hoos, C. M. Britten, C. Huber, and J. O'Donnell-Tormey. A methodological framework to enhance the clinical success of cancer immunotherapy. *Nature Biotechnology*, 29(10):867–70, 2011.

[52] Institute of Medicine. Evaluation of Biomarkers and Surrogate Endpoints in Chronic Disease, 2010.
http://www.iom.edu/~/media/Files/Report%20Files/2010/Evaluation-of-Biomarkers-and-Surrogate-Endpoints-in-Chronic-Disease/Evaluation%20of%20Biomarkers%20-%202010%20Report%20Brief%20v2.pdf.

[53] S. Janetzki, K. S. Panageas, L. Ben-Porat, J. Boyer, C. M. Britten, T. M. Clay, M. Kalos, H. T. Maecker, P. Romero, J. Yuan, W. M. Kast, and A. Hoos. Results and harmonization guidelines from two large-scale international elispot proficiency panels conducted by the cancer vaccine consortium (cvc/svi). *Cancer Immunology, Immunotherapy*, 57(3):303–15, 2008.

[54] R. W. Jang, P. K. Isogai, N. Mittmann, P. A. Bradbury, F. A. Shepherd, R. Feld, and N. B. Leighl. Derivation of utility values from European Organization for Research and Treatment of Cancer Quality of Life-Core 30 questionnaire values in lung cancer. *Journal of Thoracic Oncology*, 5(12):1953–1957, 2010.

[55] T. G. Karrison, M. L. Maitland, W. M. Stadler, and M. J. Ratain. Design of phase II cancer trials using a continuous endpoint of change in tumor size: application to a study of sorafenib and erlotinib in non-small cell lung cancer. *Journal of the National Cancer Institute*, 99(19):1455–1461, 2007.

[56] A. Kay, J. Higgins, A. Day, R. Meyer, and C. Booth. Randomized controlled trials (RCTs) in the era of molecular oncology: Methodology, biomarkers, and endpoints. In *ASCO Annual Meeting Proceedings*, volume 29, page 6049, 2011.

[57] L. E. Kazis, J. J. Anderson, and R. F. Meenan. Effect sizes for interpreting changes in health status. *Medical Care*, 27(3 Suppl):S178–89, 1989.

[58] F. Kobayashi and M. Kuroki. A new proportion measure of the treatment effect captured by candidate surrogate endpoints. *Statistics in Medicine*, 33(19):3338–53, 2014.

[59] R. L. Korn and J. J. Crowley. Overview: progression-free survival as an endpoint in clinical trials with solid tumors. *Clinical Cancer Research*, 19(10):2607–2612, 2013.

[60] M. N. Lassere. The biomarker-surrogacy evaluation schema: a review of the biomarker-surrogate literature and a proposal for a criterion-based, quantitative, multidimensional hierarchical levels of evidence schema for evaluating the status of biomarkers as surrogate endpoints. *Statistical Methods in Medical Research*, 17(3):303–340, 2008.

[61] P. T. Lavin. An alternative model for the evaluation of antitumor activity. *Cancer Clinical Trials*, 4(4):451–457, 1980.

[62] L. J. Lesko and A. Atkinson, Jr. Use of biomarkers and surrogate endpoints in drug development and regulatory decision making: criteria, validation, strategies 1. *Annual Review of Pharmacology and Toxicology*, 41(1):347–366, 2001.

[63] J. M. Llovet, A. M. Di Bisceglie, J. Bruix, B. S. Kramer, R. Lencioni, A. X. Zhu, M. Sherman, M. Schwartz, M. Lotze, J. Talwalkar, et al. Design and endpoints of clinical trials in hepatocellular carcinoma. *Journal of the National Cancer Institute*, 100(10):698–711, 2008.

[64] S. J. Mandrekar, M.-W. An, J. Meyers, A. Grothey, J. Bogaerts, and D. J. Sargent. Evaluation of alternate categorical tumor metrics and cut points for response categorization using the RECIST 1.1 data warehouse. *Journal of Clinical Oncology*, pages JCO–2013, 2014.

[65] U. A. Matulonis, A. M. Oza, T. W. Ho, and J. A. Ledermann. Intermediate clinical endpoints: A bridge between progression-free survival and overall survival in ovarian cancer trials. *Cancer*, 121(11):1737–1746, 2015.

[66] L. M. McShane, S. Hunsberger, and A. A. Adjei. Effective incorporation of biomarkers into phase II trials. *Clinical Cancer Research*, 15(6):1898–905, 2009.

[67] L. K. Mell and J.-H. Jeong. Pitfalls of using composite primary end points in the presence of competing risks. *Journal of Clinical Oncology*, 28(28):4297–4299, 2010.

[68] L. C. Michaelis and M. J. Ratain. Measuring response in a post-RECIST world: from black and white to shades of grey. *Nature Reviews Cancer*, 6(5):409–414, 2006.

[69] G. Molenberghs, M. Buyse, H. Geys, D. Renard, T. Burzykowski, and A. Alonso. Statistical challenges in the evaluation of surrogate endpoints in randomized trials. *Controlled Clinical Trials*, 23(6):607–625, 2002.

[70] R. J. Motzer, T. E. Hutson, P. Tomczak, M. D. Michaelson, R. M. Bukowski, O. Rixe, S. Oudard, S. Negrier, C. Szczylik, S. T. Kim, et al. Sunitinib versus interferon alfa in metastatic renal-cell carcinoma. *New England Journal of Medicine*, 356(2):115–124, 2007.

[71] M. Nishino, A. Giobbie-Hurder, M. Gargano, M. Suda, N. H. Ramaiya, and F. S. Hodi. Developing a common language for tumor response to immunotherapy: immune-related response criteria using unidimensional measurements. *Clinical Cancer Research*, 19(14):3936–43, 2013.

[72] G. R. Oxnard, M. J. Morris, F. S. Hodi, L. H. Baker, M. G. Kris, A. P. Venook, and L. H. Schwartz. When progressive disease does not mean treatment failure: reconsidering the criteria for progression. *Journal of the National Cancer Institute*, page djs353, 2012.

[73] K. S. Panageas, L. Ben-Porat, M. N. Dickler, P. B. Chapman, and D. Schrag. When you look matters: the effect of assessment schedule on progression-free survival. *Journal of the National Cancer Institute*, 99(6):428–432, 2007.

[74] H. Pang and S. H. Jung. Sample size considerations of prediction-validation methods in high-dimensional data for survival outcomes. *Genetic Epidemiology*, 37(3):276–82, 2013.

[75] D. L. Patrick, L. B. Burke, C. J. Gwaltney, N. K. Leidy, M. L. Martin, E. Molsen, and L. Ring. Content validity-establishing and reporting the evidence in newly developed patient-reported outcomes (PRO) instruments for medical product evaluation: ISPOR PRO Good Research Practices Task Force report: part 2-assessing respondent understanding. *Value Health*, 14(8):978–88, 2011.

[76] R. Pazdur. Endpoints for assessing drug activity in clinical trials. *The Oncologist*, 13(Supplement 2):19–21, 2008.

[77] A. S. Pickard, J. W. Shaw, H. W. Lin, P. C. Trask, N. Aaronson, T. A. Lee, and D. Cella. A patient-based utility measure of health for clinical trials of cancer therapy based on the European Organization for the Research and Treatment of Cancer Quality of Life Questionnaire. *Value Health*, 12(6):977–88, 2009.

[78] R. L. Prentice. Surrogate endpoints in clinical trials: definition and operational criteria. *Statistics in Medicine*, 8(4):431–440, 1989.

[79] M. J. Ratain, T. Eisen, W. M. Stadler, K. T. Flaherty, S. B. Kaye, G. L. Rosner, M. Gore, A. A. Desai, A. Patnaik, H. Q. Xiong, et al. Phase II placebo-controlled randomized discontinuation trial of sorafenib in patients with metastatic renal cell carcinoma. *Journal of Clinical Oncology*, 24(16):2505–2512, 2006.

[80] P. Rezai, M. J. Pisaneschi, C. Feng, and V. Yaghmai. A radiologist's guide to treatment response criteria in oncologic imaging: anatomic imaging biomarkers. *American Journal of Roentgenology*, 201(2):237–45, 2013.

[81] R. P. Riechelmann, S. Chin, L. Wang, I. F. Tannock, D. R. Berthold, M. J. Moore, and J. J. Knox. Sorafenib for metastatic renal cancer: the Princess Margaret experience. *American Journal of Clinical Oncology*, 31(2):182–187, 2008.

[82] A. G. Robinson, C. M. Booth, and E. A. Eisenhauer. Progression-free survival as an end-point in solid tumours–perspectives from clinical trials and clinical practice. *European Journal of Cancer*, 50(13):2303–2308, 2014.

[83] P. Royston and M. K. Parmar. The use of restricted mean survival time to estimate the treatment effect in randomized clinical trials when the proportional hazards assumption is in doubt. *Statistics in Medicine*, 30(19):2409–21, 2011.

[84] L. Rubinstein, J. Crowley, P. Ivy, M. LeBlanc, and D. Sargent. Randomized phase II designs. *Clinical Cancer Research*, 15(6):1883–1890, 2009.

[85] L. V. Rubinstein, E. L. Korn, B. Freidlin, S. Hunsberger, S. P. Ivy, and M. A. Smith. Design issues of randomized phase II trials and a proposal for phase II screening trials. *Journal of Clinical Oncology*, 23(28):7199–7206, 2005.

[86] E. D. Saad and M. Buyse. Overall survival: patient outcome, therapeutic objective, clinical trial end point, or public health measure? *Journal of Clinical Oncology*, 30(15):1750–1754, 2012.

[87] D. J. Sargent, H. S. Wieand, D. G. Haller, R. Gray, J. K. Benedetti, M. Buyse, R. Labianca, J. F. Seitz, C. J. O'Callaghan, G. Francini, et al. Disease-free survival versus overall survival as a primary end point for adjuvant colon cancer studies: individual patient data from 20,898 patients on 18 randomized trials. *Journal of Clinical Oncology*, 23(34):8664–8670, 2005.

[88] M. Schemper, S. Wakounig, and G. Heinze. The estimation of average hazard ratios by weighted Cox regression. *Statistics in Medicine*, 28(19):2473–89, 2009.

[89] M. R. Sharma, M. L. Maitland, and M. J. Ratain. RECIST: no longer the sharpest tool in the oncology clinical trials toolbox—point. *Cancer Research*, 72(20):5145–5149, 2012.

[90] F. A. Shepherd, J. Rodrigues Pereira, T. Ciuleanu, E. H. Tan, V. Hirsh, S. Thongprasert, D. Campos, S. Maoleekoonpiroj, M. Smylie, R. Martins, et al. Erlotinib in previously treated non-small cell lung cancer. *New England Journal of Medicine*, 353(2):123–132, 2005.

[91] Q. Shi and D. J. Sargent. Meta-analysis for the evaluation of surrogate endpoints in cancer clinical trials. *International Journal of Clinical Oncology*, 14(2):102–111, 2009.

[92] A. Shields and P. Price. *In Vivo Imaging of Cancer Therapy.* Humana Press. Totawa, NJ, USA, 2007.

[93] E. M. Smith, H. Pang, C. Cirrincione, S. Fleishman, E. D. Paskett, T. Ahles, L. R. Bressler, C. E. Fadul, C. Knox, N. Le-Lindqwister, P. B. Gilman, and C. L. Shapiro. Effect of duloxetine on pain, function, and quality of life among patients with chemotherapy-induced painful peripheral neuropathy: a randomized clinical trial. *Journal of the American Medical Association*, 309(13):1359–67, 2013.

[94] W. D. Stein, J. Wilkerson, S. T. Kim, X. Huang, R. J. Motzer, A. T. Fojo, and S. E. Bates. Analyzing the pivotal trial that compared sunitinib and ifn-α in renal cell carcinoma, using a method that assesses tumor regression and growth. *Clinical Cancer Research*, 18(8):2374–2381, 2012.

[95] A. Stone, W. Bushnell, J. Denne, D. Sargent, O. Amit, C. Chen, R. Bailey-Iacona, J. Helterbrand, and G. Williams. Research outcomes and recommendations for the assessment of progression in cancer clinical trials from a PhRMA working group. *European Journal of Cancer*, 47(12):1763–1771, 2011.

[96] T. Sugimoto, T. Sozu, T. Hamasaki, and S. R. Evans. A logrank test-based method for sizing clinical trials with two co-primary time-to-event endpoints. *Biostatistics*, 14(3):409–421, 2013.

[97] P. Therasse, S. Arbuck, E. Eisenhauer, J. Wanders, R. Kaplan, L. Rubinstein, J. Verweij, M. Van Glabbeke, A. Van Oosterom, M. Christian, et al. European Organization for Research and Treatment of Cancer, National Cancer Institute of the United States, National Cancer Institute of Canada. New guidelines to evaluate the response to treatment in solid tumors. *Journal of the National Cancer Institute*, 92(3):205–216, 2000.

[98] U.S. Food and Drug Administration. Guidance for Industry: Clinical Trial Endpoints for the Approval of Cancer Drugs and Biologics, 2007. http://www.fda.gov/downloads/Drugs/{\protect\newline}GuidanceComplianceRegulatoryInformation/Guidances/ucm071590.pdf.

[99] U.S. Food and Drug Administration. Patient-reported Outcome Measures: Use in Medical Product Development to Support Labeling Claims, 2009.
http://www.fda.gov/downloads/Drugs/Guidances/UCM193282.pdf.

[100] U.S. Food and Drug Administration. Guidance for Industry (draft): Clinical Trial Endpoints for the Approval of Non-Small Cell Lung Cancer Drugs and Biologics, 2011.
http://www.fda.gov/Drugs/GuidanceComplianceRegulatoryInformation/Guidances/default.htm.

[101] U.S. Food and Drug Administration. Guidance for Industry: Standards for Clinical Trial Imaging Endpoints, 2011.
http://www.fda.gov/Drugs/GuidanceComplianceRegulatoryInformation/Guidances/default.htm.

[102] U.S. Food and Drug Administration. Guidance for industry scientific considerations in demonstrating biosimilarity to a reference product, 2012.
http://www.fda.gov/downloads/Drugs/{\protect\newline}
GuidanceComplianceRegulatoryInformation/Guidances/UCM291128.pdf.

[103] Y. Wang, C. Sung, C. Dartois, R. Ramchandani, B. Booth, E. Rock, and J. Gobburu. Elucidation of relationship between tumor size and survival in non-small cell lung cancer patients can aid early decision making in clinical drug development. *Clinical Pharmacology & Therapeutics*, 86(2):167–174, 2009.

[104] J. E. Ware, Jr. and C. D. Sherbourne. The MOS 36-item short-form health survey (SF-36). I. Conceptual framework and item selection. *Medical Care*, 30(6):473–83, 1992.

[105] C. J. Weir and R. J. Walley. Statistical evaluation of biomarkers as surrogate endpoints: a literature review. *Statistics in Medicine*, 25(2):183, 2006.

[106] M. K. Wilson, D. Collyar, D. T. Chingos, M. Friedlander, T. W. Ho, K. Karakasis, S. Kaye, M. K. Parmar, M. R. Sydes, I. F. Tannock, et al. Outcomes and endpoints in cancer trials: bridging the divide. *Lancet Oncology*, 16(1):e43–e52, 2015.

[107] M. K. Wilson, K. Karakasis, and A. M. Oza. Outcomes and endpoints in trials of cancer treatment: the past, present, and future. *Lancet Oncology*, 16(1):e32–e42, 2015.

[108] J. D. Wolchok, A. Hoos, S. O'Day, J. S. Weber, O. Hamid, C. Lebbé, M. Maio, M. Binder, O. Bohnsack, G. Nichol, et al. Guidelines for the

evaluation of immune therapy activity in solid tumors: immune-related response criteria. *Clinical Cancer Research*, 15(23):7412–7420, 2009.

[109] World Health Organization and others. WHO handbook for reporting results of cancer treatment, 1979.

[110] F. Xia, S. L. George, and X. Wang. A multi-state model for designing clinical trials for testing overall survival allowing for crossover after progression. *Statistics in Biopharmaceutical Research*, 2015 (in press).

2

Use of Historical Data

Simon Wandel

Heinz Schmidli

Beat Neuenschwander

CONTENTS

2.1 Introduction

The use of historical data in clinical trials has attracted interest in recent years, although its origin is much older. Incorporation of historical controls was originally proposed in the 1970s [6, 47], continued throughout the 1980s [49, 67], and has become increasingly important ever since [9, 22, 36, 43, 46, 55, 58, 68]. Concurrently, substantial methodological work was developed for incorporation of historical data in non-clinical toxicology studies [23, 28, 31, 51, 59, 60, 72]. However, the topic would likely have remained a niche area if there were not several fundamental changes happening in technology, statistics, and in the medical community during the 1990s.

An important technical change was the increased availability of personal computers. Using computers, many analytically intractable problems were reduced to numerical problems which could be solved rapidly. In their daily work, statisticians began to use computationally involved methods, e.g., maximum likelihood, multi-level or mixed models, and nonlinear models. At the same time, Bayesian statistics experienced a dramatic revival due to the availability of powerful computational tools such as WinBUGS [34, 35]. Models could be fitted without the need to write one's own Gibbs sampler or Metropolis-Hastings algorithm. And finally, the emergence of Evidence Based Medicine (EBM) led to the acceptance of and an increased demand for systematic reviews and meta-analyses [14]. Clearly, the medical field is in the middle of a paradigm shift, moving away from the fragmentary single-study view to a more comprehensive perspective.

These changes initiated a number of new directions regarding the use of historical data in clinical trials. Meta-analysis added to a better understanding of how to use historical data in clinical trials. The availability of flexible statistical software offered the possibility of formally incorporating historical data in all kinds of statistical models. Additionally, the increased computational power allowed the assessment of frequentist metrics of clinical trials with historical data.

The simplest yet non-statistical approach is the *informal* use of historical data. In this setting *informal* means that historical data are used to provide a context for discussing the design and the results of the actual trial, but without any formal analysis. This approach is commonly used in the decision-making process, but it lacks a formal assessment of uncertainty and is clearly subjective. Therefore, it lacks transparency and a formal perspective.

For clinical trials, the first truly statistical approach is the bias model proposed by Pocock in 1976 [47]. Since then, other statistical approaches have been developed, mostly within the Bayesian framework [7, 27, 43, 58], but frequentist methods have also been proposed (e.g., test-then-pool [68]). These developments stimulated the interest of academic institutions, pharmaceutical companies, and regulatory agencies in using historical data in clinical trials. For example, in their *Guideline on clinical trials in small populations*, the Committee for Medicinal Products for Human Use (CHMP) of the European Medicines Agency encourages the use of innovative approaches [16] which allow incorporating historical data. The Center for Devices and Radiological Health (CDRH) of the United States' Federal Drug Administration (FDA) released a *Guidance for the Use of Bayesian Statistics in Medical Device Clinical Trials* in 2010 [64]. Several academic institutions and pharmaceutical companies are performing clinical trials incorporating historical data.

As attractive as the incorporation of historical data in clinical trials is, it comes with caveats when implemented in practice. All of the aforementioned statistical approaches require strong statistical expertise and a close collaboration with clinical colleagues. Based on our experience we will focus on the incorporation of historical data using robust meta-analytic-predictive priors.

The chapter is organized as follows. In Section 2.2 we will give an overview of the main approaches for using historical data in clinical trials, with a focus on the meta-analytic-predictive approach. We will discuss important concepts when using priors from historical data including prior robustness and prior effective sample size. In Section 2.3, we will present three applications of the meta-analytic-predictive approach. The first application focuses on a phase II trial, the second on a phase I dose-escalation trial, and the third on the derivation of a non-inferiority margin for a biosimilar study. We conclude with a discussion in Section 2.4.

2.2 Overview of Approaches for Incorporating Historical Data

2.2.1 Introduction

We now provide an overview of the main approaches to using historical data, which are: the bias model, power priors, commensurate priors, meta-analytic-combined (*MAC*) analyses, and meta-analytic-predictive (*MAP*) priors. Although these approaches are all meta-analytic in nature, we discuss *MAP* priors separately and in more detail in Section 2.2.2 and 2.2.3. It is important to note that the approaches are similar, since they account for the hierarchical structure of the data and thereby lead to discounting of historical data relative to the data in the new trial.

To facilitate the overview, we introduce basic notation. We index by $j = 1, \ldots, J, \star$ the J historical studies and the new study, respectively, with sample sizes n_j for which data on the control treatment $Y_j = \{y_{j,1}, \ldots, y_{j,n_j}\}$ are available. Note that at the design stage $Y_\star$ is not yet observed. The main parameters are denoted by $\theta_j, j = 1, \ldots J, \star$. In the Bayesian setting, $p(\theta)$ will be used for the prior distribution, $p(Y|\theta)$ for the likelihood, and $p(\theta|Y)$ for the posterior distribution.

Pocock's bias model

Pocock's bias model [47] is a hierarchical model which assumes that the historical parameters are a biased sample of the actual parameter [58]. The differences between the parameter in the actual study ($\theta_\star$) and the respective parameters in the historical studies (θ_j) are defined in a hierarchical manner: for $j = 1, \ldots, J$

$$\theta_j = \theta_\star + \delta_j, \quad \delta_j|\tau_\delta \sim N(0, \tau_\delta^2) \tag{2.1}$$

For $\tau_\delta = 0$, a common effect model with $\theta_\star = \theta_1 = \theta_2 = \ldots = \theta_J$ is obtained, and for $\tau_\delta = \infty$ a stratified model. Values for τ_δ between these extremes will result in different amounts of borrowing from historical data. When the number of historical studies is small, the posterior of τ_δ is sensitive to the prior. The choice of the prior distribution for τ_δ therefore plays a critical role. In equation (2.1), a priori the bias is centered at 0, assuming no systematic biases between the parameters of the historical and the new study. This does not need to be the case. For example, if study design characteristics between the actual and the historical studies differ, this may lead to a systematic over- or underestimation of the treatment effect [53] and may justify centering at a value other than 0.

Power priors

Power priors were proposed by Ibrahim and Chen in 2000 [7]. They do not explicitly model the different study parameters, but rather discount the historical data directly by taking the likelihood of the historical data to the power α, with $0 \leq \alpha \leq 1$. The first version of power priors assumes fixed α_j for each study

$$p(\theta_\star | Y_1, \ldots, Y_J) \propto \left(\prod_{j=1}^{J} p(Y_j | \theta_\star)^{\alpha_j} \right) p_0(\theta_\star) \tag{2.2}$$

Here, $p_0(\theta_\star)$ is the initial (usually weakly-informative) prior distribution for $\theta_\star$. While the interpretation of α_j (as a fraction of historical data entering the analysis of the new trial) makes the power prior attractive, it is also clear that the choice of α_j can be challenging. Therefore, in many situations treating the α_j as parameters is favored. However, (2.2) is then no longer valid, as the normalizing constant depends on the power parameters α_j. The correct use of power priors is then much more involved and challenging in practice; see [13, 40, 42]. In addition, power priors violate the likelihood principle [13].

Commensurate prior

Carlin and Hobbs [26, 27] introduce commensurate priors as a way to incorporate historical information into the actual study. They propose a parameterization separating the historical and the new study. For one historical study the commensurate prior for $\theta_\star$ is defined as follows:

$$p(\theta_\star | Y_1) \propto p(Y_1 | \theta_1) p(\theta_\star | \theta_1, \tau) p_0(\theta_\star) p(\tau) \tag{2.3}$$

Here, $p_0(\theta_\star)$ is the initial (usually weakly-informative) prior distribution for $\theta_\star$. Two observations are important concerning (2.3). First, the relationship between the parameter of the historical study (θ_1) and of the actual study ($\theta_\star$) is expressed by $p(\theta_\star | \theta_1, \tau)$. Second, commensurability between the parameters θ_1 and $\theta_\star$ is modeled by τ, which is a measure of variability (e.g., standard deviation). For multiple historical studies, the proposal by Hobbs et al. [27] is to use a common effect model for historical data,

$$\theta = \theta_1 = \theta_2 = \ldots = \theta_J \tag{2.4}$$

TABLE 2.1: Example with control data of two historical trials and two hypothetical data scenarios for the new trial; analyses for the control parameter in the new trial $\theta_\star$ refer to the *MAP* prior, and the scenario analyses under *MAP* and *MAC*.

	Data r/n	(%)	95%-interval (%)
historical trial 1: Y_1	4/17	23.5	7.3-44.2
historical trial 2: Y_2	2/26	7.7	1.2-20.5
new trial (scenario 1): $Y_\star$	3/20	15.0	3.6-32.6
new trial (scenario 2): $Y_\star$	9/20	45.0	23.5-64.3
MAP and MAC analyses for response rate in new trial ($\theta_\star$)			
		median	95%-interval (%)
MAP prior		13.3	2.9-41.4
MAP prior + new data 1	3/20	14.0	5.9-27.1
MAC for new data 1	3/20	13.9	5.7-27.1
MAP prior + new data 2	9/20	33.7	17.5-56.8
MAC for new data 2	9/20	34.0	17.4-56.6

for which the commensurate prior is defined as

$$p(\theta_\star|Y_1,\ldots,Y_J) \propto \left(\prod_{j=1}^{J} p(Y_j|\theta)\right) p(\theta_\star|\theta,\tau)p_0(\theta_\star)p(\tau) \tag{2.5}$$

2.2.2 Meta-analytic Approaches

We now provide a formal meta-analytic framework for historical data as complementary information in the analysis of a clinical trial. We will see that the historical data can be accounted for in two ways: the *meta-analytic-combined (MAC)* approach uses the historical data as additional data when analyzing the data of the new trial; alternatively, the *meta-analytic-predictive (MAP)* approach uses a prior distribution for the parameter in the new trial (predicted from historical data), which is then combined with the new trial data in a Bayesian way.

Formally, we assume J historical trials with data $Y_1,\ldots,Y_J$, and let $Y_\star$ be the data of the new trial, either already observed or yet to be observed, referring to retro- or prospective cases, respectively. An example with control data for two historical trials is shown in Table 2.1. The data will be used in Section 2.3.1 as complementary information for the control rate in a randomized phase II trial.

Since the data structure is hierarchical, the following model will be applicable in many situations. First, there is the statistical model (likelihood), which, in its simplest form, assumes approximately normally distributed estimates

$$Y_j|\theta_j \sim N(\theta_j, s_j^2), \quad j = 1,\ldots,J,\star \tag{2.6}$$

with standard error s_j. Of course, depending on the underlying data, the likelihood of trial-specific parameters can be more complex; for example, individual data instead of summary data may be used, and there may be nuisance parameters beyond the main parameters θ_j. In the example of Table 2.1, the likelihood is binomial, $r_j|\pi_j \sim \text{Binomial}(\pi_j, n_j)$; for two applications with more complex likelihoods see Section 2.3.

In order to make use of historical data, a parameter model linking the trials is needed. The simplest parameter model allowing for different degrees of similarity across parameters assumes exchangeability, which is a reasonable assumption if no relevant predictors are available

$$\theta_j|\mu, \tau \sim N(\mu, \tau^2), \quad j = 1, \ldots, J, \star \tag{2.7}$$

The partial exchangeability extension $\mu_j = X_j\beta$ can be considered for trial-specific predictors X_j such as trial duration, patient population, year of study start, region, etc. Another extension of (2.7) allows for differential discounting of historical data. For example, if one wants to account for two qualitatively different sets of historical data (e.g., randomized vs. observational data), respective parameters τ_1 and τ_2 could be used; see also WinBUGS code in the Appendix 2.5 for this option.

Under the *MAC* approach, inference for the parameter in the new trial $\theta_\star$ can be likelihood-based or Bayesian. The important difference from standard meta-analysis is that the parameter of interest is $\theta_\star$ rather than μ. Thus, Bayesian inference results in the posterior distribution of $\theta_\star$ from all the data

$$\theta_\star|Y_1, \ldots, Y_J, Y_\star \tag{2.8}$$

whereas a non-Bayesian analysis would comprise a point estimate, standard error, and confidence interval. On the other hand, the two-step *MAP* approach first derives the meta-analytic-predictive prior from historical data

$$\theta_\star|Y_1, \ldots, Y_J \tag{2.9}$$

In a second step, this prior will be combined with the new trial data $Y_\star$.

It is important to note that the *MAC* and *MAP* analyses give the same results [55]. Beyond this equivalence, however, there are advantages and disadvantages for the two approaches. The statistical analysis for the retrospective *MAC* approach is easier. On the other hand, *MAP* requires a formal prior derivation, which may be mandatory in certain situations, but can be beneficial also for other reasons. Not only are historical data explicitly quantified, it may also influence the trial design, by, for example, decreasing the sample size of the control group; see Application 1 in Section 2.3.

The main challenge when incorporating historical data is finding an appropriate weight relative to the new trial data, thus avoiding extreme pooling or stratification. The weight depends on the between-trial heterogeneity, the parameter τ in (2.7).

How does τ influence the analysis for the parameter $\theta_\star$ in the new trial? This can be seen explicitly for the normal-normal hierarchical model (2.6), (2.7): for fixed τ and a non-informative prior on μ, the trial-specific posterior distributions for θ_k are [58]

$$\theta_k|Y_1,\ldots,Y_J \sim N\left(B_k \sum_{j=1}^{J} \frac{w_j}{w_+} Y_j + (1-B_k)Y_k,\, B_k(\tau^2 + \frac{B_k}{w_+})\right) \tag{2.10}$$

where w_j and B_k are inverse-variance weights and shrinkage factors,

$$w_j = \frac{1}{s_j^2 + \tau^2}, \quad B_k = \frac{s_k^2}{s_k^2 + \tau^2} \tag{2.11}$$

and $w_+ = \sum_{j=1}^{J} w_j$ is the posterior precision (inverse of variance) of μ. If the new trial is included with no data ($s_\star^2 = \infty, w_\star = 0, B_\star = 1$) in the above equations, it follows that

$$\theta_\star|Y_1,\ldots,Y_J \sim N\left(\sum_{j=1}^{J} \frac{w_j}{w_+} Y_j,\, \frac{1}{w_+} + \tau^2\right) \tag{2.12}$$

For the special case of one historical trial, the variance of $\theta_\star$ becomes $s_1^2 + 2\tau^2$. From (2.12) it follows that the posterior variance of the *MAP* prior is the sum of two terms: the posterior variance of μ and the between-trial variance τ^2. The first decreases with increasing amounts of historical data, whereas the second term does not — on the contrary, adding more and more historical trials bears the risk of including increasingly heterogeneous populations. In summary, the additive between-trial variance τ^2 of trial parameters strongly influences the weight of historical data.

Not knowing τ complicates the situation, in particular if the number of trials is small; precisely estimating the variance τ^2 from a few estimated parameters is not feasible. In this case, prior judgment about the similarity of trial parameters and the data at hand will provide information for τ. If one wants to be weakly-informative for τ, we advise using prior distributions that span a wide range of plausible values; half-normal, half-t, and half-Cauchy distributions have been suggested in this context [21, 48, 58]. For instance, in the binary case τ values of 0.5 and 1 on the log-odds scale represent substantial to large between-trial heterogeneity. In the example, we used a half-normal prior with scale parameter 0.5, which has median 0.34 and 95%-interval (0.016,1.12) and thus covers small to large between-trial heterogeneity. If one wants to be even more conservative, a half-normal prior with scale 1 could be used. Even though the prior for τ can influence considerably the weight of historical data, since these data are usually selected under fairly stringent conditions, it seems reasonable to use priors that allow for non-negligible borrowing from historical data.

When using the two-step *MAP* approach, it is important to note that the *MAP* prior cannot be derived analytically, which makes MCMC analysis necessary; code for the binary example is given in the Appendix. Moreover, looking at the MCMC prior for the example (histogram in Figure 2.1), we see that an approximation by a standard distribution can be poor. Here, the approximations by a Beta distribution, Beta(1.84,10.15), or Beta(2.21,11.94) using moment-matching or maximum-likelihood are fairly similar but deliver disappointing fits.

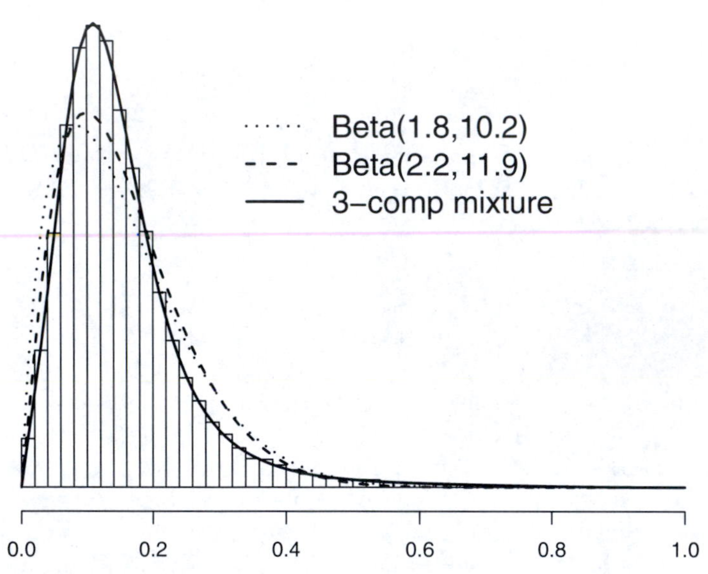

FIGURE 2.1: Histogram of MCMC MAP prior for example of Section 2.2.2, with best fitting moment-matching (dotted line) and MLE (dashed line) Beta distributions, and 3-component Beta mixture (solid line).

Thus, better approximations to *MAP* priors are needed. These can be obtained to any degree of accuracy by mixtures of standard distributions [10]. In the example, the following 3-component mixture (shown in Figure 2.1) gives a very good fit

$$p(\theta_\star|Y_1, Y_2) = 0.52\,\text{Beta}(2.1, 11.7) + 0.43\,\text{Beta}(5.3, 34.2) + 0.05\,\text{Beta}(1.8, 3.2) \tag{2.13}$$

The advantages of the mixture representation are two-fold. First, in conjugate settings, analytical solutions exist for mixtures of conjugate priors, with posterior mixture weights depending on the prior mixture weights and the marginal likelihood of the data for each mixture component [44]. Second, and more importantly, *MAP* priors are often quite robust, due to the fact that one of the mixture components is typically weakly-informative. How to further robustify *MAP* priors is discussed in Section 2.2.3.

In the example of Table 2.1, the *MAP* analyses for the two data scenarios were obtained under prior (2.13). The results show minimal differences between *MAP* and *MAC*, which are due to using the mixture approximation rather than the actual *MAP* prior.

2.2.3 Robust Meta-analytic-predictive Priors and Prior-data Conflict

The main assumption when using historical data is that they are relevant for the current clinical study. Through careful selection of the historical studies, the risk of conflict between historical and current study information can be minimized [47]. Nevertheless, one has to consider the possibility that for unforeseen reasons, historical data are not relevant. If we acknowledge this, and denote the probability of this happening by $1-p_R$, then the prior information to use is

$$p_{HR}(\theta_\star) = p_R \, p_H(\theta_\star) + (1-p_R) \, p_V(\theta_\star) \tag{2.14}$$

where $p_H(\theta_\star)$ is the *MAP* prior from historical data and $p_V(\theta_\star)$ is a vague prior that would be used if no historical data were available.

The robust historical prior $p_{HR}(\theta_\star)$ is heavy-tailed, which has the consequence that the informative component $p_H(\theta_\star)$ is adaptively discarded in case of prior-data conflict [45]. To illustrate this, we consider the prior from the example in Section 2.2.2 using moment-matching, $p_{Beta}(\theta_\star) = \text{Beta}(1.8, 10.2)$. If we judge that the historical data may not be relevant for the current trial with a probability of $1 - p_R = 0.5$, then the robust prior $p_{HR}(\theta_\star) = 0.5 p_{Beta}(\theta_\star) + 0.5\text{Beta}(1,1)$ would be appropriate.

Figure 2.2 shows the posterior distribution for two data scenarios with 3/20 (15%) or 15/20 (75%) responders in the control group, using either the historical prior $p_{Beta}(\theta_\star)$ or the robust historical prior $p_{HR}(\theta_\star)$. When prior and data are consistent (3/20), the posteriors are similar for both priors. However, in case of prior-data conflict, the behavior for the priors $p_H(\theta_\star)$ and $p_{HR}(\theta_\star)$ is very different. While for the conjugate historical prior the posterior is always a compromise between prior and data, the robust historical prior essentially leads to a discarding of the historical information in case of clear prior-data conflict.

As mentioned in Section 2.2.2, meta-analytic-predictive priors are typically heavy-tailed. Hence, even without further robustification, such priors will be downweighted if the data are in conflict with the prior. Further robustifying these priors by adding a vague component will lead to a more rapid reaction to prior-data conflict [55]. Although we considered here priors derived from historical data, robustification of priors may also be used if they were obtained through elicitation from experts [20].

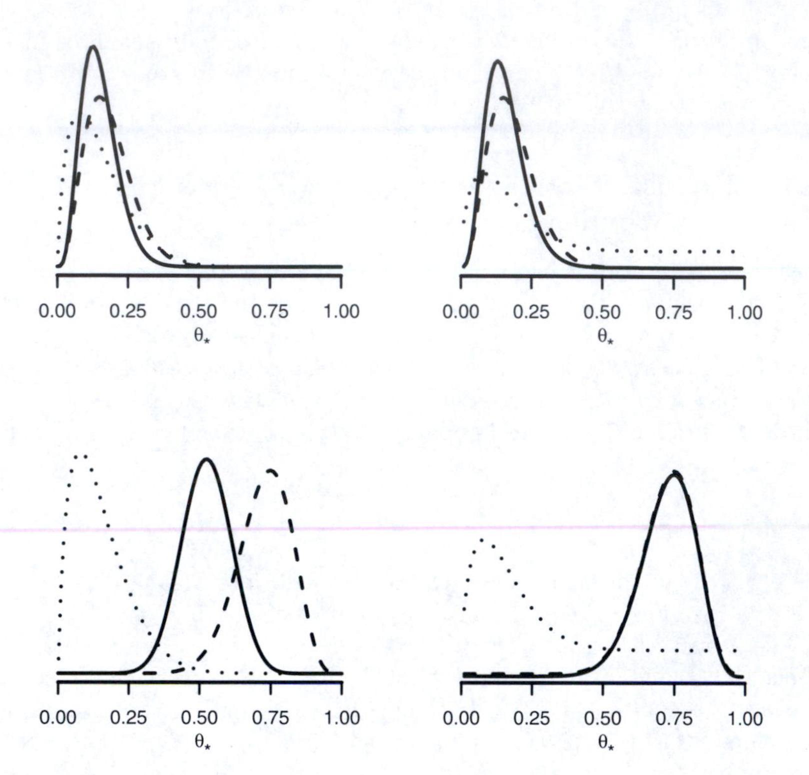

FIGURE 2.2: Prior (dotted line), normalized likelihood (dashed line), and posterior (solid line) for four scenarios. The left panels show results for the conjugate Beta(1.8, 10.2) prior, and the right panels for the robust prior 0.5Beta(1.8, 10.2) + 0.5Beta(1, 1). The upper panels correspond to prior-data consistency (3/20 responders), the lower panels to prior-data conflict (15/20 responders).

2.2.4 Prior Effective Sample Size

When using an informative prior in the Bayesian analysis of a clinical study, it is important to quantify how much this prior information is worth in number of patients, i.e., the (prior) effective sample size (*ESS*). The *ESS* is relevant for communication, but also for the design of the clinical study. For example, in a randomized controlled study one may want to reduce the number of patients randomized to control using historical control information (see Application 1 in Section 2.3).

The calculation of *ESS* is straightforward for conjugate priors [5]. For example if the endpoint is binary, a conjugate Beta(a, b) prior has an *ESS* of $a+b$. However, priors derived through meta-analytic-predictive approaches are non-conjugate priors, and for these only an approximate correspondence of a prior to a sample size can be established. A general approach was proposed by Morita et al. [37], where the ESS is the number of patients such that the expected information of the posterior under a non-informative prior is the same as the information of the informative prior; the calculation of the ESS assumes approximate normality of prior and posterior. If the prior is a conjugate prior, e.g., Beta(1.8, 10.2), then $ESS = 12$ using this approach, as desired. If the prior is non-conjugate, e.g., the mixture prior 0.5Beta(1.8, 10.2)+0.5Beta(1, 1), then $ESS = 5$.

Simpler approaches, based on the assumption that variances of estimates are inversely proportional to sample sizes, were given in [36, 43, 46]. For example, under complete homogeneity, with variance V_0 for $\theta_\star$, the ESS is the sum of the historical control patients: $ESS = N = \sum_{j=1}^{J} n_j$. On the other hand, under heterogeneity the respective variance V_τ of $\theta_\star$ is larger than V_0, providing the following ESS:

$$ESS = \frac{V_0}{V_\tau} N \tag{2.15}$$

The respective ESS for the two prior distributions mentioned before can be found using the normal approximation on the logit-scale. The respective numbers are $ESS = 10$ for the conjugate prior, and $ESS = 3$ for the mixture prior. At this point, it may also be interesting to derive the ESS for the mixture approximation (2.13) to the meta-analytic-predictive prior derived in Section 2.2.2. Using the approach by Morita et al., the respective ESS is found as 25; for the variance ratio approach the ESS is 15. These differences are due to the different approximations which are used by the approaches.

2.3 Applications

2.3.1 Application 1: A Randomized Phase II Trial Using Historical Control Data

In this application, we extend the example from Section 2.2.2 to the design of a randomized phase II study with a new treatment (T) and standard of care (P); for the latter we will use historical data as described in Section 2.2.2. The number of responders are denoted by $r_\star^T$ and $r_\star^P$, respectively, and the likelihood is given by

$$r_\star^T | \pi_\star^T \sim \text{Binomial}(n_\star^T, \pi_\star^T), \quad r_\star^P | \pi_\star^P \sim \text{Binomial}(n_\star^P, \pi_\star^P) \tag{2.16}$$

The measure of interest is the difference in response rates $\delta_\star = \pi_\star^T - \pi_\star^P$. Study success is defined as at least 95% posterior probability that the new treatment is better than the standard of care, i.e., $P(\delta_\star > 0 | r_\star^T, r_\star^P) \geq 0.95$.

Without historical data, this study should have about 90% power using

1 : 1 randomization and assuming an alternative for the treatment difference $\delta_\star = 0.3$, which could be achieved with 40 patients per group. Since historical data are available, we will reduce the required number of patients in the control arm.

In Section 2.2.4, we have assessed the *ESS* of the *MAP* prior (2.13) as being approximately 15 to 25 patients. Even after robustification, the prior will still contain valuable information for the control rate. Therefore, it seems realistic to reduce the number of patients in the control arm by 50% to 20 patients. In order to ensure this design still has the desired properties, we will assess its operating characteristics.

When evaluating Bayesian designs, there are two design characteristics which should be considered. The first refers to data scenarios. They are used to illustrate analyses based on hypothetical on-study data. In Section 2.2.2 two data scenarios have been presented (for the control group), and we will not investigate these further. However, evaluation of data scenarios helps to understand inferential outcomes and communicate potential trial results.

The second characteristic is the frequentist properties of a design (operating characteristics), such as type I error and power. For a traditional study not using prior information, we would assess the type I error and power by calculating the probability of declaring study success given the null hypothesis ($\delta_\star = 0$) and the alternative hypothesis ($\delta_\star = 0.3$). However, when using historical control information, we would also like to assess these metrics for varying response rates in the control arm. This will provide insight into the performance in the case of a potential prior-data conflict.

For the treatment arm, we use a Beta$(0.176, 1)$ prior which is weakly-informative with mean 0.15 and 95% probability interval $(0.00, 0.87)$. For the control arm, in order to illustrate the properties of the robust *MAP* prior, we also assessed the non-robustified *MAP* prior (2.13) and the moment-matching Beta distribution. Additionally, we compared the design against two trials without historical data. The first is a 2:1 randomized study with 40 and 20 patients in the treatment and control arm, respectively, and the second a 1:1 randomized study with 40 patients per arm. The prior distributions for the control and treatment response rate are chosen as Beta$(0.176, 1)$. This leads to the following five cases:

	$n_\star^T$ / $n_\star^C$	$p(\theta_\star^T)$	$p(\theta_\star^C)$
1 – Hist: p_{Mix}	40/20	Beta(0.176, 1)	$0.5p_{MAP} + 0.5\text{Beta}(1, 1)$
2 – Hist: p_{MAP}	40/20	Beta(0.176, 1)	MAP prior from (2.13)
3 – Hist: p_{Beta}	40/20	Beta(0.176, 1)	Beta(1.8, 10.2)
4 – No hist: 40/20	40/20	Beta(0.176, 1)	Beta(0.176, 1)
5 – No hist: 40/40	40/40	Beta(0.176, 1)	Beta(0.176, 1)

Table 2.2 presents the results based on 10,000 simulated trials. We first discuss the results for the design using historical data. When there is high agreement between the historical and the actual control rate, the type I error

TABLE 2.2: Type I error and power (%) under different control rates $\theta_\star^P$ and treatment effects $\delta_\star$ for different study designs (see text of Application 1).

$\theta_\star^P$	Hist:p_{Mix}	Hist:p_{MAP}	Hist:p_{Beta}	No hist:40/20	No hist:40/40
			No treatment effect ($\delta_\star = 0$)		
0.15	2.6	2.8	3.8	5.0	6.0
0.25	7.9	11.5	8.1	4.9	5.2
0.30	9.0	15.4	11.6	4.7	5.1
			Treatment effect ($\delta_\star = 0.3$)		
0.15	87	94	91	80	92
0.25	80	93	92	74	87
0.30	77	91	94	70	85

is well controlled for all of the priors. By design, we would expect around 5% type I error; the maximum observed is 3.8%. With increasing difference between the historical and actual control rate, type I errors increase. The most extreme inflation is for prior 2, but also prior 3 has considerable inflation. The lowest inflation in type I error is observed for prior 1. It should be noted though that such a scenario is highly unlikely given the historical evidence on the control rate.

Regarding power, we have similar performance of priors 2 and 3, whereas prior 1 reacts to a potential prior-data conflict. Overall, the p_{Mix} prior shows good performance with well controlled type I error and close to 90% power for the consistent scenario.

Finally, when comparing to the randomized studies without historical data (cases 4 and 5), a few observations are of interest. Both designs control the type I error; however, case 4 has only about 80% power which is substantially below the desired 90%. Case 5, on the other hand, reaches the 90% threshold. It has slightly higher power than case 1, but numbers are close showing that the chosen reduction of sample size by 50% for case 1 is reasonable.

2.3.2 Application 2: Design of a Japanese Dose Escalation Study Incorporating Data from Western Patients

In this application we present the design of a Japanese phase I dose escalation study which incorporates historical data from a dose escalation study in Western patients. The main goal of phase I dose escalation studies in Oncology is to assess the relationship between dose and toxicity. This is usually done by identifying the maximum tolerated dose (MTD) based on adverse events known as dose-limiting toxicities (DLT) [15]. Dose escalation happens sequentially, enrolling cohorts of 3 to 6 patients to the current dose. Based on the prespecified decision criteria and depending on the observed DLT data (and other relevant information, such as exposure and adverse event data), the next cohort of patients is assigned to a higher, lower, or to the same dose. Escalation continues until the MTD is reached or until a lower dose with favorable efficacy and safety is identified.

Most dose escalation studies are conducted globally. However, based on the guideline on global clinical trials [29] of Japan's Pharmaceuticals and Medical Devices Agency (PMDA), stand-alone dose escalation studies are regularly conducted in Japanese patients only. Most often, at the time when the Japanese study is designed, considerable data from Western patients are already available. Therefore, it is of interest to incorporate these data into the design of the Japanese study.

A Bayesian logistic regression model with overdose control (EWOC) will guide the dose escalation [3, 41, 73]. The model is defined as follows: for dose d, the number of patients with a DLT (r_d) in a cohort of size n_d is binomial

$$r_d|\pi_d \sim \text{Binomial}(n_d, \pi_d) \tag{2.17}$$

and the log-odds of DLT is given by

$$\text{logit}(\pi_d) = \log(\alpha) + \beta \log(d/d^\star) \tag{2.18}$$

where $d^\star$ re-scales the doses, with the interpretation that α is the odds of a DLT at $d^\star$. Prior distributions for $\theta = (\log(\alpha), \log(\beta))$ are specified as bivariate normal

$$\theta \sim N_2(m, S) \tag{2.19}$$

with prior means $m = (m_1, m_2)$ and prior covariance matrix S composed of standard deviations s_1, s_2 and correlation cor. If no relevant prior information is available, we use a weakly-informative prior distribution given by $m_1 = \log(0.5), m_2 = 0, s_1 = 2, s_2 = 1, cor = 0$ [73]. The inferential part of dosing recommendations is based on the posterior distribution of π_d. Statistics such as mean, standard deviation and interval probabilities are of interest. We will use the following intervals, which have gained wide acceptance by various review boards:

$$\begin{aligned} \pi_d &< 0.16 && \text{underdosing (UD)} \\ 0.16 \le \pi_d &< 0.33 && \text{targeted toxicity (TT)} \\ \pi_d &\ge 0.33 && \text{overdosing (OD)} \end{aligned}$$

Following escalation with overdose control [3], only doses with $P(\pi_d \ge 0.33) < 0.25$ are eligible for the next cohort. This is a commonly accepted boundary to control the risk to which patients are exposed.

Since the majority of decision makers in a dose escalation meeting are not statisticians, it is important to illustrate these metrics in an easily readable way. Graphical illustrations have proven useful in the communication to non-statisticians. For example, consider the top row in Figure 2.3. On the left-hand side, the mean and 95% probability intervals are shown, and on the right-hand side, the probability of underdosing, targeted dosing, and overdosing;

the bars for overdosing are highlighted in black. Non-statisticians immediately understand these doses are considered too toxic for patients given the available evidence. In this application, the figures will also be used to illustrate various aspects of the design.

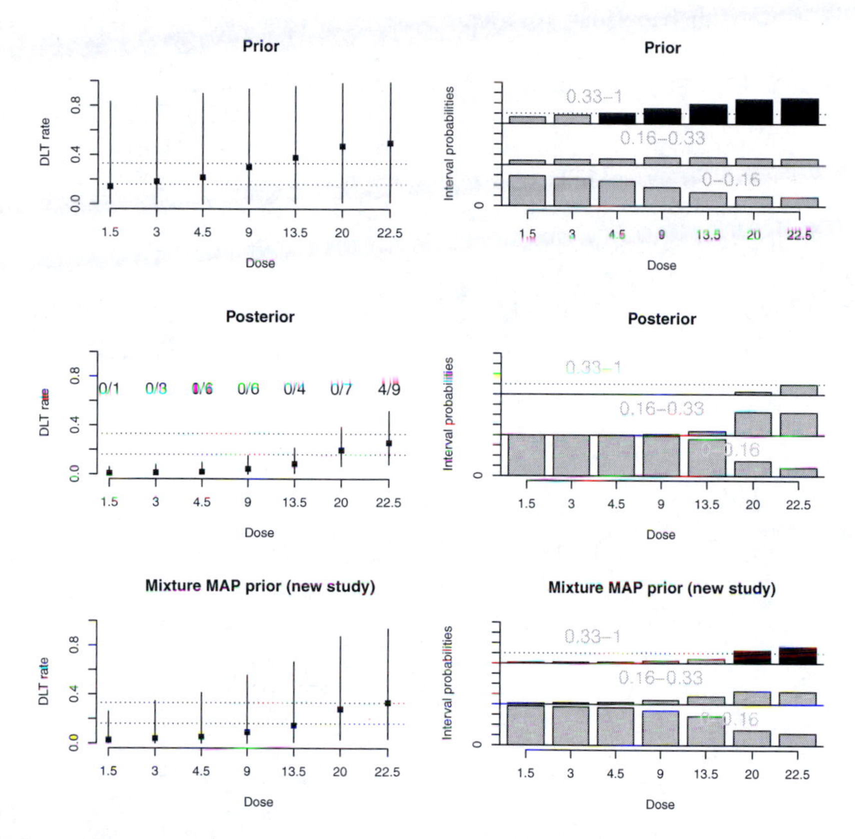

FIGURE 2.3: Western single-agent trial: mean and 95% intervals (left panels) for DLT rates, with interval probabilities of underdosing, targeted toxicity, overdosing (right panels), for prior (top row), posterior (middle row), and *MAP* mixture prior for Japan (bottom row).

We will incorporate historical information using the meta-analytic-predictive approach described in Section 2.2.2. For the aforementioned logistic model, the respective meta-analytic-predictive prior is found using a hierarchical model for $\theta_j, \theta_\star$:

$$\begin{aligned} r_{d,j}|\pi_{d,j} &\sim \text{Binomial}(n_{d,j}, \pi_{d,j}) \qquad (2.20) \\ \text{logit}(\pi_{d,j}) &= \log(\alpha_j) + \beta_j \log(d/d^*) \\ \theta_j|\mu_1, \mu_2, \Psi &\sim N_2((\mu_1, \mu_2), \Psi) \\ \theta_\star|\mu_1, \mu_2, \Psi &\sim N_2((\mu_1, \mu_2), \Psi) \end{aligned}$$

with

$$\Psi = \begin{pmatrix} \tau_1^2 & \rho\tau_1\tau_2 \\ \rho\tau_1\tau_2 & \tau_2^2 \end{pmatrix} \tag{2.21}$$

Normal prior distributions are used for μ_1, μ_2, log-normal prior distributions for τ_1, τ_2, and a uniform prior distribution for ρ.

When designing the Japanese study, considerable data from the Western dose escalation study were available (see top row of Table 2.3). As often the case in dose escalation trials, no DLTs were seen at lower cohorts, and DLTs only occurred near the MTD. These data are used to derive the meta-analytic-predictive prior based on the model described before, with the following prior specifications:

- $\mu_1 \sim N(0, 2^2)$, $\mu_2 \sim N(0, 1)$
- $\tau_1 \sim LN(\log(0.5), \log(2)/1.96)$, $\tau_2 \sim LN(\log(0.25), \log(2)/1.96)$
- $\rho \sim Unif(-1, 1)$

The priors are weakly-informative for μ_1, μ_2, reflect substantial between-trial variability (median) with 95%-interval from moderate to large for τ_1, τ_2, and are non-informative for ρ.

TABLE 2.3: Western data and two data scenarios for Japanese study.

	Doses						
	1.5	3.0	4.5	9.0	13.5	20.0	22.5
Western	0/1	0/3	0/6	0/6	0/4	0/7	4/9
Japan S–1	–	–	0/3	0/3	1/3	–	–
Japan S–2	–	–	0/3	2/3	–	–	–

Since Western and Japanese dose-DLT profiles for the drug are expected to be similar, it is reasonable to assume substantial (with range from moderate to large) between-trial variability, reflected in the priors for τ_1, τ_2. An important question, however, remains: what happens if the DLT profiles are dissimilar? In this case, it would be better to reduce the amount of borrowing from the historical data. Therefore, we define our prior as a mixture of the informative (MAP) prior and a second, weakly-informative component in order to make it robust (see Section 2.2.3). The mixture prior will help to borrow from the historical data if the two DLT profiles are similar, whilst it will discount the historical data in case of dissimilarity (prior-data conflict). The prior mixture weights were chosen as 90% for the MAP component and 10% for the weakly-informative component, resulting in the following prior for $\theta_\star$:

$$p(\theta_\star) = 0.9 \times N_{2,MAP} + 0.1 \times N_{2,V} \tag{2.22}$$

Figure 2.3 illustrates the derivation of the prior distribution. In the top row, the weakly-informative prior distribution for the Western study is shown. In the middle row, the posterior distribution, and in the bottom row, the mixture *MAP* prior (2.22). Based on this prior distribution, one could start with a dose as high as 13.5 mg: the overdose probability is clearly below 25%, which can also be seen in Figure 2.3 (overdose probability bar shown in light gray). However, based on additional non-DLT information, the starting dose for the Japanese study was chosen as 4.5 mg.

In order to illustrate the on-study behavior of the statistical model, we present two data scenarios: a first scenario where the Japanese and Western dose-DLT profiles are similar, and a second scenario where they are dissimilar. The respective data can be found in the middle and bottom row of Table 2.3. The inferential results of the analyses are shown in Figure 2.4. For scenario 1, the hypothetical data are in good agreement with the historical data, and borrowing from the Western data is fairly strong. The posterior distribution would allow re-testing at the dose of 13.5 mg. The mixture weights are updated to 94% for the *MAP* component and to 6% for the weakly-informative component, respectively.

For scenario 2, the situation is different. The observed dose-DLT profiles are considerably dissimilar with an increased toxicity for the Japanese patients. This would be of potential concern if re-testing at 9 mg was allowed. However, this is not the case: the overdose probability at 9 mg is above the 25% threshold requiring a de-escalation to 4.5 mg. It is important to note that the mixture prior plays an important role in this scenario: the mixture weights are updated to 76% for the *MAP* component, and 24% for the weakly-informative component, reflecting the dissimilarity between the historical and the actual data. This is not unexpected: under the *MAP* prior, the predicted probability of observing 2 or more DLTs in 3 patients is 3%, pointing towards a disagreement between the historical and the actual data. We also observe that for this scenario, the posterior uncertainty (95% probability intervals) is slightly larger than the mixture prior uncertainty. This is due to the fact that more weight is given to the weakly-informative component, reflecting that the *MAP* prior should be less relevant for the data observed.

Finally, we note that a thorough evaluation of the model should include frequentist operating characteristics (see Application 1). This can be done by simulations based on assumed true dose-DLT profiles; for an example see [73].

In conclusion, using the meta-analytic-predictive prior to incorporate adequately discounted historical data and making the prior robust by adding a weakly-informative mixture component offers a promising approach for phase I dose escalation trials.

2.3.3 Application 3: Non-inferiority and Biosimilar Trials

To establish the efficacy of a test drug, a clinical study comparing the test drug to placebo is often the preferred option. Such a design allows a direct evaluation within the study on whether the test drug is superior to placebo,

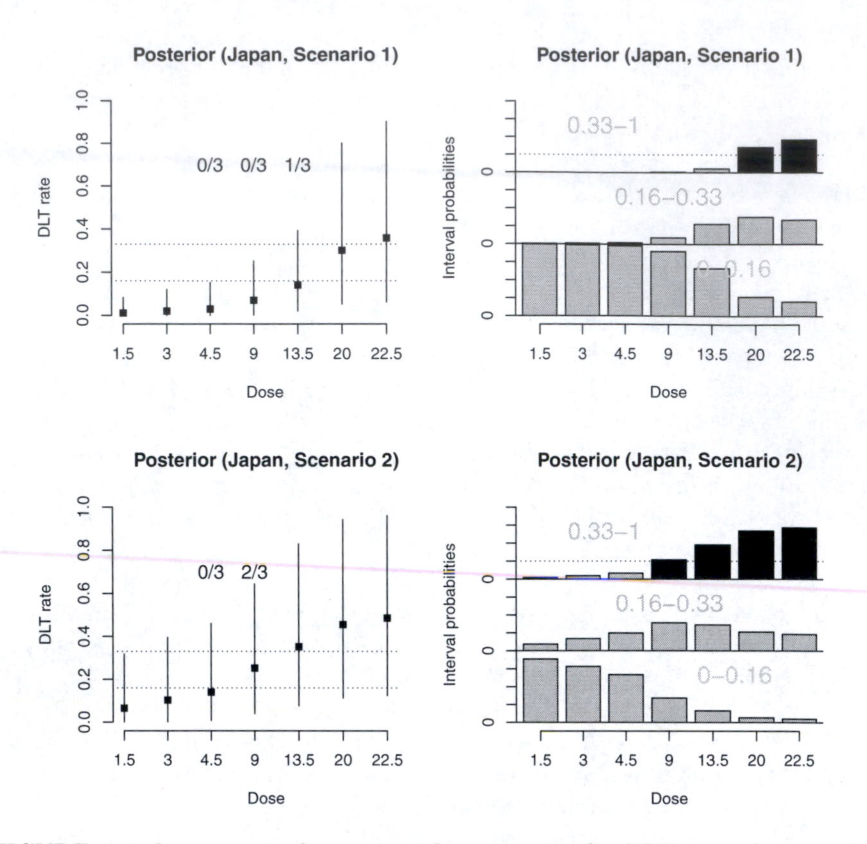

FIGURE 2.4: Japanese single-agent trial: summaries for DLT rates for two data scenarios.

which is the minimal efficacy requirement for approval by health authorities. However, for serious diseases where a treatment is already available, use of placebo may not be ethical, and then a non-inferiority study comparing the test drug with an active-control drug may be considered [61]. Such studies cannot provide direct evidence on whether the test drug is superior to placebo, and hence require external historical information to address the minimal efficacy requirement. Similar considerations also apply to biosimilar studies, where a test biosimilar is compared to a biologic drug.

To address the minimal efficacy requirement in a non-inferiority trial comparing test drug (T) with placebo (P), we consider the simplest setup, where J historical trials comparing the active control (C) with placebo are available. Formally, we assume that the non-inferiority trial also contains a placebo arm, for which, however, no data are available. We denote the efficacy parameters in the non-inferiority trial for the three arms as $\theta_\star^T$, $\theta_\star^C$, and $\theta_\star^P$. The test drug is superior to placebo if $\theta_\star^T - \theta_\star^P > 0$, assuming here that larger values of θ

correspond to better efficacy. We can express the difference between test drug and placebo as:

$$\theta_\star^T - \theta_\star^P = (\theta_\star^T - \theta_\star^C) + (\theta_\star^C - \theta_\star^P) \tag{2.23}$$

Information on $\theta_\star^T - \theta_\star^C$ is directly obtained from the non-inferiority trial, while for information on $\theta_\star^C - \theta_\star^P$ external data from the J historical trials are required. We denote the efficacy parameters in the j-th historical trial by θ_j^C, and θ_j^P.

To make use of the historical information, a model linking the parameters of the historical trials and the non-inferiority trial is needed. Following the methodology of Section 2.2.2, we use a random-effects model:

$$(\theta_\star^C - \theta_\star^P), (\theta_1^C - \theta_1^P), \ldots, (\theta_J^C - \theta_J^P) | \mu_{CP}, \tau^2 \sim N(\mu_{CP}, \tau^2) \tag{2.24}$$

where μ_{CP} is the population mean difference of control and placebo, and τ is the between-trial standard deviation. An analysis of the historical data with this model provides inference on $(\theta_\star^C - \theta_\star^P)$, and, hence, on whether the test drug is superior to placebo.

We considered here a basic setup, where several historical placebo-controlled clinical trials with the active control are available. More complex settings can be handled using evidence synthesis models. For example, if only single arm trials on placebo may be available, then models for historical controls can be used; see Section 2.2.2. Often several historical trials are available which are directly or indirectly linked to either active-control or placebo, and this information can be used for inference in the non-inferiority trial [56, 57], using network meta-analytic methods [24, 32, 52]. In some cases, meta-regression models are needed to relate the parameters of the historical trials and the non-inferiority trial [71].

Biosimilar trial

We now consider a biosimilar trial in cancer patients which will compare the test biosimilar (T) to the active-control (C), a biologic drug, with $n_\star^T$ and $n_\star^C$ patients in the two treatment arms. Denoting the number of responders by $Y_\star^T$ and $Y_\star^C$, respectively, we assume that $Y_\star^T | \pi_\star^T \sim \text{Binomial}(n_\star^T, \pi_\star^T)$ and $Y_\star^C | \pi_\star^C \sim \text{Binomial}(n_\star^C, \pi_\star^C)$. The response rate of the putative placebo (P) in this biosimilar trial is denoted by $\pi_\star^P$ (placebo here actually corresponds to standard chemotherapy).

The minimal efficacy requirement for the test treatment is that it would have been superior to placebo, had placebo been included in this biosimilar trial; this corresponds to a comparison between $\pi_\star^T$ and $\pi_\star^P$. However, as no placebo arm is included in the biosimilar trial, indirect evidence from historical clinical trials in the same patient population involving C and/or P is needed to address this question. For the biosimilar trial, the historical data in the population of interest are shown in Figure 2.5. It should be noted that of these 10 historical trials, all except the first are single-arm trials.

We assume that $j = 1, \cdots, J$ historical studies involving C and/or P are

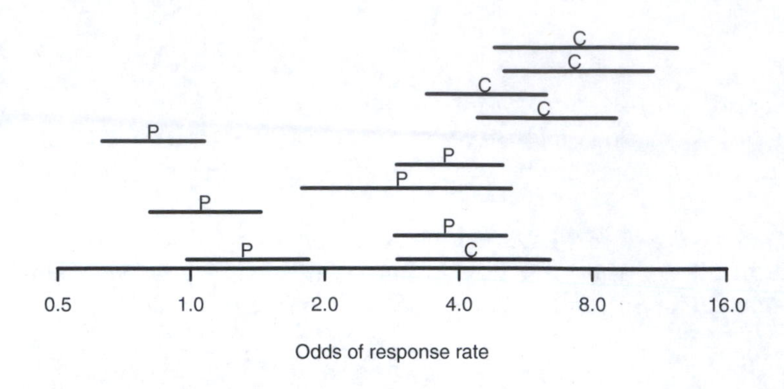

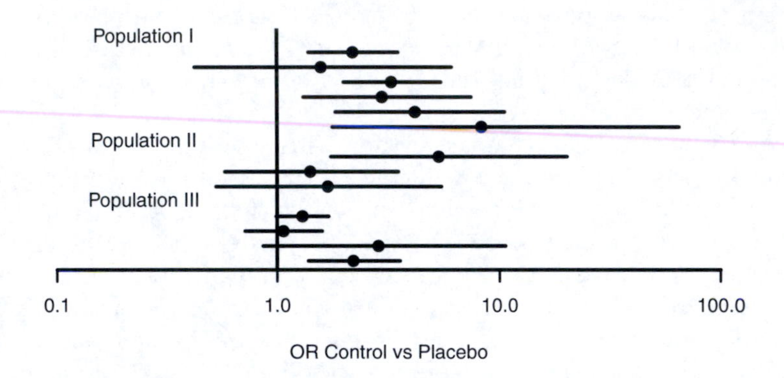

FIGURE 2.5: Biosimilar trial: the upper panel shows the odds of the response rates with 95% probability intervals for 10 historical trials (C=control, P=Placebo). The lower panel shows odds ratios with 95% probability intervals for 13 historical trials in three related populations, denoted by I, II, and III.

available, with n_j^C and n_j^P patients on the control and placebo arm, respectively (n_j^C or n_j^P are 0 for single-arm studies). The corresponding number of responders are denoted by Y_j^T and Y_j^C, and it is assumed that for $j = 1, \ldots, J$:

$$Y_j^C|\pi_j^C \sim \text{Binomial}(n_j^C, \pi_j^C), \quad Y_j^P|\pi_j^P \sim \text{Binomial}(n_j^P, \pi_j^P)$$

with response rates π_j^C and π_j^P (either Y_j^C or Y_j^P are missing for single-arm studies).

To make use of the historical trials to address the minimal efficacy requirement, assumptions linking the true response rates in the biosimilar trial and the historical trials have to be made. To specify these links, the log-odds scale commonly considered in the meta-analytic literature will be used. The log-odds of the response rates is denoted by $\theta_j^i = \text{logit}(\pi_{\text{j}}^{\text{i}})$ for $j = \star, 1, \ldots, J$ and $i = T, C, P$.

The first link uses a random-effects model for the log-odds of the response rates in the control group

$$\theta_j^C | \mu_C, \tau_C^2 \sim N(\mu_C, \tau_C^2), \quad j = \star, 1, \dots, J \tag{2.25}$$

where μ_C is the population mean, and τ_C is the between-trial standard deviation. This assumption allows to incorporate information from single-arm trials, appropriately discounted due to between-trial variability.

The second link is established by assuming a random-effects model for the log-odds ratios,

$$\delta_j^{CP} = \theta_j^C - \theta_j^P | \mu_{CP}, \tau_\delta^2 \sim N(\mu_{CP}, \tau_\delta^2), \quad j = \star, 1, \dots, J \tag{2.26}$$

where μ_{CP} is the population mean, and τ_δ is the between-trial standard deviation. If τ_δ were zero, a common effect model would be obtained, where the odds ratios are all identical in the biosimilar trial and the historical trials, i.e., $\theta_\star^C - \theta_\star^P = \theta_1^C - \theta_1^P = \dots = \theta_J^C - \theta_J^P$.

To estimate τ_δ, the historical trials must include at least two randomized trials comparing C and P. In our case, only one randomized historical trial is available (see Figure 2.5). Hence either a plausible value of τ_δ can be assumed, or it can be assumed that τ_δ is the same as in related patient populations, where C and P have been used, and where several randomized historical trials are available [24]. A random-effects analysis of these historical randomized trials in the different patient population will then provide a prior distribution for τ_δ.

In our case, 13 historical randomized trials in three related populations (denoted by I, II, and III) are shown in Figure 2.5. The random-effects model assumes that the population means are different for each of these populations and the population of interest, but that the between-trial standard deviation τ_δ is the same for each of these populations, and also for the population of interest. The Bayesian meta-analysis of these 13 trials with weakly-informative priors provides a posterior distribution for τ_δ which can be approximated by a Normal distribution truncated at zero: $N_0(0.125, 0.13^2)$. This posterior is then used as a prior for the analysis of the historical data in the population of interest (Figure 2.5). The resulting Bayesian analysis gives the posterior distribution for the odds-ratio of control against placebo in the biosimilar trial, summarized by the median 3.2 and 95% probability interval (1.8, 5.7). Once the biosimilar results are available, this information will allow to derive the posterior distribution for the odds-ratio of the test biosimilar against placebo. Alternatively, an equivalence margin could be obtained, e.g., 1.8, the lower limit of the 95% probability interval (margin approach).

2.4 Discussion

There has been growing interest in the use of historical data in clinical trials in recent years. This trend will likely continue, driven by ongoing changes in the health care environment. Ever-increasing drug development costs [1, 12, 39], narrower patient populations based on individualized treatment regimens [65], and challenging pricing and reimbursement negotiations [8] put continuous pressure on the pharmaceutical industry. In addition, especially in life-threatening diseases such as cancer, it may be more ethical to conduct studies which incorporate historical information [63]. Clinical teams are challenged to design studies which are smaller, quicker, more flexible, and cost-effective. Therefore, it is important for all parties, including statisticians, to become more flexible and implement novel approaches in practice.

In this chapter, we have described different approaches to incorporate historical data in clinical studies. This is one of several important elements in making clinical trials more efficient and, depending on the situation, more ethical. The examples illustrating the meta-analytic-predictive approach are based on real clinical studies; at Novartis Oncology alone, there are more than 100 phase I/II studies within 20 drug programs which have incorporated historical data [73]. Evidently, the added value of studies incorporating historical data was recognized not only by statisticians, but also by clinical teams implementing the studies, by the management endorsing them, and by external stakeholders approving them. This holds true for studies in other disease areas: for example, Baeten et al. [4] conducted a randomized trial in patients with ankylosing spondylitis enriching the control group with historical data, Walley et al. [69] presented a case study in chronic kidney disease, and several study groups have implemented the approach proposed by French et al. [19]. These are encouraging signals that clinical trials incorporating historical data are becoming more popular in practice.

Historical data play an essential role in evidence synthesis and in health economics. Most models for evidence synthesis rely on meta-analytic approaches including (random) effects meta-analysis, meta-regression, network meta-analysis [33] (also known as mixed treatment comparisons [32]), and similar models for individual data. The major concern in this area is therefore not the question of whether to include historical data or not, but rather which data should be included (e.g., from randomized studies, observational studies, registries) and how they should be included. Additionally, especially when data are sparse or the number of available studies is small, the question of incorporating external evidence to inform model parameters is of major importance. For example, including external evidence to inform the between-trial heterogeneity as proposed in [24] is also recommended in the NICE DSU Technical Support Document 2 [11].

Another area where historical data play an important role is diagnostic test studies. As high as the sensitivity and specificity of a diagnostic test may be, its positive and negative predictive values depend on the underlying disease prevalence. In their seminal paper in 1995, Joseph et al. [30] described the added value of incorporating historical (or concurrent) data when investigating a diagnostic test. Ang et al. [2] use the approach combined with historical information from meta-analyses on the sensitivity and specificity of diagnostic tests. Especially in the absence of a gold standard, the approach is frequently applied in diagnostic test studies.

Finally, one field where historical data are regularly used is statistical modelling. Especially in population pharmacokinetic (PK) (see, e.g., [50]) and pharmacodynamic (PD) modelling, historical data are important. Population PK/PD models integrate the available evidence across studies and therefore use actual and historical data simultaneously. One could even argue that from the viewpoint of a population PK/PD model, all data are actual since the model is continuously updated. Weber and colleagues [70] extend this approach developing a drug-disease model which integrates internal and external evidence, again showing that in some situations the distinction between actual and historical evidence may be less relevant than the distinction between internal and external evidence.

Another important subject which we have not discussed here is pediatric studies. Pediatric patients are a vulnerable subgroup and they need to be protected from undue risk [17]. Incorporating relevant information from adult patients (usually available at the time a pediatric indication is studied) may help to mitigate this risk [66]. For example, the same approach as described in Application 2 in Section 2.3 can be used to incorporate data from adult patients in a pediatric dose escalation study.

Whilst the benefits of incorporating historical data in clinical trials have been outlined, there are also challenges one has to overcome when implementing these trials in practice. The potentially biggest hurdle is to change the *status quo*. Many clinical teams, including statisticians, still perceive historical data as something which can, at best, be used for sample size calculation. To convince colleagues and management of an alternative approach which incorporates historical data in the actual study may not be simple. However, a clinical trial design which is potentially more ethical, requires fewer patients, and still has favorable statistical properties is a clear competitive advantage.

Another hurdle when incorporating historical data is the identification and preparation of the historical evidence. It is beyond the scope of this chapter to provide thorough guidance on this topic. However, in our experience, the required resources are often underestimated. Preparation of the historical evidence requires close collaboration between statisticians and clinicians. Judgment on the relevance of historical studies, on inclusion and exclusion criteria and on other aspects to avoid potential bias have to be made. Good guidance to successfully complete this task is given in the *Cochrane Handbook for Systematic Reviews of Interventions* [25], which is also available online (http://www.cochrane.org/handbook).

Finally, it is clear that not all phases of clinical development are open to clinical trials which incorporate historical data. In early development, especially for phase I and II studies, there are many opportunities for using historical data. The same is true for phase IV studies, where historical data are too often ignored. However, the situation is more complicated for phase III trials. With historical data, strict type I error control can generally not be guaranteed, and this may preclude the use of historical data for pivotal studies. However, it should be noted that this depends on the actual case [18, 54]; for example, in rare diseases, it is possible to propose alternative study designs to regulatory agencies. Adaptive designs that incorporate historical data and adjust decisions for prior-data conflict at the times of interim analyses [55] are particularly attractive. It is clear though that discussing such designs with regulatory agencies at an early stage is required.

Last but not least, many topics which we discussed are still developing as the field is growing. *ESS* calculation is being actively researched [37, 38, 62] and additional models to incorporate historical information (e.g., for survival data) are being developed. We are looking forward to an interesting future with an increased use of all relevant data in a prospective way, for the good of patients in need of novel therapies.

Acknowledgments

We would like to thank Satrajit Roychoudhury and Sebastian Weber for fruitful discussions on statistical-technical subjects, and Yulan Li and Shu-Fang Hsu-Schmitz for their contribution to the examples.

2.5 Appendix

WinBUGS code for the analysis is given below, including results for scenario 1 of the example in Section 2.2.2 (see Table 2.1).

```
model{
# prior for mean parameter of exchangeability distribution (*mu*)
   Prior.mu.prec <- pow(Prior.mu[2], -2)
   mu ~ dnorm(Prior.mu[1], Prior.mu.prec)

# Prior(s) for between trial standard deviation(s) tau
# for *Ntau* exchangeability distributions
 for (j in 1:Ntau){
    tau2.prec[j] <- pow(Prior.tau[j,2], -2)
```

```
    tau[j] ~ dnorm(Prior.tau[j,1], tau2.prec[j])I(0,)
    tau.prec[j] <- pow(tau[j], -2)
                        }
# likelihood/sampling model
# tau.index: a vector of length (Nstudy +1)
 for (h in 1:Nstudy) {
    r[h] ~ dbin(p[h], n[h])
    theta[h] <- mu + theta1[h]
    theta1[h] ~ dnorm(0, tau.prec[tau.index[h]])
    logit(p[h]) <- theta[h]
                        }
# Prediction for new trial
 theta.pred ~ dnorm(mu, tau.prec[tau.index[Nstudy+1]])
 logit.p.pred <- theta.pred
 logit(p.pred) <- theta.pred

# Optional (for graph using Inference-Compare): add exch mean
# and prediction in postilions Nstudy+1 and Nstudy+2
 logit(p[Nstudy+1]) <- mu
 theta[Nstudy+1] <- mu
 logit(p[Nstudy+2]) <- theta.pred
 theta[Nstudy+2] <- theta.pred
}

# ---------------------------------------------------------
# Data (for scenario 1)
# ---------------------------------------------------------

# Data list
list(
  Ntau          = 1,
  Prior.mu      = c(0,10000),
  Prior.tau     = structure(.Data= c(0, 0.5), .Dim=c(1, 2)),
# Prior.tau     = structure(.Data= c(0, 0.25, 0, 0.5), .Dim=c(2, 2)),
# actual data: number of cohorts, administered dose of the respective
# cohort, number of responses, number of patients in different studies
# for data scenarios, change input in this part only
  Nstudy =3,
  tau.index  =c(1,1,1,1),
  r = c( 4, 2, 3),
  n = c(17,26,20)
)

# initial values for 4 chains
list(mu = 0, tau = c(0.5))
list(mu = -0.2, tau = c(0.5))
list(mu = 0.2, tau = c(0.5))
list(mu = 0, tau = c(0.25))
```

```
# results, 4 chains, 10'000 burn-in, followed by 15'000 updates
node      mean    sd   MC error   2.5%   median  97.5%  start  sample
mu      -1.850 0.454   0.0029   -2.794  -1.834  -0.997  10001   60000
p[1]     0.166 0.065   0.0004    0.068   0.156   0.322  10001   60000
p[2]     0.126 0.049   0.0003    0.044   0.122   0.233  10001   60000
p[3]     0.146 0.055   0.0002    0.058   0.139   0.271  10001   60000
p[4]     0.144 0.055   0.0003    0.058   0.138   0.270  10001   60000
p[5]     0.152 0.082   0.0004    0.039   0.138   0.357  10001   60000
p.pred   0.152 0.082   0.0004    0.039   0.138   0.357  10001   60000
tau[1]   0.364 0.270   0.0033    0.013   0.312   1.003  10001   60000
```

Bibliography

[1] C. P. Adams and V. V. Brantner. Spending on new drug development. *Health Economics*, 19(2):130–141, 2010.

[2] M. Ang, W. L. Wong, S. Y. Kiew, X. Li, and S. P. Chee. Prospective head-to-head study comparing 2 commercial Interferon Gamma release assays for the diagnosis of tuberculous uveitis. *American Journal of Ophthalmology*, 157(6):1306–1314, 2014.

[3] J. Babb, A. Rogatko, and S. Zacks. Cancer phase I clinical trials: efficient dose escalation with overdose control. *Statistics in Medicine*, 17(10):1103–1120, 1998.

[4] D. Baeten, X. Baraliakos, J. Braun, J. Sieper, P. Emery, D. van der Heijde, I. McInnes, J. M. van Laar, R. Landewé, P. Wordsworth, J. Wollenhaupt, H. Kellner, J. Paramarta, J. Wei, A. Brachat, S. Bek, D. Laurent, Y. Li, Y. A. Wang, A. P. Bertolino, S. Gsteiger, A. M. Wright, and W. Hueber. Anti-interleukin-17A monoclonal antibody secukinumab in treatment of ankylosing spondylitis: a randomised, double-blind, placebo-controlled trial. *Lancet*, 382(9906):1705–1713, 2013.

[5] J. M. Bernardo and A. F. M. Smith. *Bayesian Theory*. Wiley, 1994.

[6] R. H. Browne. Reducing sample sizes when comparing experimental and control groups. *Archives of Environmental Health*, 31(3):169–170, 1976.

[7] M. H. Chen and J. G. Ibrahim. Power prior distributions for regression models. *Statistical Science*, 15(1):46–60, 2000.

[8] J. Cohen, A. Malins, and Z. Shahpurwala. Compared to US practice, evidence-based reviews in Europe appear to lead to lower prices for some drugs. *Health Affairs (Millwood)*, 32(4):762–770, 2013.

[9] L. Di Scala, J. Kerman, and B. Neuenschwander. Collection, synthesis, and interpretation of evidence: a proof-of-concept study in COPD. *Statistics in Medicine*, 32(10):1621–1634, 2013.

[10] P. Diaconis and D. Ylvisaker. Quantifying prior opinion. *Bayesian Statistics (Proceedings of the Second Valencia International Meeting)*, 2:133–148, 1984.

[11] S. Dias, N. J. Welton, A. J. Sutton, and A. E. Ades. NICE DSU Technical Support Document 2: A generalised linear modelling framework for pairwise and network meta-analysis of randomised controlled trials, 2011. http://www.nicedsu.org.uk.

[12] J. A. DiMasi, R. W. Hansen, and H. G. Grabowski. The price of innovation: new estimates of drug development costs. *Journal of Health Economics*, 22(2):151–185, 2003.

[13] Y. Y. Duan, K. Ye, and E. P. Smith. Evaluating water quality using power priors to incorporate historical information. *Environmetrics*, 17(1):95–106, 2006.

[14] M. Egger, G. D. Smith, and D. G. Altman. *Systematic Reviews in Health Care: Meta-analysis in Context.* BMJ Publishing Group, 1995.

[15] E. A. Eisenhauer, C. Twelves, and M. Buyse. *Phase I Cancer Trials - A Practical Guide.* Oxford University Press, 2006.

[16] EMEA's Committee for Medicinal Products for Human Use (CHMP). Guideline on Clinical Trials in Small Populations, 2006. http://www.ema.europa.eu/docs/en_GB/document_library/Scientific_guideline/2009/09/WC500003615.pdf.

[17] EMEA's Committee for Proprietary Medicinal Products (CPMP). Note for Guidance on Clinical Investigation of Medicinal Products in the Paediatric Population, 2001. http://www.ema.europa.eu/docs/en_GB/document_library/Scientific_guideline/2009/09/WC500002926.pdf.

[18] J. A. French, N. R. Temkin, B. F. Shneker, A. E. Hammer, P. T. Caldwell, and J. A. Messenheimer. Lamotrigine XR conversion to monotherapy: first study using a historical control group. *Neurotherapeutics*, 9(1):176–184, 2012.

[19] J. A. French, S. Wang, B. Warnock, and N. Temkin. Historical control monotherapy design in the treatment of epilepsy. *Epilepsia*, 51(10):1936–1943, 2010.

[20] P. H. Garthwaite, J. B. Kadane, and A. O'Hagan. Statistical Methods for Eliciting Probability Distributions. *Journal of the American Statistical Association*, 100(470):680–701, 2005.

[21] A. Gelman. Prior distributions for variance parameters in hierarchical models. *Bayesian Analysis*, 1(3):515–534, 2006.

[22] S. Gsteiger, B. Neuenschwander, F. Mercier, and H. Schmidli. Using historical control information for the design and analysis of clinical trials with overdispersed count data. *Statistics in Medicine*, 32(21):3609–3622, 2013.

[23] J. K. Haseman, J. Huff, and G. A. Boorman. Use of historical control data in carcinogenicity studies in rodents. *Toxicologic Pathology*, 12(2):126–135, 1984.

[24] J. P. Higgins and A. Whitehead. Borrowing strength from external trials in a meta-analysis. *Statistics in Medicine*, 15(24):2733–2749, 1996.

[25] J. P. T. Higgins and S. Green, editors. *Cochrane Handbook for Systematic Reviews of Interventions*. Wiley, 2008.

[26] B. P. Hobbs, B. P. Carlin, S. J. Mandrekar, and D. J. Sargent. Hierarchical commensurate and power prior models for adaptive incorporation of historical information in clinical trials. *Biometrics*, 67(3):1047–1056, 2011.

[27] B. P. Hobbs, D. J. Sargent, and B. P. Carlin. Commensurate Priors for Incorporating Historical Information in Clinical Trials Using General and Generalized Linear Models. *Bayesian Analysis*, 7(3):639–674, 2012.

[28] D. G. Hoel and T. Yanagawa. Incorporating historical controls in testing for a trend in proportions. *Journal of the American Statistical Association*, 81(396):1095–1099, 1986.

[29] Japan's Pharmaceuticals and Medical Devices Agency (PMDA). Basic principles on Global Clinical Trials, 2007. http://www.pmda.go.jp/kijunsakusei/file/guideline/new_drug/GlobalClinicalTrials_en.pdf.

[30] L. Joseph, T. W. Gyorkos, and L. Coupal. Bayesian estimation of disease prevalence and the parameters of diagnostic tests in the absence of a gold standard. *American Journal of Epidemiology*, 141(3):263–272, 1995.

[31] Y. Kikuchi and T. Yanagawa. Incorporating historical information in testing for a trend in Poisson means. *Annals of the Institute of Statistical Mathematics*, 40(2):367–379, 1988.

[32] G. Lu and A. E. Ades. Combination of direct and indirect evidence in mixed treatment comparisons. *Statistics in Medicine*, 23(20):3105–3124, 2004.

[33] T. Lumley. Network meta-analysis for indirect treatment comparisons. *Statistics in Medicine*, 21(16):2313–2324, 2002.

[34] D. J. Lunn, C. Jackson, N. Best, A. Thomas, and D. Spiegelhalter. *The BUGS Book: A Practical Introduction to Bayesian Analysis.* Chapman & Hall/CRC Texts in Statistical Science, 2012.

[35] D. J. Lunn, A. Thomas, N. Best, and D. Spiegelhalter. WinBUGS - a Bayesian modelling framework: concepts, structure, and extensibility. *Statistics and Computing*, 10:325–337, 2000.

[36] D. Malec. A closer look at combining data among a small number of binomial experiments. *Statistics in Medicine*, 20(12):1811–1824, 2001.

[37] S. Morita, P. F. Thall, and P. Müller. Determining the effective sample size of a parametric prior. *Biometrics*, 64(2):595–602, 2008.

[38] S. Morita, P. F. Thall, and P. Müller. Prior Effective Sample Size in Conditionally Independent Hierarchical Models. *Bayesian Analysis*, 7(3):561–614, 2012.

[39] B. Munos. Lessons from 60 years of pharmaceutical innovation. *Nature Reviews Drug Discovery*, 8:959–968, 2009.

[40] B. Neelon and A. J. O'Malley. Bayesian analysis using power priors with application to pediatric quality of care. *Journal of Biometrics & Biostatistics*, 1:103, 2010.

[41] B. Neuenschwander, M. Branson, and T. Gsponer. Critical aspects of the Bayesian approach to phase I cancer trials. *Statistics in Medicine*, 27(13):2420–2439, 2008.

[42] B. Neuenschwander, M. Branson, and D. J. Spiegelhalter. A note on the power prior. *Statistics in Medicine*, 28(28):3562–3566, 2009.

[43] B. Neuenschwander, G. Capkun-Niggli, M. Branson, and D. J. Spiegehalter. Summarizing historical information on controls in clinical trials. *Clinical Trials*, 7(1):5–18, 2010.

[44] A. O'Hagan and J. J. Forster. *Kendall's Advanced Theory of Statistics Vol 2B Bayesian Inference.* Arnold, 2004.

[45] A. O'Hagan and L. Pericchi. Bayesian heavy-tailed models and conflict resolution: a review. *Brazilian Journal of Probability and Statistics*, 26(4):372–401, 2012.

[46] G. Pennello and L. Thompson. Experience with reviewing Bayesian medical device trials. *Journal of Biopharmaceutical Statistics*, 18(1):81–115, 2008.

[47] S. J. Pocock. The combination of randomized and historical controls in clinical trials. *Journal of Chronic Diseases*, 29(3):175–188, 1976.

[48] N. G. Polson and J. G. Scott. On the half-Cauchy prior for a global scale parameter. *Bayesian Analysis*, 7(4):887–902, 2012.

[49] A. Racine, A. P. Grieve, H. Flühler, and A. F. M. Smith. Bayesian methods in practice: experiences in the pharmaceutical industry. *Journal of the Royal Statistical Society: Series C*, 35(2):93–150, 1986.

[50] A. Racine-Poon and J. Wakefield. Statistical methods for population pharmacokinetic modelling. *Statistical Methods in Medical Research*, 7(1):63–84, 1998.

[51] L. Ryan. Using historical controls in the analysis of developmental toxicity data. *Biometrics*, 49(4):1126–1135, 1993.

[52] G. Salanti, J. P. T. Higgins, A. E. Ades, and J. P. A. Ioannidis. Evaluation of networks of randomized trials. *Statistical Methods in Medical Research*, 17(3):279–301, 2008.

[53] J. Savoviċ, H. Jones, D. Altman, R. Harris, P. Jüni, J. Pildal, B. Als-Nielsen, E. Balk, C. Gluud, L. Gluud, J. Ioannidis, K. Schulz, R. Beynon, N. Welton, L. Wood, D. Moher, J. Deeks, and J. Sterne. Influence of reported study design characteristics on intervention effect estimates from randomized, controlled trials. *Annals of Internal Medicine*, 157(6):429–438, 2012.

[54] H. Schmidli, F. Bretz, and A. Racine-Poon. Bayesian predictive power for interim adaptation in seamless phase II/III trials where the endpoint is survival up to some specified timepoint. *Statistics in Medicine*, 26(27):4925–4938, 2007.

[55] H. Schmidli, S. Gsteiger, S. Roychoudhury, A. O'Hagan, D. Spiegelhalter, and B. Neuenschwander. Robust meta-analytic-predictive priors in clinical trials with historical control information. *Biometrics*, 70(4):1023–32, 2014.

[56] H. Schmidli, S. Wandel, and B. Neuenschwander. The network meta-analytic-predictive approach to non-inferiority trials. *Statistical Methods in Medical Research*, 22(2):219–240, 2013.

[57] R. Simon. Bayesian design and analysis of active control clinical trials. *Biometrics*, 55(2):484–487, 1999.

[58] D. J. Spiegelhalter, K. R. Abrams, and J. P. Myles. *Bayesian Approaches to Clinical Trials and Health-Care Evaluation.* Wiley, 2004.

[59] R. E. Tarone. The use of historical control information in testing for a trend in Poisson means. *Biometrics*, 38(2):457–462, 1982.

[60] R. E. Tarone. The use of historical control information in testing for a trend in proportions. *Biometrics*, 38(1):215–220, 1982.

[61] R. Temple and S. S. Ellenberg. Placebo-controlled trials and active-control trials in the evaluation of new treatments. Part 1: Ethical and scientific issues. *Annals of Internal Medicine*, 133(6):455–463, 2000.

[62] P. F. Thall, R. C. Herrick, H. Q. Nguyen, J. J. Venier, and J. C. Norris. Effective sample size for computing prior hyperparameters in Bayesian phase I-II dose-finding. *Clinical Trials*, 11(6):657–666, 2014.

[63] U.S. Food and Drug Administration (FDA). Guidance E 10 Choice of Control Group and Related Issues in Clinical Trials, 2001. http://www.fda.gov/downloads/drugs/{\protect\newline} guidancecomplianceregulatoryinformation/guidances/ucm073139.pdf.

[64] U.S. Food and Drug Administration (FDA). Guidance for the Use of Bayesian Statistics in Medical Device Clinical Trials, 2010. http://www.fda.gov/downloads/MedicalDevices/ DeviceRegulationandGuidance/GuidanceDocuments/ucm071121.pdf.

[65] U.S. Food and Drug Administration (FDA). Paving the Way for Personalized Medicine: FDA's Role in a New Era of Medical Product Development, 2013. http://www.fda.gov/downloads/ScienceResearch/SpecialTopics/ PersonalizedMedicine/UCM372421.pdf.

[66] U.S. Food and Drug Administration (FDA). Leveraging Existing Clinical Data for Extrapolation to Pediatric Uses of Medical Devices. Draft Guidance for Industry and Food and Drug Administration Staff, 2015. http://www.fda.gov/downloads/MedicalDevices/ DeviceRegulationandGuidance/GuidanceDocuments/UCM444591.pdf.

[67] J. Van Ryzin. Designing for nonparametric Bayesian survival analysis using historical controls. *Cancer Treatment Reports*, 64(2-3):503–506, 1980.

[68] K. Viele, S. Berry, B. Neuenschwander, B. Amzal, F. Chen, N. Enas, B. Hobbs, J. G. Ibrahim, N. Kinnersley, S. Lindborg, S. Micallef, S. Roychoudhury, and L. Thompson. Use of historical control data for assessing treatment effects in clinical trials. *Pharmaceutical Statistics*, 13(1):41–54, 2014.

[69] R. J. Walley, C. L. Smith, J. D. Gale, and P. Woodward. Advantages of a wholly Bayesian approach to assessing efficacy in early drug development: a case study. *Pharmaceutical Statistics*, 14(3):205–215, 2015.

[70] S. Weber, B. Carpenter, D. Lee, FY. Bois, A. Gelman, and A. Racine. Bayesian Drug Disease Model with Stan - Using published longitudinal data summaries in population models, 2014. http://www.page-meeting.org/pdf_assets/2669-Bayesian_Drug_Disease_ Model_with_Stan_PAGE14_final_pub.pdf.

[71] S. Witte, H. Schmidli, A. O'Hagan, and A. Racine. Designing a non-inferiority study in kidney transplantation: a case study. *Pharmaceutical Statistics*, 10(5):427–432, 2011.

[72] T. Yanagawa and D. G. Hoel. Use of historical controls for animal experiments. *Environmental Health Perspectives*, 63:217–224, 1985.

[73] W. Zhao and H. Yang, editors. *Statistical Methods in Drug Combination Studies.* Chapman & Hall/CRC Biostatistics, 2015.

3

Multiplicity

Dong Xi

Ekkehard Glimm

Frank Bretz

CONTENTS

3.1 Introduction to Multiplicity Issues

This chapter describes statistical methods for addressing multiplicity issues faced in cancer clinical trials, with a focus on confirmatory phase III clinical trials. Often in such confirmatory trials, multiple inferences are made using hypothesis testing approaches. Based on such inferences, the success of the trial is judged. False positive claims play an important role in this judgment and an adequate control of the Type I error rate then becomes mandatory while making such inferences. In order to adequately control the Type I error rate in situations where multiple inferences are made at one or multiple time points, appropriate multiplicity adjustments must be performed.

This chapter contains a brief description of the sources of multiplicity, explains why multiplicity is a problem that needs to be addressed, and proposes some recommendations on how to address such issues. It is important to note that multiplicity is not a problem that can be resolved by statisticians alone. While there exist many statistical methods that could provide a satisfactory solution, the decision on which method to use depends largely on collaborative discussions between statisticians and their clinical partners. It is critical that important inputs are taken from every stakeholder before a decision is made on the method that is used to deal with this issue. For a more detailed exposure to the theory of multiple testing and its applications, we refer the interested readers to the following literature [11, 25, 49, 55].

3.1.1 Sources of Multiplicity

Clinical trials with multiple objectives are becoming more prominent in clinical development. Much of this stems from the idea that investigators want to learn as much as possible from every clinical trial and have more than one way of claiming success. Some of the common sources of multiplicity seen in cancer trials include

- testing multiple endpoints in the same trial, e.g., both progression-free survival (PFS) and overall survival (OS);
- investigating multiple treatment groups, e.g., comparing several doses of a new compound against placebo on top of the standard of care;
- repeated hypothesis testing at multiple interim analyses, where each test can potentially lead to success;
- investigating different subpopulations;
- combined non-inferiority and superiority testing in the presence of other sources of multiplicity.

In some cases, there can be a combination of some of the sources mentioned above which then lead to increased levels of multiplicity. For example, if a new compound is investigated for both PFS and OS in two populations at an interim and a final analysis, three levels of multiplicity are involved.

Other sources of multiplicity exist, which are less commonly encountered in or controlled for in cancer trials, but which also should be kept in mind when designing trials. These include measuring endpoints at multiple time-points (e.g., PFS rate at 6, 8, and 12 weeks), using different statistical tests on the same data, and using different analysis sets for the same endpoint (e.g., full analysis set and per protocol set).

3.1.2 Types of Error Rates

When testing multiple null hypotheses, the overall Type I error rate can be measured in different ways. Examples of error rates that have traditionally been considered include [101]

- the error rate per comparison, defined as the proportion of incorrect statements, among infinitely many statements made;
- the familywise error rate, defined as the proportion of families with at least one incorrect statement, among infinitely many families.

Here, a family is defined as a collection of inferences for which it is meaningful to take into account some combined measure of error.

Controlling an error rate can be done either in a weak or in a strong sense. Weak control is defined as controlling the error rate only under the assumption that all null hypotheses are true. In the example of testing multiple doses against placebo, weak control would mean controlling the error rate only under the assumption that all doses are ineffective. Strong control, on the other hand, is defined as controlling the error rate under any configuration of true and false null hypotheses. In the multiple doses example, strong control would imply Type I error rate control even under the assumption that some of the doses are effective.

It follows from the previous definitions that an error rate control in the strong sense is more desirable to have than in the weak sense. For confirmatory clinical trials, strong control of the familywise error rate (FWER) is therefore mandated by regulatory agencies [34, 35]. That is, the probability of incorrectly rejecting at least one true null hypothesis has to be controlled at a prespecified significance level α regardless of the configuration of the true and false null hypotheses under consideration.

More recently, the false discovery rate (FDR), defined as the expected proportion of falsely rejected hypotheses among the rejected hypotheses [4], has become popular in discovery studies. As this chapter focuses on multiplicity issues arising in confirmatory clinical trials, the FDR and its variants will not be considered further in this chapter. The interested readers are referred to the literature [28, 32] for details.

3.1.3 Why Multiplicity Adjustment

Multiple comparisons allow a trial to succeed in more than one way. For example, if a new compound is investigated in three disjoint populations, each at a one-sided significance level of 2.5%, the chance of having at least one false positive finding increases to $1-(1-2.5\%)^3 = 7.31\%$. Similarly, if in a trial five interim analyses for efficacy are performed, each at 2.5% nominal significance level, then the chance of succeeding in one of the interim analyses or the final analysis is considerably larger than 2.5%. Thus, the FWER increases with the number of tests performed and a multiplicity adjustment using an appropriate multiple comparison procedure is mandatory in order to adequately control the FWER at a specified significance level α.

3.1.4 A Motivating Example

In this section we describe the BELLE-2 trial to motivate the need for multiplicity adjustments. This example will be re-visited later to illustrate some of the methods described in this chapter.

The BELLE-2 trial [ClinicalTrials.gov ID: NCT01610284] is a placebo-controlled phase III trial to investigate BKM120 with fulvestrant in post-menopausal patients with hormone receptor positive HER2-negative locally advanced or metastatic breast cancer. The primary trial objective is to demonstrate an improvement of PFS in the overall and a biomarker-positive $B+$ populations. PFS is defined as the time from the date of randomization until the date of the first radiologically documented disease progression or death due to any cause. The secondary trial objective is to demonstrate an improvement of OS in the same two populations, where OS is defined as the time from date of randomization to the date of death from any cause. BELLE-2 is thus a two-armed trial exhibiting two levels of multiplicity, with four null hypotheses resulting from the comparison of BKM120 against placebo for two endpoints (PFS and OS) in two populations (overall and $B+$). A short discussion of some of the statistical issues faced in the BELLE-2 trial can be found in [41].

To illustrate the methodologies in the following sections, we keep the BELLE-2 design as a conceptual example for now with H_1, H_2 denoting the null hypotheses for PFS in the overall and the $B+$ populations, respectively, and H_3, H_4 the null hypotheses for OS in the same populations. The final trial design is shown in Section 3.4.1 along with the discussion on clinical considerations and the rationale. There, we will illustrate some of the advanced multiple comparison procedures described in Section 3.3.

3.2 Common Multiple Comparison Procedures

In this section, we introduce general concepts concerning multiple testing and selected ways to construct multiple comparison procedures (MCPs). In Section 3.2.1, we discuss relevant concepts and methods to construct MCPs including single-step and stepwise procedures and the closure principle. We then summarize commonly used MCPs based on univariate p-values. Methods presented in Section 3.2.2 include the Bonferroni test, the Simes test, and their improvements. In Section 3.2.3, we review MCPs with additional parametric assumptions including the Dunnett test and multiple comparisons in linear models.

3.2.1 General Concepts

Single-step and stepwise procedures

MCPs can be categorized into single-step and stepwise procedures. Single-step procedures are methods for which the rejection or non-rejection of a null hypothesis is not influenced by the decisions on any other hypothesis. A well-known example of single-step procedures is the Bonferroni test. For stepwise procedures, the rejection or non-rejection of a null hypothesis may depend on the decision about other hypotheses. For example, the Holm procedure is a stepwise extension of the Bonferroni test [50] (see Section 3.2.2.1).

For single-step procedures, the order in which the hypotheses are tested is not important. In contrast, stepwise procedures are further classified into step-down and step-up procedures. Step-down procedures start with the most significant p-value while step-up procedures adopt the reversed order and start with the least significant p-value. The Holm procedure in Section 3.2.2.1 and the Hochberg procedure in Section 3.2.2.2 are examples of step-down and step-up procedures, respectively [47, 50].

Union-intersection and intersection-union tests

Union-intersection [82] and intersection-union [6] tests are two ways to construct MCPs for the intersection and union of elementary hypotheses, respectively. Let H_i denote the i-th null hypothesis and K_i the i-th alternative hypothesis, $i = 1, \ldots, m$. The union-intersection method tests the intersection of null hypotheses against the union of alternative hypotheses, that is, $H = \bigcap_{i=1}^{m} H_i$ versus $K = \bigcup_{i=1}^{m} K_i$. In contrast, the intersection-union method tests $H' = \bigcup_{i=1}^{m} H_i$ versus $K' = \bigcap_{i=1}^{m} K_i$. The union-intersection test integrates nicely with many MCPs and therefore it is taken as the construction method for the procedures described in this chapter.

Closure principle and closed test procedures

The closure principle and the closed test procedure play a key role in constructing MCPs that lead to stepwise procedures [68]. For simplicity, we

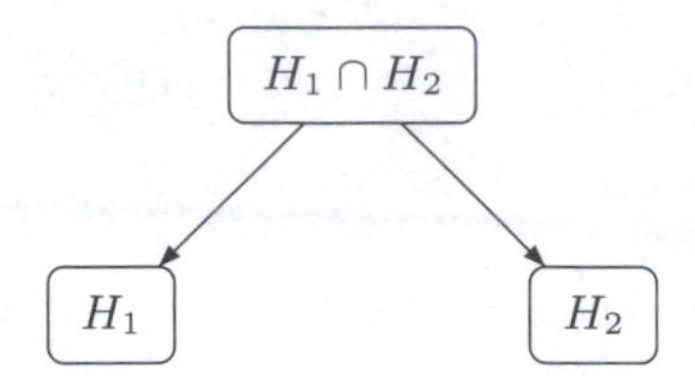

FIGURE 3.1: Visualization of the closed test procedure for H_1 and H_2.

consider a case of two null hypotheses $H_i : \theta_i \leq 0,\ i = 1, 2$, where θ_i denotes the mean effect difference between treatment $i = 1, 2$ and control.

To construct the closed test procedure for H_1 and H_2, we first define the closure family consisting of all possible intersection null hypotheses: $H_1 \cap H_2$, H_1, and H_2. The closure principle allows a suitable union-intersection test for each intersection hypothesis at the local significance level α. The resulting MCP rejects an elementary hypothesis if all intersection hypotheses contained therein are rejected locally at level α. For instance, the closed test procedure rejects $H_1(H_2)$ if both $H_1 \cap H_2$ and $H_1(H_2)$ are rejected at level α, respectively. Visualization of this process is shown in Figure 3.1.

For the general case of testing m null hypotheses $H_1, \ldots, H_m$, the closed test procedure rejects any $H_j,\ j \in \{1, \ldots, m\}$, if all $H_I = \bigcap_{i \in I} H_i$ for $j \in I \subseteq \{1, \ldots, m\}$ are rejected locally at level α. This closed test procedure controls the FWER in the strong sense at level α [68]. Many MCPs are in fact closed test procedures including, but not limited to, step-down procedures [50, 87], step-up procedures [42, 47], the Hommel procedure [51], fixed sequence procedures [73, 104], fallback procedures [107, 108], gatekeeping procedures [3, 22, 26, 27, 53, 92, 104, 111], and graphical approaches [13, 15, 17, 70].

One disadvantage of closed test procedures is the computational burden because up to $2^m - 1$ intersection hypotheses may have to be tested for m elementary hypotheses. Thus it is helpful to derive stepwise procedures in at most m or m^2 steps for implementation and communication purposes. We refer to [7, 43, 53, 80, 105] for further details.

Coherence and consonance

Coherence is an essential requirement for MCPs. A coherent procedure has the property that if H_J is rejected, then any H_I with $I \supseteq J$ is rejected as well [39]. Interpretation problems may arise if coherence is not satisfied. Closed test procedures are coherent by construction. Note that any non-coherent MCP can be replaced by a coherent procedure which is uniformly at least as powerful [90].

An MCP is called consonant if the rejection of H_I with $|I| > 1$ always leads to the rejection of at least one H_J with $J \subset I$ [39]. Consonance is a desirable property of MCPs which implies that the rejection of H_I leads to the rejection of at least one elementary hypothesis H_i, $i \in I$. A more detailed discussion of consonance can be found in [7].

Adjusted p-values

Adjusted p-values are defined as the smallest significance level for which one can reject the elementary hypotheses H_i, $i = 1, \ldots, m$, given the MCP [106]. In contrast, univariate raw p-values are called unadjusted p-values. It is often helpful in practice to use adjusted p-values because they capture the multiplicity adjustment and the underlying decision strategy. As a result, an elementary hypothesis can be rejected if its adjusted p-value is less than α while controlling the FWER.

Point estimation and simultaneous confidence intervals

Point estimation of treatment effects in clinical trials with multiple hypotheses is a challenging problem. If, for example, several treatment regimens are compared with the standard of care, the estimate of the treatment effect in the best-performing regimen will tend to overestimate the true effect of this selected regimen. Unfortunately, it is very difficult to correct for this selection bias. For example, in a single-stage trial with normal endpoints, an unbiased estimate of the treatment effect in the best-performing treatment does not even exist [20, 91]. A discussion of the issue can be found in [2, 16].

Simultaneous confidence intervals provide a natural extension to the confidence intervals for univariate hypothesis testing problems [36, 46]. Simultaneous confidence intervals can be obtained for many single-step procedures but are difficult to derive for stepwise procedures. We refer to the following references for recent results and discussions [44, 45, 92].

Power and sample size

Power calculation may become complex with multiple hypotheses because the sample size have to be calculated to ensure a certain probability of achieving the primary objective and/or key secondary objectives. For example, in a cancer trial where PFS is the primary endpoint and the OS is the secondary endpoint, the sample size calculation may be needed to ensure not only a high power to reject the hypothesis for PFS but also a reasonable power to reject the one for OS, given the appropriate multiplicity adjustment. The calculation could be even more complicated by different distributions of endpoints, complex logical restrictions among the hypotheses, early stopping at interim analyses, and other factors. A unified approach is usually difficult to achieve [86], but many software packages (including ADDPLAN®, EAST®, nQuery®, PASS®, and others) provide practical calculation of sample size for various situations.

3.2.2 Methods Based on Univariate p-Values

Multiplicity adjustment based on univariate p-values is common in clinical trials because it is easy to understand and communicate. We will focus on two single-step tests: the Bonferroni test and the Simes test. Their stepwise extensions will be also discussed to demonstrate the advantages of the underlying closed test procedure.

3.2.2.1 Methods Based on the Bonferroni Test

The Bonferroni test is a single-step procedure, which compares the unadjusted univariate p-values with a common threshold. In the problem of investigating m hypotheses at a significance level α, the Bonferroni test rejects H_i if $p_i \leq \alpha/m$. The adjusted p-values are calculated as $\tilde{p}_i = \min\{mp_i, 1\}$ and thus the Bonferroni test rejects H_i if $\tilde{p}_i \leq \alpha$. Strong control of the FWER (see Section 3.1.2) follows from the Bonferroni inequality

$$\text{FWER} = P\left[\bigcup_{i \in M_0} (p_i \leq \alpha/m)\right] \leq \sum_{i \in M_0} P(p_i \leq \alpha/m) \leq m_0\alpha/m,$$

where M_0 denotes the set of $m_0 = |M_0|$ true null hypotheses. Note that in reality M_0 is unknown and m is used as the upper bound of m_0.

Although the Bonferroni test is simple to use and valid for any joint distribution of the test statistics, it is conservative in the sense that there are other procedures which reject at least as many hypotheses as the Bonferroni test at the expense of additional complexity or assumptions.

Holm procedure

The Holm procedure is a step-down procedure which applies the Bonferroni test repeatedly from the most significant p-value to the least significant one [50]. Let $p_{(1)} \leq \cdots \leq p_{(m)}$ denote the ordered unadjusted p-values and $H_{(1)}, \ldots, H_{(m)}$ the corresponding hypotheses. The Holm procedure is carried out in m steps as follows:

- Step $i = 1, \ldots, m$. If $p_{(i)} \leq \alpha/(m-i+1)$, reject $H_{(i)}$ and go to Step $i+1$ until Step m; otherwise stop testing and fail to reject $H_{(i)}, \ldots, H_{(m)}$.

The Holm procedure is more powerful than the Bonferroni test because it increases the threshold from α/m successively to test the ordered hypotheses. The adjusted p-value is $\tilde{p}_{(1)} = \min\{1, mp_{(1)}\}$ for $H_{(1)}$ and $\tilde{p}_{(i)} = \min\left\{\max\left[(m-i+1)p_{(i)}, \tilde{p}_{(i-1)}\right], 1\right\}$ for $H_{(2)}, \ldots, H_{(m)}$.

Another way to construct the Holm procedure is to utilize the closure principle in Section 3.2.1. When there are no logical dependences among the null hypotheses, it can be shown that the Holm procedure is a shortcut to the closed test procedure in which the intersection hypotheses are tested locally using the Bonferroni test [50]. This serves as a proof that the Holm procedure controls the FWER strongly and also an example of how to improve MCPs using the closure principle.

3.2.2.2 Methods Based on the Simes Test

The Simes test modifies the Bonferroni test to test the intersection hypothesis $H = \bigcap_{i=1}^{m} H_i$. Let $p_{(1)} \leq \cdots \leq p_{(m)}$ denote the ordered unadjusted p-values and $H_{(1)}, \ldots, H_{(m)}$ the corresponding hypotheses. The Simes test rejects H if $p_{(i)} \leq i\alpha/m$ for at least one $i \in \{1, \ldots, m\}$ [88]. Note that the Simes test does not reject the elementary hypothesis $H_{(i)}$ if $p_{(i)} \leq i\alpha/m$ [51].

The Simes test uses all ordered p-values instead of just $p_{(1)}$ and thus if H is rejected by the Bonferroni test, it is also rejected by the Simes test but not vice versa. However, this power advantage comes at the expense of additional assumptions on the joint distribution of $p_1, \ldots, p_m$. It has been proved that the Type I error rate is exactly α if $p_1, \ldots, p_m$ are independent [88]. In the case of one-sided tests, it is shown that the Simes test preserves the Type I error rate if the test statistics satisfy a certain type of positive dependence. For further details, we refer to [83, 84].

Hochberg procedure

The Hochberg procedure is a step-up extension of the Simes test, which makes inference on elementary hypotheses $H_1, \ldots, H_m$ [47]. This procedure can also be seen as a Holm procedure in the reversed order. The Hochberg procedure is carried out in m steps as follows:

- Step $i = 1, \ldots, m$. If $p_{(m-i+1)} > \alpha/i$, do not reject $H_{(m-i+1)}$ and go to Step $i + 1$ until Step m; otherwise stop and reject $H_{(m-i+1)}, \ldots, H_{(1)}$.

The Hochberg procedure controls the FWER under the same conditions as the Simes test controls the Type I error rate. Moreover, this procedure is more powerful than the Holm procedure. The adjusted p-values of the Hochberg procedure are $\tilde{p}_i = \min\left\{ \min\left[(m - i + 1)p_{(i)}, \tilde{p}_{(i+1)}\right], 1\right\}$.

Hommel procedure

The Hommel procedure is a shortcut to a closed test procedure that applies the Simes test to each intersection hypothesis [51]. The Hommel procedure is carried out as follows:

- Step 1. If $p_{(m)} > \alpha$, do not reject $H_{(m)}$ and go to the next step; otherwise stop and reject all hypotheses.

- Step $i = 2, \ldots, m$. If $p_{(m-j+1)} > (i-j+1)\alpha/i$ for $j = 1, \ldots, i$, do not reject $H_{(m-i+1)}$ and go to Step $i + 1$ until Step m; otherwise stop and reject all among $H_{(m-i+1)}, \ldots, H_{(1)}$ for which the unadjusted p-values $\leq \alpha/(i - 1)$.

The Hommel procedure controls the FWER under the same condition as the Simes test controls the Type I error rate. It can be shown that it rejects at least as many hypotheses as the Hochberg procedure [52]. However, the Hommel procedure requires at most m^2 thresholds to identify all rejected hypotheses and the Hochberg procedure only requires at most m thresholds. The adjusted p-values of the Hommel procedure are given in [110].

TABLE 3.1: Comparison of the Bonferroni test and the Holm, Hochberg and Hommel procedures for $m = 4$ hypotheses at $\alpha = 0.025$.

Hyp.	p-value	Threshold	Adjusted p-value			
(i)	$p_{(i)}$	$\alpha/(4-i+1)$	Bonferroni	Holm	Hochberg	Hommel
1	0.005	0.00625	0.02*	0.02*	0.02*	0.016*
2	0.01	0.00833	0.04	0.03	0.024*	0.02*
3	0.012	0.0167	0.048	0.03	0.024*	0.024*
4	0.03	0.025	0.12	0.03	0.03	0.03

* The adjusted p-values significant at $\alpha = 0.025$.

3.2.2.3 Numerical Illustration

Consider the example in Section 3.1.4 with $m = 4$ hypotheses tested at the level $\alpha = 0.025$. To apply the procedures in this section, we modify the example by treating all hypotheses equally without the logical restrictions.

Let $p_1 = 0.012$, $p_2 = 0.01$, $p_3 = 0.005$, and $p_4 = 0.03$ be the unadjusted p-values. The Bonferroni test rejects H_3 because $p_{(1)} = p_3 = 0.005 \leq 0.00625 = \alpha/4$ but $p_{(2)} = p_2 = 0.01 > 0.00625$. The Holm procedure rejects H_3 since $p_{(1)} = p_3 = 0.005 \leq 0.00625$ but $p_{(2)} = p_2 = 0.01 > 0.00833 = \alpha/3$. The Hochberg procedure rejects H_3, H_2, H_1 since $p_{(4)} = p_4 = 0.03 > 0.025 = \alpha$ but $p_{(3)} = p_1 = 0.012 \leq 0.0125 = \alpha/2$. The Hommel procedure rejects H_3, H_2, H_1 since $p_{(4)} = p_4 = 0.03 > 0.025 = \alpha$ but $p_{(3)} = p_1 = 0.012 \leq 0.0167 = 2\alpha/3$. Table 3.1 summarizes the procedures with the associated adjusted p-values.

There are many further topics on methods based on univariate p-values. An alternative way to view the Holm, Hochberg, and Hommel procedures is given in [66]. A version of the Holm procedure accounting for logical restrictions among the null hypotheses was proposed in [87]. When some hypotheses are deemed more important, weighted versions of the procedures were proposed, such as the weighted Bonferroni test [81], the weighted Holm procedures [5, 50], and the weighted Simes test and its extensions [5, 8, 48, 94].

3.2.3 Parametric Methods

Parametric methods utilize parametric assumptions on the joint distribution of the test statistics to improve upon the methods based on univariate p-values, which are discussed in Section 3.2.2. In a dose finding study with normal outcomes, the correlation between test statistics for multiple dose-control comparisons can be calculated and the well-known Dunnett test [29] is derived in this setting.

3.2.3.1 Dunnett Test

To introduce the Dunnett test, we assume in a one-way layout that the response for the j-th observation in the i-th treatment group is

$$y_{ij} = \mu_i + \epsilon_{ij},$$

where μ_i denotes the mean effect of treatment group $i = 0, 1, \ldots, m$ and ϵ_{ij}, $j = 1, \ldots, n_i$, are independently normally distributed errors following $N(0, \sigma^2)$. The control group is denoted as $i = 0$.

To test the null hypotheses $H_i : \theta_i \leq 0$ versus $K_i : \theta_i > 0$ with $\theta_i = \mu_i - \mu_0$, $i = 1, \ldots, m$, the pairwise t statistics are given by

$$t_i = \frac{\bar{y}_i - \bar{y}_0}{s\sqrt{\frac{1}{n_i} + \frac{1}{n_0}}},$$

where $\bar{y}_i$ denotes the sample mean in the i-th treatment group and s the pooled sample standard deviation. Then $\boldsymbol{t} = (t_1, \ldots, t_m)$ follows an m-multivariate t distribution with the number of degrees of freedom $\nu = \sum_{i=0}^{m} n_i - (m + 1)$ and the correlation between t_i and t_j being $\rho_{ij} = \sqrt{\frac{n_i}{n_i+n_0}}\sqrt{\frac{n_j}{n_j+n_0}}$ for $i \neq j$.

The Dunnett test is a single-step test which rejects H_i if $t_i \geq q_\alpha(m, \nu)$ [29]. The critical threshold $q_\alpha(m, \nu)$ is calculated numerically by solving $P\left[\bigcup_{i=1}^{m} (t_i \geq x)\right] = \alpha$ for x. This also justifies FWER control of the Dunnett test. The threshold of the Dunnett test is smaller than the one of the Bonferroni test and therefore the Dunnett test is more powerful. To see this, consider the example in Section 3.1.4 but treating the four hypotheses as comparing four treatment groups with a control group. Assume an equal allocation of 30 subjects in each group. The correlation between the test statistics is then 0.5. Thus the Dunnett threshold is $q_{0.025}(4, 145) = 2.47$ and the Bonferroni threshold is 2.53, which is the upper 0.025/4 quantile of the univariate t distribution with 145 degrees of freedom.

3.2.3.2 Multiple Testing in Linear Models

In this section, we extend the Dunnett test and construct MCPs in linear models. The general theory is covered, among others, in [11, 49, 55]. Consider the linear model

$$\boldsymbol{y} = \boldsymbol{X\beta} + \boldsymbol{\epsilon},$$

where $\boldsymbol{y}$ denotes an $n \times 1$ response vector, $\boldsymbol{X}$ a fixed and known $n \times p$ design matrix, $\boldsymbol{\beta}$ a $p \times 1$ vector of unknown parameter and $\boldsymbol{\epsilon}$ an $n \times 1$ vector of independent normally distributed errors with mean 0 and unknown variance σ^2.

Assume that we are interested in m comparisons among p unknown parameters $\boldsymbol{\beta}$ resulting in m elementary hypothesis testing problems,

$$H_i : \boldsymbol{c}_i^\top \boldsymbol{\beta} \leq a_i \text{ versus } K_i : \boldsymbol{c}_i^\top \boldsymbol{\beta} > a_i, \ i = 1, \ldots, m,$$

where $\boldsymbol{c}_i$ denotes a $p \times 1$ vector of known constants and a_i a fixed number.

The least square estimates of $\boldsymbol{\beta}$ and σ are given by $\hat{\boldsymbol{\beta}} = \left(\boldsymbol{X}^\top \boldsymbol{X}\right)^- \boldsymbol{X}^\top \boldsymbol{y}$ and $\hat{\sigma} = \left(\boldsymbol{y} - \boldsymbol{X}\hat{\boldsymbol{\beta}}\right)^\top \left(\boldsymbol{y} - \boldsymbol{X}\hat{\boldsymbol{\beta}}\right)/\nu$, where $\left(\boldsymbol{X}^\top \boldsymbol{X}\right)^-$ is the generalized inverse of $\boldsymbol{X}^\top \boldsymbol{X}$ and $\nu = n - \text{rank}(\boldsymbol{X})$ is the number of degrees of freedom. Then H_i can be tested using the test statistic $t_i = \left(\boldsymbol{c}_i^\top \hat{\boldsymbol{\beta}} - a_i\right)/s_i$, where $s_i = \hat{\sigma}\sqrt{\boldsymbol{c}_i^\top \left(\boldsymbol{X}^\top \boldsymbol{X}\right)^- \boldsymbol{c}_i}$. It can be shown that the joint distribution of $t_1, \ldots, t_m$ is a multivariate t distribution with ν degrees of freedom and correlation matrix $\boldsymbol{D}\boldsymbol{C}^\top \left(\boldsymbol{X}^\top \boldsymbol{X}\right)^- \boldsymbol{C}\boldsymbol{D}$, where $\boldsymbol{D} = \left\{\text{diag}\left[\boldsymbol{c}_i^\top \left(\boldsymbol{X}^\top \boldsymbol{X}\right)^- \boldsymbol{c}_i\right]\right\}^{-1/2}$ and $\boldsymbol{C}$ is a $p \times m$ matrix with $\boldsymbol{c}_i$ in the i-th column.

Using this general framework, we are able to illustrate the single-step Dunnett test in Section 3.2.3.1 for comparing m treatment groups versus control. Let $\boldsymbol{\beta} = (\mu_0, \mu_1, \ldots, \mu_m)^\top$ denote the unknown parameter vector and μ_0 the effect in the control group. In this case, $p = m + 1$ and the vector of known constants $\boldsymbol{c}_i^\top = (-1, 0, \ldots, 0, 1, 0, \ldots, 0)$ such that $\boldsymbol{c}_i^\top \boldsymbol{\beta} = \mu_i - \mu_0$.

In addition to the Dunnett test, this general framework includes the Tukey test [99], various trend tests [67, 109], and other procedures [10]. An extension to other parametric and semi-parametric models relying on asymptotic multivariate normal assumptions was proposed [54]. Note that in Section 3.2.3.1 and 3.2.3.2 we focused on single-step procedures. It is possible to develop stepwise parametric procedures including the step-down Dunnett procedures [30, 68, 76] and the step-up Dunnett procedure [31]. A systematic discussion on this topic was provided in [11].

3.3 Advanced Multiple Comparison Procedures

Early MCPs focused primarily on adjustments which treated all hypotheses equally: The methods discussed in Section 3.2 do not use different significance levels for the various elementary hypotheses H_i. In many applications, however, elementary hypotheses are of differing importance. In addition, certain hypotheses may be related to each other, giving rise to hierarchies or partial hierarchies of hypotheses. In a cancer trial, two different doses of a new drug may be tested versus the standard of care and treatment success may be characterized by the effects on PFS and objective response rate (ORR), which is the proportion of patients with reduction in tumor burden. In this case, PFS will usually be the more important outcome. ORR is then relevant only after a PFS benefit has been established (Figure 3.2). Any MCP used to test these four hypotheses should adequately take account of these considerations.

The simplest method for dealing with hypotheses of different importance

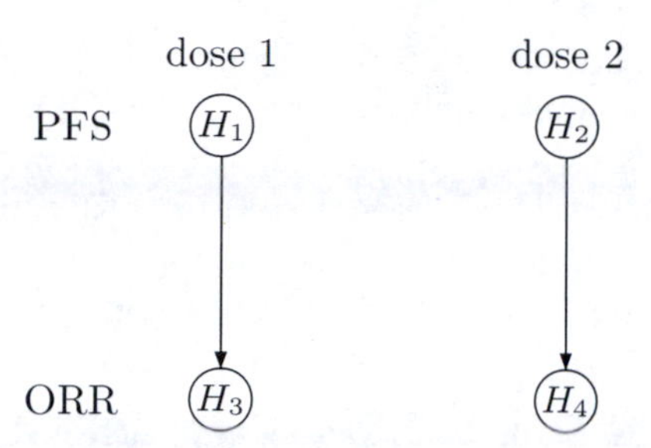

FIGURE 3.2: Two doses of a treatment with two endpoints.

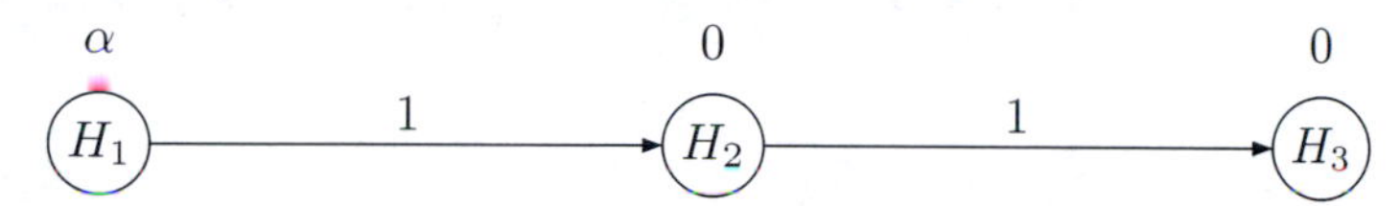

FIGURE 3.3: Graphical visualization of the hierarchical test ($m = 3$).

is a strictly hierarchical approach. This approach tests the elementary hypotheses H_i in a predefined fixed order [73, 104]. Assume that the elementary hypotheses are labeled $H_1, H_2, \ldots, H_m$ according to the order in which they are tested. The hierarchical test can then be seen as a closed test procedure where each intersection hypothesis H_I is rejected if H_i is rejected locally at level α with $i = \min\{j \in I\}$. A graphical representation of the hierarchical test with three hypotheses is shown in Figure 3.3.

Procedures designed as a compromise between a strictly hierarchical approach and the Holm procedure (like, e.g., fallback procedures [107, 108]) triggered the development of more general graphical approaches [13] and gatekeeping procedures [23]. We will focus on these procedures in Sections 3.3.1 and 3.3.2, respectively.

Cancer trials are often performed as group sequential trials (i.e., trials where a hypothesis is tested repeatedly in time). Hence, there is a need to combine methods for multiple testing of several hypotheses with repeated testing in time. Section 3.3.3 deals with this important question. It also discusses some complications arising from the use of time-to-event endpoints (such as PFS or OS) in group sequential trials. Finally, Section 3.3.4 discusses adaptive designs. These can be seen as a generalization of group sequential trials allowing modifications of an ongoing trial such as sample size reassessment or subpopulation selection based on interim results.

3.3.1 Graphical Approaches

The graphical approach to multiple testing allows to represent closed test procedures based on the Bonferroni test by a weighted directed graph [13]. Formally, the graphical MCP consists of a vector $\alpha = (\alpha_1, \ldots, \alpha_m)$ of initial levels for the elementary hypotheses $H_i, i = 1, \ldots, m$, and an $m \times m$ transition matrix $\boldsymbol{G} = (g_{ij})$ which determines how significance levels are propagated in case of rejection of hypotheses. An updating algorithm is provided to perform hypothesis testing [13]. It starts by comparing the unadjusted p-values p_i of all elementary hypotheses with the respective original levels α_i. If $p_i \leq \alpha_i$, H_i is rejected and its significance level is "released" and propagated to increase the levels of the not-yet-rejected hypotheses. The precise rule for this propagation is determined by the transition matrix $\boldsymbol{G}$.

To state the updating algorithm, some notation is needed. Let $M = \{1, \ldots, m\}$ denote the index set of elementary hypotheses, $I \subseteq M$ a subset of M with complement $I^c = M \setminus I$. Further, let $\alpha_i = \alpha w_i$ with $0 \leq w_i \leq 1$ for $\sum_{i=1}^m w_i = 1$ and $0 \leq g_{ij} \leq 1$, $g_{ii} = 0$, with $\sum_{j=1}^m g_{ij} \leq 1$ for all $i, j \in I$. The weights w_i determine at which fraction of the significance level α the hypothesis H_i is initially tested. As hypotheses get rejected, these weights increase. For a given set $I \subseteq M$, we denote the corresponding weights by $w_i(I)$, such that $w_i = w_i(M)$. The updating algorithm is then given by

Algorithm: Weighted Bonferroni Test

1. Select a $j \in I$ such that $p_j \leq w_j(I)\alpha$ and reject H_j; otherwise stop.
2. Update the graph:

$$I \to I \setminus \{j\}$$

$$w_\ell(I) \to \begin{cases} w_\ell(I) + w_j(I) g_{j\ell}, & \ell \in I \\ 0, & \text{otherwise} \end{cases}$$

$$g_{\ell k} \to \begin{cases} \frac{g_{\ell k} + g_{\ell j} g_{jk}}{1 - g_{\ell j} g_{j\ell}}, & \ell, k \in I, \ell \neq k, g_{\ell j} g_{j\ell} < 1 \\ 0, & \text{otherwise.} \end{cases}$$

3. If $|I| \geq 1$, go to step 1; otherwise stop.

It has been shown that an MCP defined by a graph in conjunction with the updating algorithm uniquely defines a closed test procedure based on the Bonferroni test [13]. Hence, the graphical MCP keeps the FWER at level α and is consonant. Furthermore, the weights $w_j(I), j \in I$, do not depend on the sequence in which hypotheses $H_j, j \in I^c$, are rejected. Hence, the ultimate decision about rejection or non-rejection of the hypothesis H_i does not depend on which of the eligible hypothesis H_j is rejected in step 1.

Figure 3.4 provides an example of a graphical MCP. Together with the significance level α, this graph is the visual representation of the mathematical description just given. Hypotheses are represented by vertices and propagations by edges. To return to the example in Figure 3.2, assume that H_1 and

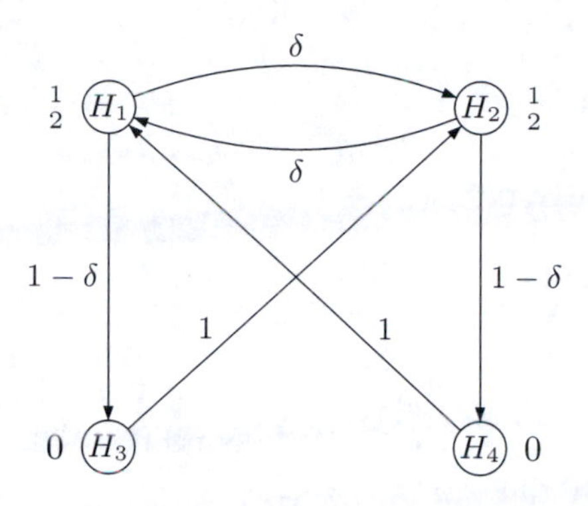

FIGURE 3.4: Graphical display of weighting strategy for a graphical MCP.

H_2 are the hypotheses of no treatment effect on PFS for two different doses of a new treatment and H_3 and H_4 are the hypotheses of no treatment effect on ORR for these doses. The graph allows to arrange the multiple comparison problem in such a way that these relations are highlighted and the statistical tests focus on relevant combinations of statements about the drug's effect. For example, the initial weights $w_3 = w_4 = 0$ in conjunction with the absence of edges between H_3 and H_4 make sure that a test for ORR is performed only if a PFS benefit was established before. The weights $w_1 = w_2 = 1/2$ indicate that there is no prior preference for either of the two doses. The propagation factor δ can be chosen based on clinical considerations. If, for example, it would be most desirable to show a benefit of at least one dose on both endpoints, $\delta = 0$ would be a sensible choice. Note that several extensions of the graphical approach are available [14], including group sequential designs described in Section 3.3.3 [71] and adaptive designs in the form of Section 3.3.4 [60, 93].

3.3.2 Gatekeeping Procedures

The graphical approach just described is closely related to the class of gatekeeping procedures, which gained popularity in recent years. Gatekeeping procedures use a grouping of the elementary hypotheses into families F_i which are tested in sequence (e.g., "primary" and "secondary" families). The word "gatekeeping" refers to the fact that hypotheses in family F_{i_2} are tested only if family F_{i_1} had been tested before when $i_1 < i_2$. The FWER is controlled at level α across all families $\bigcup F_i$.

For simplicity, assume that there are only two families F_1 (primary hypotheses) and F_2 (secondary hypotheses). Depending on whether rejection of all, of only some, or of only one hypothesis in the primary family is required for testing of secondary hypotheses, different classes of gatekeeping methods have been introduced. For example, serial gatekeeping is a generalization of the hierarchical test which tests F_1 first, moving on to testing F_2 if and only if all hypotheses in F_1 had been rejected before [3, 73, 104]. In contrast, parallel gatekeeping allows tests of F_2 if at least one hypothesis in F_1 can be rejected by using a specific form of closed test procedures based on the weighted Bonferroni test [22]. Tree gatekeeping unifies and generalizes serial and parallel gatekeeping [26]. Furthermore, a general multistage gatekeeping procedure was introduced to address arbitrary parallel gatekeeping problems using component procedures for each family [27]. Then the gatekeeping procedure is constructed by performing the component procedure sequentially starting with F_1. An important condition is that the significance level is not fully exhausted by F_1, a property called separability. Then the k-out-of-n gatekeeping unifies the serial and the parallel gatekeeping procedures by allowing the test of F_2 if at least k out of n hypotheses in F_1 can be rejected [111].

Other developments in gatekeeping procedures include the mixture parallel gatekeeping procedures [24] which can be more powerful than general multistage parallel gatekeeping procedures. Many gatekeeping procedures as well as the chain procedures [74] can be visualized using the graphical approach from Section 3.3.1 [13–15, 70].

3.3.3 Group Sequential Procedures

Cancer trials are very often performed in a group sequential manner. This means that at one or several preplanned points in time, an interim analysis of the available trial data is performed. Typically, group sequential cancer trials have a time-to-event endpoint (PFS or OS) and are event-driven which means that the interim analysis is done when a certain number of events have been observed. A typical example would be a two-stage trial where the interim analysis is performed after 300 PFS events had been observed. If the trial is continued, the final analysis is planned after 600 events.

Group sequential trials were originally developed to facilitate early testing of a drug for efficacy [58]. At any interim time point, investigators would decide to either stop the trial for efficacy or futility or to continue to the next stage. Any other decision (including modifications of sample sizes, treatment, or subpopulation selection) is not foreseen and would convert the group sequential design into a so-called adaptive design. Although in theory, group sequential trials can be set up in such a way that the Type I error rate control encompasses both stopping for futility and for efficacy of the experimental drug, it is widespread practice to disregard futility in the calculation of the Type I error rate (so called "non-binding" futility stopping). This does not preclude the possibility of actually stopping a trial if results are disappointing at an interim analysis; it merely means that this possibility is not used to modify critical values for efficacy claims. We will thus restrict the subsequent discussion to group sequential designs that foresee stopping of a trial for efficacy only.

In the following, we discuss group sequential designs based on asymptotically normal test statistics. This theory is most relevant in the context of randomized clinical phase III trials. In addition to these general approaches, there is a large body of literature on single arm cancer phase II trials. Essentially, this literature discusses group sequential trials for binary endpoints (tumor response), either working directly with the binomial distribution or with normal approximations tailored to the binomial distribution. These methods play an important role in phase II trials and we refer to Chapter 7 of the book for a detailed discussion. The interested readers are also referred to the following references [33, 37, 69, 85, 89].

Let $\boldsymbol{t} = (t_1, \ldots, t_s)$ be (asymptotically) multivariately normally distributed test statistics, where s denotes the total number of analysis time points. For simplicity, we restrict the discussion to testing a one-sided hypothesis H_0 of no treatment effect. Under H_0, the distribution is assumed to be $N(\boldsymbol{0}, \boldsymbol{R})$ where $\boldsymbol{R}$ is a completely known correlation matrix, i.e., it has diagonal elements 1 and correlations that are determined by the information fractions; see [58, Chapter 3] for details. The Type I error rate of the repeated testing of H_0 is controlled by determining critical values $c_1, \ldots, c_s$ in such a way that

$$\begin{aligned} 1 - P_{H_0}(t_1 < c_1, \ldots, t_s < c_s) &= \alpha \text{ if large } t_i \text{ reject } H_0 \text{ or,} \\ 1 - P_{H_0}(t_1 > c_1, \ldots, t_s > c_s) &= \alpha \text{ if small } t_i \text{ reject } H_0. \end{aligned} \quad (3.1)$$

We mention both versions of the one-sided test here, because the vast majority of statistics textbooks introduces one-sided tests that reject H_0 for large values of the test statistic. In cancer trials, however, the primary endpoint is usually a hazard ratio (for PFS or OS) and small values of its estimate are indicative of a significant treatment effect and lead to the rejection of H_0.

The critical values $c_1, \ldots, c_s$ for the test statistics can be transformed into critical values for the p-values $p_{t_k} = 1 - \Phi^{-1}(t_k)$, $k = 1, \ldots, s$. Note that any set of values $(c_1, \ldots, c_s)$ fulfilling (3.1) defines a valid group sequential testing procedure. Many suggestions have been made regarding functions to calculate $(c_1, \ldots, c_s)$ [62, 77, 78].

3.3.3.1 Group Sequential Procedures with Multiple Hypotheses

Conventional group sequential trials test only a single hypothesis H_0, albeit this is done repeatedly in time. If several hypotheses are tested simultaneously in a group sequential trial, a number of complications arise. To give a simple, instructive example, consider the situation of a primary hypothesis H_1 and a secondary H_2 which are tested hierarchically. For example, consider that H_1 is tested with a group sequential design at a single interim analysis after 50% of observations were obtained. We claim to use a strictly hierarchical approach and test H_2 if and only if H_1 has been rejected. Assume this test of H_2 is done at the full significance level α at the interim or the final analysis time point, depending on when significance was achieved for H_1. Then, the FWER is not preserved in general [56].

In the following, we focus on multiple comparisons which use only the m marginal test statistics for the elementary hypotheses $H_i, i = 1, \ldots, m$ in all tests for any intersection hypothesis $H_I = \bigcap_{i \in I} H_i, I \subseteq \{1, \ldots, m\}$. Such tests have been called "max-T" or "min-p" tests [106]. Using such tests, the problem of properly combining group sequential and multiplicity adjustment is solved by structurally separating these two aspects of the design:

1. The MCP is set up in exactly the same way as for any usual, non-group sequential set of hypotheses.
2. For each α_i that can arise in the MCP, we choose a group sequential approach.

Following this simple principle results in a group sequential MCP which guarantees FWER control: As soon as a hypothesis H_i is rejected, its significance level is propagated to the remaining hypotheses as determined by the MCP. However, the levels at which a remaining hypothesis H_i is subsequently tested follow the pre-defined group sequential approach. There is no "retrieving of α" from previous analysis time points.

The validity of this approach rests on one additional restriction [64, 71] which is easy to establish in practice. Assume that p-values are used as the test statistics. Then all group sequential components of the design must be such that all possible critical values $c_i(\alpha_j, t)$ fulfill the condition

$$c_i(\alpha, t) \leq c_i(\alpha', t) \text{ for all hypotheses } H_i, \text{ all } \alpha \leq \alpha', \text{ and all times } t. \quad (3.2)$$

In other words: no critical value is allowed to decrease at any analysis time point when a hypothesis receives the additional significance level from the rejection of another hypothesis. This condition is easy to check and fulfilled for most popular group sequential approaches, e.g., Pocock or O'Brien and Fleming [71].

Example

Assume that PFS and OS are the two endpoints in a clinical trial and are to be tested with the Bonferroni-Holm procedure. There are only two hypotheses H_{PFS} and H_{OS} of no treatment benefit, but they are tested repeatedly at different points in time. Assume that there are 3 analysis time points and the significance level is 2.5%. The information fractions (i.e., the time points of the interim analyses relative to the total information gathered in the trial; see Section 3.3.3.2) are fixed at 0.5 and 0.75 for the two interim analyses. For the sake of illustration, we assume here that the information fractions for PFS and OS are the same. Note that in practice, this is very unrealistic, as the time point for an interim analysis will typically be determined by the number of events in only one of these endpoints, and the information fraction for the two endpoints at this point in time will almost never be the same. We will come back to this topic with a brief discussion in Section 3.3.3.2. A more dedicated exposition can be found in Chapter 10 on data monitoring.

It is decided to use O'Brien-Fleming-like Lan-DeMets-α-spending (OF) for OS and Pocock-like Lan-DeMets-α-spending (PK) for PFS [62]. The p-values of logrank tests are used as test statistics. This means that we reject H_{PFS} if $p_{t_k,\text{PFS}} \leq c_{\text{PFS}}(1.25\%, t_k)$ at any look $k = 1, 2, 3$ or if $p_{t_k,\text{PFS}} \leq c_{\text{PFS}}(2.5\%, t_k)$ and $p_{t_k,\text{OS}} \leq c_{\text{OS}}(1.25\%, t_k)$ at any look $k = 1, 2, 3$ (ditto for H_{OS}). In this context, the p-value $p_{t_k,i}$ of the logrank test is used as the test statistic and formula (3.1) states that $c_i(\alpha, t_k)$ fulfill

$$1 - P_{H_0}\left[p_{t_1,i} > c_i(\alpha', t_1),\ p_{t_2,i} > c_i(\alpha', t_2),\ p_{t_3,i} > c_i(\alpha', t_3)\right] = \alpha'$$

for $\alpha' = \alpha/2,\ \alpha$ and $i = \text{PFS, OS}$.

For the OF and the PK group sequential α-spending with information fractions $t_1 = 0.5, t_2 = 0.75$, and $t_3 = 1$, $[c_i(\alpha, t_1), c_i(\alpha, t_2), c_i(\alpha, t_3)]$ are given by:

- (0.1%, 0.4%, 1.1%) for OF and $\alpha = 1.25\%$,
- (0.2%, 0.9%, 2.2%) for OF and $\alpha = 2.5\%$,
- (0.8%, 0.5%, 0.5%) for PK and $\alpha = 1.25\%$,
- (1.6%, 1.0%, 1.0%) for PK and $\alpha = 2.5\%$.

By the MCP approach, we set out with a significance level of 1.25% per hypothesis. At interim analysis 1, we test PFS at 0.8% and OS at 0.1%. Assume that none of these two tests is significant. We would then move on to interim analysis 2 and test PFS at 0.5% and OS at 0.4% with the updated data. Assume now that PFS is significant. Hence, H_{PFS} can be rejected and does not need to be tested again at the final analysis. Regarding OS, we switch to an overall level of 2.5% according to the propagation of the significance level (see Section 3.3.1) and test OS at a level of 0.9% (which is the local level at an information fraction of 0.75 from the O'Brien-Fleming-like Lan-deMets approach for an overall α of 2.5%). If this is not significant, we test OS again at the final analysis at the level of 2.2%. Notice that in theory, we could go back to the first interim analysis result and see if this had been significant at a level of 0.2% to reject H_{OS} after the rejection of H_{PFS} at interim analysis 2. In practice, however, this is not done. Notice also that a recalculation of critical values for the remaining two tests of H_{OS}, assuming that only 0.1% have been spent at the first interim analysis on H_{OS}, would not control the FWER in general (for instance, see [40, 72, 95, 112]).

Applying the closed test principle, it is easy to see that the outlined approach keeps the FWER. In contrast, attempts to split or double "local" levels (or other critical values for test statistics) will usually fail and are not easily generalizable to weighted Bonferroni-Holm approaches or to other overall significance levels. In the situation here, replacing $c_i(\alpha/2, t)$ by $c_i(\alpha, t)/2$ leads to a liberal test that does not control the FWER, whereas replacing $c_i(\alpha, t)$ by $2c_i(\alpha/2, t)$ produces a conservative procedure which can uniformly be improved by an α-spending approach that fixes $c_i(\alpha/2, t)$ and recalculates all

$c_i(\alpha, t)$ such that they fulfill $c_i(\alpha, t) > 2c_i(\alpha/2, t)$. Due to these issues, MCPs which represent adjustments as functions of ratios or differences of local critical values in group sequential trials are often of very limited practical value.

We note in passing that the approach does not make use of the correlation between the test statistics for PFS and OS. In a typical application, this correlation could be highly positive and ignoring it might lead to a loss of power. A potential improvement of the approach presented here may be achieved if this correlation is estimated and a parametric test from Section 3.2.3 is used for the MCP part of the design. The main difficulties with this are the impact of the correlation estimate on the FWER in finite samples, the fact that the correlation estimate changes from interim analysis to interim analysis, and the fact that for many non-normally distributed endpoints, parameters which have an impact on the response also affect the correlation, such that correlation estimation and treatment effect estimation cannot be separated as in the case of normally distributed response.

3.3.3.2 Group Sequential Procedures with a Time-to-event Endpoint

Most cancer trials use time-to-event endpoints. In case of the simple comparison of two treatment groups with a logrank test, the sequence of test statistics has been shown to have an approximate joint normal distribution with correlations depending on the number of events per group [98]. This fact is used for the construction of group sequential time-to-event designs which almost always use an α-spending approach to determine the critical values $(c_1, \ldots, c_s)$ [62]. To be more precise, assume that there are s time points at which the event in question has occurred. For simplicity, we assume that all these event times are distinct. In an event-driven group sequential trial, the k-th (interim) analysis is performed after a fixed number of d_k events. If there are two treatment groups (experimental and control, say), then let $\delta_{d_k} \in \{0, 1\}$ be the indicator of event occurrence in the experimental group at the time of the d_k-th event. The statistic of the logrank test at the k-th interim analysis is given by

$$t_k = \frac{\sum_{h=1}^{d_k} (\delta_h - p_h)}{\sqrt{\sum_{h=1}^{d_k} p_{h1}(1 - p_{h1})}} \tag{3.3}$$

where $p_{h1} = \frac{r_{h1}}{r_h}$, r_{h1} is the number of patients at risk in the experimental group at the time of the h-th event, and r_h is the total number of patients at risk at that time. Under the null hypothesis of no difference between the two treatments, the vector $(t_1, \cdots, t_s)^\top$ of logrank test statistics has approximately a $N(\mathbf{0}, \boldsymbol{R})$-distribution where $\boldsymbol{R}$ is a correlation matrix with diagonal elements 1 and off-diagonal elements

$$v_{k_1,k_2} = \frac{\sqrt{\sum_{h=1}^{d_{k_1}} p_{h1}(1 - p_{h1})}}{\sqrt{\sum_{h=1}^{d_{k_2}} p_{h1}(1 - p_{h1})}} \text{ for } 1 \leq k_1 < k_2 \leq s. \tag{3.4}$$

The correlations $v_{k,s}$ of the interim test statistic t_k with the final test statistic t_s are also called information fractions in the context of group sequential trials. In a sense, they are the "time units" used in group sequential time-to-event trials.

According to [38] "typical presentations of the proportional-hazards model involve a lot of hand-waving." We agree with this assessment, and the hand-waving continues with extensions of the logrank test to group sequential versions. The literature on the group sequential logrank test (e.g., [58, Chapter 13]) typically gives formula (3.4) and then proceeds to recommend the use of some α-spending approach to derive critical values $(c_1, \ldots, c_s)$ such that equation (3.1) is fulfilled, where $P_{H_0}(t_1 < c_1, \ldots, t_s < c_s)$ is the cumulative distribution function of the multivariate normal distribution with mean $\mathbf{0}$ and correlation matrix from (3.4). The α-spending approach is used to calculate the information fraction at the time t_k of interim analysis k (relative to a planned total accrued information which is $\sum_{h=1}^{d_s} p_{h1}(1 - p_{h1})$ and which is of course not known until the final analysis is actually reached) and to obtain the corresponding critical value c_k based on how much level was spent before (i.e., fulfilling (3.1) with the previously calculated $c_1, \ldots, c_{k-1}$ and the assumed putative $c_{k+1}, \ldots, c_s$ based on the planned future α-spending). For the sake of planning the trial, the information fractions must be approximated. Under H_0, we expect $p_{h1} = 1/2,\ h = 1, \ldots, d_s$. If H_0 is true, v_{k_1,k_2} is approximately equal to $\sqrt{\frac{d_{k_1}}{d_{k_2}}}$. These are the numbers typically used at the planning stage of the trial: $(c_1, \ldots, c_s)$ are calculated from (3.1) under the assumption of a multivariate normal distribution with correlations $\sqrt{\frac{d_{k_1}}{d_{k_2}}}$ instead of v_{k_1,k_2} and power calculations or trial simulations are performed using these numbers. Note that the simplification of using observed $\sqrt{\frac{d_{k_1}}{d_{k_2}}}$ instead of observed v_{k_1,k_2} for the calculation of critical values from the multivariate normal distribution with correlation from (3.4) can also be used in the actual analysis of the data.

Impact of event-driven interim analyses on multiple hypotheses

If multiple hypotheses are tested simultaneously in an event-driven group sequential trial with time-to-event endpoints, several complications arise from the fact that rejections of hypotheses can occur at different points in time. The complications are similar, but slightly different depending on whether the multiple hypotheses relate to different event types, or whether they concern different subpopulations or treatment arms.

As an example of the first situation, consider a two-stage group sequential trial with PFS and OS as the two endpoints. The protocol foresees that the interim analysis is performed after 200 PFS events and the final analysis after 400 PFS events. This means that for OS, the information fraction observed at the interim analysis is a random number. Formula (3.4) allows us to calculate actual information fractions, but only after the trial has been completed. Hence, in order to implement the design, we have to speculate about the expected number of deaths at the time of 200 (400) PFS events and calculate critical values for OS in such a way that (3.1) is fulfilled for these expected numbers. Once the final analysis is reached, we must recalculate the final critical value c_2^* for OS in such a way that $1 - P_{H_0}(t_1 < c_1, t_2 < c_2^*) = \alpha$ is fulfilled for the actually observed information fraction v_{t_1,t_2}, whereas c_1 was based upon an assumed information fraction at the beginning of the trial.

More seriously, it remains unclear how to proceed with H_{OS} in the situation where H_{PFS} can already be rejected at interim.

We could keep on monitoring PFS to determine the time point of the final analysis. Having rejected H_{PFS} already, however, it seems wasteful to do this and would also beg the question whether H_{PFS} must be retested at the final analysis.

In practice, this dilemma is often solved by a hierarchical approach. The interim analysis is triggered by a fixed number of PFS events. At this point in time, PFS is tested. The trial continues if and only if H_{PFS} is significant at this analysis (i.e., the interim analysis is the "final analysis for PFS"). If this is the case, the time point of the final analysis is determined by a fixed number of OS events. The method outlined above can be used to calculate information fractions for OS.

This approach generalizes to the situation with more than two interim analyses and/or parallel, non-hierarchical testing of PFS and OS in a natural way:

The design is set up such that interim analyses $1, \ldots, q$ occur after fixed numbers of PFS events. Analysis q is the final analysis for PFS. Subsequent analysis time points $q+1, \ldots, s$ are determined by fixed numbers of OS events. Let $d_{\text{PFS},k}$ and $d_{\text{OS},k}$ be the number of PFS and OS events at analysis k, respectively. All $d_{\text{PFS},k}, k = 1, \ldots, q$ and all $d_{\text{OS},k}, k = q+1, \ldots, s$ are fixed. The $d_{\text{OS},k}, k = 1, \ldots, q$ are random. In theory, it could happen that $d_{\text{OS},k} > d_{\text{OS},q+1}$, but in practice, interim analyses are usually timed in such a way that this is ruled out. The one aspect that needs to be considered is the case where H_{PFS} can be rejected at analysis $k < q$. If that happens, there must be an alternative criterion of a number of OS events that triggers interim analyses $k+1, \ldots, s$ instead of the originally planned PFS-based criterion.

If PFS and OS are tested in parallel rather than in a hierarchical structure, the recalculation of critical values for OS at the PFS-driven interim analyses proceeds as described above, potentially for the different significance levels that can arise from α-propagation in the context of the MCP. It is then important that condition (3.2) is fulfilled not only for a discrete, pre-planned number of time points t, but for the entire continuum of time points (or, to be more precise, information fractions) which can arise from the random number of OS events which are available at the time of the interim analysis.

In the case that several treatment arms are compared in an event-driven group sequential trial, problems are similar in the sense that if a hypothesis can be rejected at the interim analysis, the number of events for later stages of the trial may arise from a random number from remaining treatment arms. For example, a trial may be set up to compare three treatment arms tested at an interim analysis after 300 events. Rules for the final analysis could then be:

- The final analysis will be done after a total of 600 events (across both stages) in the remaining arms, or
- In treatment arms that are rejected, recruitment is stopped. The final analysis will be done after 600 events (across both stages) from all arms.

Depending on which hypotheses can be rejected at the interim analysis, the events in the second stage of the trial may be from one, two, or three treatment arms. If stopping rules are completely fixed in advance, traditional group-sequential theory [58, Chapter 7] in combination with MCPs and information fraction recalculation as outlined previously in this section can still be used. If, however, non-binding futility rules or other not completely prespecified modifications of the trial are allowed at interim analyses, assumptions of these traditional methods can be violated and selection biases can arise. For details, see [2, 57]. In this case, adaptive trial methodology must be used to handle FWER control properly.

3.3.4 Adaptive Designs

A clinical trial design is called adaptive when certain, prespecified modifications of the trial conduct are allowed after examination of the data at an interim analysis. The practically most relevant design modifications are changes to the sample size or duration of the trial, the selection of treatment arms, and the selection of subpopulations. In theory, other ways of redesigning the trial including changes of the primary endpoint or the test statistics could be considered, but this is very rarely done in practice [12].

Adaptive designs are based on ideas of combining test statistics from different stages of a trial into a single decision about a null hypothesis [1, 79]. This basic principle proved to be very useful and resulted in a number of adaptive design approaches, most notably the p-value combination approach [63] and the conditional error function approach [75].

For simplicity, we restrict attention to the p-value combination approach in a two-stage trial. Assume that p_1 and p_2 denote the stagewise p-values for a null hypothesis H_0. It is assumed that p_1 is based only on the first stage and p_2 only on the second stage data. Furthermore, there is a combination function $C(p_1, p_2)$. H_0 is rejected if either $p_1 \leq \alpha_1$ or if $C(p_1, p_2) \leq c$, where c is calculated in such a way that

$$\alpha_1 + \int_{\alpha_1}^{\infty} \int_0^1 \mathbf{1}_{[C(q_1,q_2) \leq c]} dq_1 \, dq_2 = \alpha. \tag{3.5}$$

The indicator function $\mathbf{1}_{[\cdot]}$ equals 1 if $C(p_1, p_2) \leq c$ and 0 otherwise.

Obviously, this decision criterion defines a level-α-test. The most important practically relevant implementation of this approach uses the inverse normal p-value combination function [63] given by

$$C(p_1, p_2) = 1 - \Phi\left[w_1\,\Phi^{-1}(1-p_1) + w_2\,\Phi^{-1}(1-p_2)\right], \qquad (3.6)$$

where w_1 and w_2 denote prespecified weights such that $w_1^2 + w_2^2 = 1$ and Φ denotes the cumulative distribution function of the standard normal distribution.

To give a motivation for this combination function, assume that an (asymptotically) normally distributed test statistic is used which is $N(0,1)$-distributed under H_0. Let z_i denote this test statistic calculated from n_i patients in stage $i = 1, 2$ of a two-stage trial. There is no overlap in patients between the two stages. Then $z_i \sim N(0,1)$, $i = 1, 2$ are stochastically independent and $z = \sqrt{\frac{n_1}{n}}z_1 + \sqrt{\frac{n_2}{n}}z_2 \sim N(0,1)$ under H_0 is the z-test statistic based on all $n = n_1 + n_2$ observations. Since $p_i = 1 - \Phi(z_i)$, we obtain $C(p_1, p_2) = 1 - \Phi(w_1 z_1 + w_2 z_2)$. If in addition $\alpha_1 = 0$ and $w_i = \sqrt{\frac{n_i}{n}}$, then $C(p_1, p_2) \leq c$ is equivalent to $z \leq \Phi^{-1}(1-\alpha)$. Hence, if the trial is never stopped and never modified at the interim, an ordinary z-test is performed on the data. However, if for example the sample size n_2 is changed to n_2^* based on the observations from the n_1 patients of stage 1, the test still keeps the Type I error rate, but since the combination uses $w_i = \sqrt{\frac{n_i}{n}}$ rather than $\sqrt{\frac{n_i^*}{n_1+n_2^*}}$, the test is no longer equivalent to the uniformly most powerful, fixed sample size z-test of H_0. This is the "price to pay" for a design modification which is not entirely prespecified.

A key requirement of these approaches is the independence of the stage-1 test statistic and the conditional stage-2 test statistic given the stage-1 data. This condition is called the conditional invariance principle [65]. It can sometimes be subtly undermined in practice. For example, consider a situation where the primary endpoint is the change from baseline after 12 weeks of treatment. The interim analysis is done after 50% of patients have completed 12 weeks of treatment. At this point in time, an adaptation is made based on the stage-1 data. If this contains information on the stage-2 test statistic, e.g., because safety signals are used that contain events from patients who have not yet finished 12 weeks of treatment, but are already recruited into the trial, or because the test statistics of both stages use variance estimates based on all available data or a longitudinal model is used to impute missing values, then the assumption is violated.

We have focused on adaptive designs with FWER control since these are most relevant in confirmatory phase III trials. In earlier phases, designs which target towards exploratory aims, e.g., Bayesian response-adaptive and enrichment designs, are often applied. We refer to [96, 97] and Chapter 12 of this book. Among the many approaches that we could not cover due to space restrictions are permutation and resampling methods (see e.g., [103]) and papers that deal in-depth with other sources of multiplicity than the ones discussed here (see, e.g., [9, 19, 59, 100, 102]).

3.4 Applications

3.4.1 Multiple Comparison Procedure in the BELLE-2 Trial

In this section, we revisit the BELLE-2 trial from Section 3.1.4. In this two-armed trial, there are four hypotheses accounting for two endpoints (PFS and OS) for the comparisons of BKM120 against placebo in two populations (overall and $B+$). The reason to test the biomarker $B+$ population in particular is that this gene status may be a predictor of poor prognostic outcome and thus plays a critical role in inducing resistance to current therapies. Since the $B-$ population is not the target subpopulation of interest, it is not included in the formal testing framework [41].

In addition to the given set of null hypotheses, clinical considerations often lead to a structured hypothesis testing problem subject to certain logical constraints. In cancer trials it is often reasonable to assume that PFS is to be declared significant before OS and thus PFS is considered as the primary endpoint. Therefore, for BELLE-2 the four null hypotheses can be grouped into two primary hypotheses H_1, H_2 (comparisons in the overall and the $B+$ populations for PFS) and two secondary hypotheses H_3, H_4 (comparisons in the same populations, but for OS). In addition, a success in either population is considered as important, which rules out a full hierarchy of testing first the overall and, conditional on its significance, then the $B+$ population (say). In addition, it is required that a secondary OS hypothesis is not tested without having rejected the associated primary PFS hypothesis (successiveness property). The objective is to test all four hypotheses H_1, H_2, H_3, H_4 under strong FWER control while reflecting the clinical considerations above and without leading to illogical decisions.

Common MCPs in Section 3.2, such as the procedures by Bonferroni, Holm, or Dunnett, are not suitable here, because they treat all four hypotheses equally and do not address the underlying structure of the test problem. Instead, the graphical approach in Section 3.3.1 is well suited for such a trial with complex objectives. Figure 3.5 visualizes the testing strategy for BELLE-2 in which the primary objective is to demonstrate the PFS benefit in the overall and $B+$ population. Therefore, the significance level $\alpha = 2.5\%$ (one-sided) is split into $\frac{4}{5}\alpha = 2\%$ and $\frac{1}{5}\alpha = 0.5\%$ for testing H_1 and H_2. The secondary objective is to show the OS benefit which is of interest after the PFS effect has been shown in the associated populations. For example, if PFS in the full population is significant at level 2%, this level is further split and propagated to other hypotheses according to prespecified weights and edges. In this case, OS in the full population will be tested at level $\frac{3}{5}\alpha = 1.5\%$ and PFS in the $B+$ population will be tested at level $\frac{1}{5}\alpha + \frac{1}{5}\alpha = \frac{2}{5}\alpha = 1\%$. This strategy can be easily adapted to incorporate group sequential designs, to reflect relative importance of objectives, and to evaluate power outcomes of the trial.

Sample size calculation is usually driven by a particular hypothesis in a

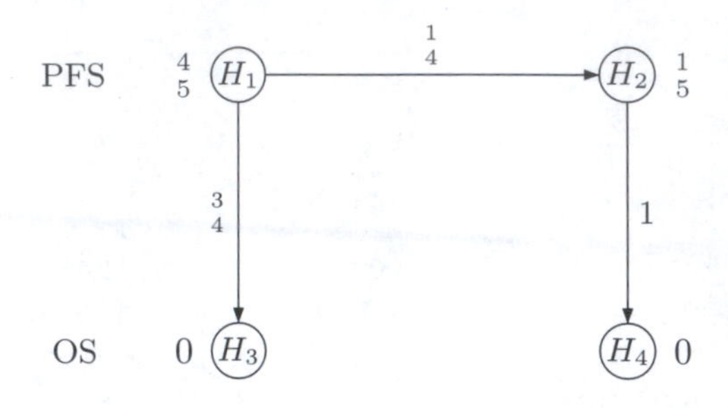

FIGURE 3.5: Graphical visualization of the multiple comparison procedure of BELLE-2 [41].

trial with complex decision strategies. Because of the event driven nature of the BELLE-2 trial, the number of events needed for a PFS hypothesis in either the overall or the $B+$ population is first calculated to achieve a certain power. Based on the accrual rate and the duration of the trial, the number of subjects needed is calculated for the overall and $B+$ populations. Then the number of events and power for all hypotheses are calculated. Further adjustment to the sample size is often helpful in practice to better reflect the importance of different hypotheses.

3.4.2 Comparison with a Common Control in Time-to-event Trials

As an example of the complications arising from testing different treatment arms on the same endpoint in event-driven time-to-event trials, we consider the comparison of two doses of a treatment with a common control group C. The two test statistics are calculated according to (3.3) from only two of the three groups in the trial (dose 1, control and dose 2, control, respectively). They do not use a variance estimate calculated from all three groups in the trial. As discussed in Section 3.2.3.1, the correlation between the test statistics is a function of sample sizes per group. In time-to-event trials, this must be replaced by numbers of events per group, which — in contrast to sample sizes — are random rather than fixed. It can be shown that the correlation between the two logrank test statistics for dose 1 versus control and dose 2 versus control at interim analysis k is

$$v^*_{k_1,k_2} = \frac{\sum_{h=1}^{d_k} p^*_{h1} p^*_{h2}}{\sqrt{\sum_{h=1}^{d_k} p^*_{h1}(1-p^*_{h1}) \times \sum_{h=1}^{d_k} p^*_{h2}(1-p^*_{h2})}} \text{ for } 1 \leq k_1 < k_2 \leq s,$$

where

$$p_{hj}^{*} = \begin{cases} \frac{r_{hj}}{r_{hj}+r_{hC}} & \text{if the } h\text{-th event occurs in group } j \text{ or in group } C, \\ 0 & \text{otherwise} \end{cases}$$

with r_{hj} and r_{hC} being the number of patients at risk in group $j = 1, 2$ and group C, respectively, at the time of the h-th event [21]. This formula is derived from the conditional distribution of the logrank test statistic given the event times and numbers of patients at risk at these event times. From this perspective, they are conditionally fixed, non-random quantities. However, unconditionally, they are of course random, even if we fix the total number of events in an event-driven time-to-event trial. Furthermore, in contrast to the usual situation described in Section 3.2.3.1, the expected values of this correlation changes depending on whether the null hypothesis of a zero log hazard ratio is true or not. Under H_0 and with equal sample sizes per group, v_{k_1,k_2}^{*} is approximately equal to 0.5. Using this correlation value in a Dunnett test applied to group sequential testing is feasible and asymptotically protects the FWER [18, 21, 61]. Still, health authorities have occasionally voiced concerns about the fact that this constitutes yet another element of approximation. A similar concern arises in the conventional Dunnett test if the originally planned sample sizes are not realized, i.e., there are deviations from the originally planned sample sizes n_0, n_1, and n_2. Interestingly, it can be shown that the Dunnett test conditional on the realized sample sizes (n_0^*, n_1^*, and n_2^*, say) controls the FWER, whereas the test using the originally planned ones does so only asymptotically for the normal approximation of the t statistics. Both of these statements require that all deviations from the originally planned sample sizes occur stochastically independent from the observed data, e.g., at random or due to operational considerations which are not triggered by the observed values of incoming results. Otherwise, if sample sizes are changed based on observed response values, the trial is adaptive and additional statistical adjustments are needed for FWER control and bias correction.

3.5 Concluding Remarks

Multiplicity adjustments are important in planning, executing, and analyzing clinical trials. Failure to do so will endanger the integrity of trial conduct and thus reduce the scientific contribution. In this chapter, we focused on procedures to control the familywise error rate, which is commonly required for confirmatory clinical trials. As can be seen, no single procedure outperforms the others. Thus it is more important to understand the merits and limitations of these methods in order to tailor an MCP to specific study objectives.

The underlying principle of the methodologies is to use the overall Type

I error rate more efficiently while reflecting the relevance and importance of hypotheses. Advanced multiple comparison methods like graphical approaches provide a flexible and transparent way to design, evaluate, and communicate alternative options. Group sequential and adaptive designs provide another dimension of flexibility which allows early termination of the trial and midway adaptations. However, challenges exist and some of them were highlighted due to the event-driven nature of many cancer trials. As we emphasized in the introduction, an informed decision on the multiplicity adjustment can only be made through collaborations between statisticians and other stakeholders of the clinical trial.

Bibliography

[1] P. Bauer and K. Köhne. Evaluation of experiments with adaptive interim analyses. *Biometrics*, 50(4):1029–1041, 1994.

[2] P. Bauer, F. König, W. Brannath, and M. Posch. Selection and bias - two hostile brothers. *Statistics in Medicine*, 29(1):1–13, 2010.

[3] P. Bauer, J. Röhmel, W. Maurer, and L. Hothorn. Testing strategies in multi-dose experiments including active control. *Statistics in Medicine*, 17(18):2133–2146, 1998.

[4] Y. Benjamini and Y. Hochberg. Controlling the false discovery rate: a practical and powerful approach to multiple testing. *Journal of the Royal Statistical Society. Series B (Methodological)*, pages 289–300, 1995.

[5] Y. Benjamini and Y. Hochberg. Multiple hypotheses testing with weights. *Scandinavian Journal of Statistics*, 24(3):407–418, 1997.

[6] R. L. Berger. Multiparameter hypothesis testing and acceptance sampling. *Technometrics*, 24(4):295–300, 1982.

[7] W. Brannath and F. Bretz. Shortcuts for locally consonant closed test procedures. *Journal of the American Statistical Association*, 105(490):660–669, 2010.

[8] W. Brannath, F. Bretz, W. Maurer, and S. Sarkar. Trimmed weighted Simes' test for two one-sided hypotheses with arbitrarily correlated test statistics. *Biometrical Journal*, 51(6):885–898, 2009.

[9] W. Brannath, E. Zuber, M. Branson, F. Bretz, P. Gallo, M. Posch, and A. Racine-Poon. Confirmatory adaptive designs with Bayesian decision tools for a targeted therapy in oncology. *Statistics in Medicine*, 28(10):1445–1463, 2009.

[10] F. Bretz, A. Genz, and A. L. Hothorn. On the numerical availability of multiple comparison procedures. *Biometrical Journal*, 43(5):645–656, 2001.

[11] F. Bretz, T. Hothorn, and P. Westfall. *Multiple Comparisons using R.* CRC Press, 2010.

[12] F. Bretz, F. König, W. Brannath, E. Glimm, and M. Posch. Adaptive designs for confirmatory clinical trials. *Statistics in Medicine*, 28(8):1181–1217, 2009.

[13] F. Bretz, W. Maurer, W. Brannath, and M. Posch. A graphical approach to sequentially rejective multiple test procedures. *Statistics in Medicine*, 28(4):586–604, 2009.

[14] F. Bretz, W. Maurer, and J. Maca. Graphical approaches to multiple testing. In W.R. Young and D.-G. Chen, editors, *Clinical Trial Biostatistics and Biopharmaceutical Applications*. Taylor & Francis, Boca Raton, FL, 2014.

[15] F. Bretz, M. Posch, E. Glimm, F. Klinglmueller, W. Maurer, and K. Rohmeyer. Graphical approaches for multiple comparison procedures using weighted Bonferroni, Simes, or parametric tests. *Biometrical Journal*, 53(6):894–913, 2011.

[16] F. Bretz and P. H. Westfall. Multiplicity and replicability: two sides of the same coin. *Pharmaceutical statistics*, 13(6):343–344, 2014.

[17] C-F. Burman, C. Sonesson, and O. Guilbaud. A recycling framework for the construction of Bonferroni-based multiple tests. *Statistics in Medicine*, 28(5):739–761, 2009.

[18] M. Carreras, G. Gutjahr, and W. Brannath. Adaptive seamless designs with interim treatment selection: a case study in oncology. *Statistics in Medicine*, 34(8):1317–1333, 2015.

[19] C. Chen and R. A. Beckman. Hypothesis testing in a confirmatory phase III trial with a possible subset effect. *Statistics in Biopharmaceutical Research*, 1(4):431–440, 2009.

[20] A. Cohen and H. B. Sackrowitz. Two stage conditionally unbiased estimators of the selected mean. *Statistics & Probability Letters*, 8(3):273–278, 1989.

[21] L. Di Scala and E. Glimm. Time-to-event analysis with treatment arm selection at interim. *Statistics in Medicine*, 30(26):3067–3081, 2011.

[22] A. Dmitrienko, W. W. Offen, and P. H. Westfall. Gatekeeping strategies for clinical trials that do not require all primary effects to be significant. *Statistics in Medicine*, 22(15):2387–2400, 2003.

[23] A. Dmitrienko and A. C. Tamhane. Gatekeeping procedures in clinical trials. In A. Dmitrienko, A. C. Tamhane, and F. Bretz, editors, *Multiple Testing Problems in Pharmaceutical Statistics.* CRC Press, Boca Raton, FL, 2010.

[24] A. Dmitrienko and A. C. Tamhane. General theory of mixture procedures for gatekeeping. *Biometrical Journal*, 55(3):402–419, 2013.

[25] A. Dmitrienko, A. C. Tamhane, and F. Bretz. *Multiple Testing Problems in Pharmaceutical Statistics.* CRC Press, Boca Raton, FL, 2010.

[26] A. Dmitrienko, A. C. Tamhane, L. Liu, and B. L. Wiens. A note on tree gatekeeping procedures in clinical trials. *Statistics in Medicine*, 27(17):3446–3451, 2008.

[27] A. Dmitrienko, A. C. Tamhane, and B.L. Wiens. General multistage gatekeeping procedures. *Biometrical Journal*, 50(5):667–677, 2008.

[28] S. Dudoit and M.J. Van Der Laan. *Multiple Testing Procedures with Applications to Genomics.* Springer, New York, 2007.

[29] C. W. Dunnett. A multiple comparison procedure for comparing several treatments with a control. *Journal of the American Statistical Association*, 50(272):1096–1121, 1955.

[30] C. W. Dunnett and A. C. Tamhane. Step-down multiple tests for comparing treatments with a control in unbalanced one-way layouts. *Statistics in Medicine*, 10(6):939–947, 1991.

[31] C. W. Dunnett and A. C. Tamhane. A step-up multiple test procedure. *Journal of the American Statistical Association*, 87(417):162–170, 1992.

[32] B. Efron. *Large-scale Inference: Empirical Bayes Methods for Estimation, Testing, and Prediction*, volume 1. Cambridge University Press, 2010.

[33] S. Englert and M. Kieser. Improving the flexibility and efficiency of phase II designs for oncology trials. *Biometrics*, 68(3):886–892, 2012.

[34] European Medicines Agency. ICH Topic E9: Notes for Guidance on Statistical Principles for Clinical Trials, 1998. http://www.cardiff.ac.uk/racdv/resgov/Resources/EMA%20ICH%20Topic%20E9.pdf.

[35] European Medicines Agency. Points to consider on multiplicity issues in clinical trials, 2002. http://www.ema.europa.eu/docs/en_GB/document_library/Scientific_guideline/2009/09/WC500003640.pdf.

[36] H. Finner and K. Strassburger. The partitioning principle: a powerful tool in multiple decision theory. *Annals of Statistics*, 30(4):1194–1213, 2002.

[37] T. R. Fleming. One-sample multiple testing procedure for phase II clinical trials. *Biometrics*, 38(1):143–151, 1982.

[38] D. A. Freedman. Survival analysis. *American Statistician*, 62(2):110–119, 2008.

[39] K. R. Gabriel. Simultaneous test procedures-some theory of multiple comparisons. *Annals of Mathematical Statistics*, 40(1):224–250, 1969.

[40] E. Glimm, W. Maurer, and F. Bretz. Hierarchical testing of multiple endpoints in group-sequential trials. *Statistics in Medicine*, 29(2):219–228, 2010.

[41] S. Goteti, S. Hirawat, C. Massacesi, N. Fretault, F. Bretz, and B. Dharan. Some practical considerations for phase III studies with biomarker evaluations. *Journal of Clinical Oncology*, 32(8):854–855, 2014.

[42] J. Gou, A. C. Tamhane, D. Xi, and D. Rom. A class of improved hybrid Hochberg-Hommel type step-up multiple test procedures. *Biometrika*, 101(4):899–911, 2014.

[43] E. Grechanovsky and Y. Hochberg. Closed procedures are better and often admit a shortcut. *Journal of Statistical Planning and Inference*, 76(1):79–91, 1999.

[44] O. Guilbaud. Simultaneous confidence regions corresponding to Holm's step-down procedure and other closed-testing procedures. *Biometrical Journal*, 50(5):678–692, 2008.

[45] O. Guilbaud. Alternative confidence regions for Bonferroni-based closed-testing procedures that are not alpha-exhaustive. *Biometrical Journal*, 51(4):721–735, 2009.

[46] A. J. Hayter and J. C. Hsu. On the relationship between stepwise decision procedures and confidence sets. *Journal of the American Statistical Association*, 89(425):128–136, 1994.

[47] Y. Hochberg. A sharper Bonferroni procedure for multiple tests of significance. *Biometrika*, 75(4):800–802, 1988.

[48] Y. Hochberg and U. Liberman. An extended Simes' test. *Statistics & Probability Letters*, 21(2):101–105, 1994.

[49] Y. Hochberg and A. C. Tamhane. *Multiple Comparison Procedures*. John Wiley & Sons, Inc., 1987.

[50] S. Holm. A simple sequentially rejective multiple test procedure. *Scandinavian Journal of Statistics*, 6(2):65–70, 1979.

[51] G. Hommel. A stagewise rejective multiple test procedure based on a modified Bonferroni test. *Biometrika*, 75(2):383–386, 1988.

[52] G. Hommel. A comparison of two modified Bonferroni procedures. *Biometrika*, 76(3):624–625, 1989.

[53] G. Hommel, F. Bretz, and W. Maurer. Powerful short-cuts for multiple testing procedures with special reference to gatekeeping strategies. *Statistics in Medicine*, 26(22):4063–4073, 2007.

[54] T. Hothorn, F. Bretz, and P. Westfall. Simultaneous inference in general parametric models. *Biometrical Journal*, 50(3):346–363, 2008.

[55] J. Hsu. *Multiple Comparisons: Theory and Methods.* CRC Press, 1996.

[56] H. M. J. Hung, S.-J. Wang, and R. O'Neill. Statistical considerations for testing multiple endpoints in group sequential or adaptive clinical trials. *Journal of Biopharmaceutical Statistics*, 17(6):1201–1210, 2007.

[57] M. Jenkins, A. Stone, and C. Jennison. An adaptive seamless phase II/III design for oncology trials with subpopulation selection using correlated survival endpoints. *Pharmaceutical Statistics*, 10(4):347–356, 2011.

[58] C. Jennison and B. W. Turnbull. *Group Sequential Methods with Applications to Clinical Trials.* CRC Press, 1999.

[59] W. Jiang, B. Freidlin, and R. Simon. Biomarker-adaptive threshold design: a procedure for evaluating treatment with possible biomarker-defined subset effect. *Journal of the National Cancer Institute*, 99(13):1036–1043, 2007.

[60] F. Klinglmueller, M. Posch, and F. König. Adaptive graph-based multiple testing procedures. *Pharmaceutical Statistics*, 13(6):345–356, 2014.

[61] F. König, W. Brannath, F. Bretz, and M. Posch. Adaptive Dunnett tests for treatment selection. *Statistics in Medicine*, 27(10):1612–1625, 2008.

[62] K. K. G. Lan and D. L. DeMets. Discrete sequential boundaries for clinical trials. *Biometrika*, 70(3):659–663, 1983.

[63] W. Lehmacher and G. Wassmer. Adaptive sample size calculations in group sequential trials. *Biometrics*, 55(4):1286–1290, 1999.

[64] Q. Liu and K.M. Anderson. On adaptive extensions of group sequential trials for clinical investigations. *Journal of the American Statistical Association*, 103(484):1621–1630,, 2008.

[65] Q. Liu, M.A. Proschan, and G.W. Pledger. A unified theory of two-stage adaptive designs. *Journal of the American Statistical Association*, 97(460):1034–1041, 2002.

[66] W. Liu. Multiple tests of a non-hierarchical finite family of hypotheses. *Journal of the Royal Statistical Society: Series B*, 58(2):455–461, 1996.

[67] R. Marcus. The powers of some tests of the equality of normal means against an ordered alternative. *Biometrika*, 63(1):177–183, 1976.

[68] R. Marcus, P. Eric, and K. R. Gabriel. On closed testing procedures with special reference to ordered analysis of variance. *Biometrika*, 63(3):655–660, 1976.

[69] L. Mariani and E. Marubini. Design and analysis of phase II cancer trials: a review of statistical methods and guidelines for medical researchers. *International Statistical Review/Revue Internationale de Statistique*, 64(1):61–88, 1996.

[70] W. Maurer and F. Bretz. Memory and other properties of multiple test procedures generated by entangled graphs. *Statistics in Medicine*, 32(10):1739–1753, 2013.

[71] W. Maurer and F. Bretz. Multiple testing in group sequential trials using graphical approaches. *Statistics in Biopharmaceutical Research*, 5(4):311–320, 2013.

[72] W. Maurer, E. Glimm, and F. Bretz. Multiple and repeated testing of primary, coprimary, and secondary hypotheses. *Statistics in Biopharmaceutical Research*, 3(2), 2011.

[73] W. Maurer, L. A. Hothorn, and W. Lehmacher. Multiple comparisons in drug clinical trials and preclinical assays: a-priori ordered hypotheses. *Biometrie in der Chemisch-pharmazeutischen Industrie*, 6:3–18, 1995.

[74] B. A. Millen and A. Dmitrienko. Chain procedures: a class of flexible closed testing procedures with clinical trial applications. *Statistics in Biopharmaceutical Research*, 3(1):14–30, 2011.

[75] H. H. Müller and H. Schäfer. Adaptive group sequential designs for clinical trials: combining the advantages of adaptive and of classical group sequential approaches. *Biometrics*, 57(3):886–891, 2001.

[76] U. D. Naik. Some selection rules for comparing p processes with a standard. *Communications in Statistics-Theory and Methods*, 4(6):519–535, 1975.

[77] P. C. O'Brien and T. R. Fleming. A multiple testing procedure for clinical trials. *Biometrics*, 35(3):549–556, 1979.

[78] S. J. Pocock. Group sequential methods in the design and analysis of clinical trials. *Biometrika*, 64(2):191–199, 1977.

[79] M. A. Proschan and S. A. Hunsberger. Designed extension of studies based on conditional power. *Biometrics*, 51(4):1315–1324, 1995.

[80] J. P. Romano and M. Wolf. Stepwise multiple testing as formalized data snooping. *Econometrica*, 73(4):1237–1282, 2005.

[81] R. Rosenthal and D. B. Rubin. Multiple contrasts and ordered Bonferroni procedures. *Journal of Educational Psychology*, 76(6):1028, 1984.

[82] S. N. Roy. On a heuristic method of test construction and its use in multivariate analysis. *Annals of Mathematical Statistics*, 24(2):220–238, 1953.

[83] S. K. Sarkar. Some probability inequalities for ordered MTP2 random variables: a proof of the Simes conjecture. *Annals of Statistics*, 26(2):494–504, 1998.

[84] S. K. Sarkar and C. K. Chang. The Simes method for multiple hypothesis testing with positively dependent test statistics. *Journal of the American Statistical Association*, 92(440):1601–1608, 1997.

[85] J. R. Schultz, F. R. Nichol, G. L. Elfring, and S. D. Weed. Multistage procedures for drug screening. *Biometrics*, 29:293–300, 1973.

[86] S. Senn and F. Bretz. Power and sample size when multiple endpoints are considered. *Pharmaceutical Statistics*, 6(3):161–170, 2007.

[87] J. P. Shaffer. Modified sequentially rejective multiple test procedures. *Journal of the American Statistical Association*, 81(395):826–831, 1986.

[88] R. Simes. An improved Bonferroni procedure for multiple tests of significance. *Biometrika*, 73(3):751–754, 1986.

[89] R. Simon. Optimal two-stage designs for phase II clinical trials. *Controlled Clinical Trials*, 10(1):1–10, 1989.

[90] E. Sonnemann and H. Finner. Vollständigkeitssätze für multiple testprobleme. In *Multiple Hypothesenprüfung/Multiple Hypotheses Testing*, pages 121–135. Springer, 1988.

[91] N. Stallard, S. Todd, and J. Whitehead. Estimation following selection of the largest of two normal means. *Journal of Statistical Planning and Inference*, 138(6):1629–1638, 2008.

[92] K. Strassburger and F. Bretz. Compatible simultaneous lower confidence bounds for the Holm procedure and other Bonferroni-based closed tests. *Statistics in Medicine*, 27(24):4914–4927, 2008.

[93] T. Sugitani, F. Bretz, and W. Maurer. A simple and flexible graphical approach for adaptive group-sequential clinical trials. *Journal of Biopharmaceutical Statistics*, pages 1–15, 2015.

[94] A. C. Tamhane and L. Liu. On weighted hochberg procedures. *Biometrika*, 95(2):279–294, 2008.

[95] A.C. Tamhane, C.R. Mehta, and L. Liu. Testing a primary and a secondary endpoint in a group sequential design. *Biometrics*, 66(4):1174–1184, 2010.

[96] S. H. Tan, D. Machin, and S. B. Tan. Bayesian Designs for Phase II Oncology Clinical Trials. In S.-C. Chow, editor, *Encyclopedia of Biopharmaceutical Statistics.* Taylor & Francis, Boca Raton, FL, third edition, 2012.

[97] P. F. Thall and R. Simon. Practical Bayesian guidelines for phase IIB clinical trials. *Biometrics*, 50(2):337–349, 1994.

[98] A. A. Tsiatis. Repeated significance testing for a general class of statistics used in censored survival analysis. *Journal of the American Statistical Association*, 77(380):855–861, 1982.

[99] J. W. Tukey. The problem of multiple comparisons. In H. I. Braun, editor, *The Collected Works of John W. Tukey*, volume 8, 1994. Chapman and Hall, New York, 1953.

[100] R. Wang, S. W. Lagakos, J. H. Ware, D. J. Hunter, and J. M. Drazen. Statistics in medicine - reporting of subgroup analyses in clinical trials. *New England Journal of Medicine*, 357(21):2189–2194, 2007.

[101] S.-J. Wang, J.C. Hsu, W. Maurer, F. Bretz, H.M.J. Hung, J. Berger, M. Posch, T. Lang, and D. Wright. Errors in multiple testing: Biomarker-clinical endpoints, primary-secondary endpoints, subgroup-overall populations. panel discussion at the 8th international conference on multiple comparison procedures. *Submitted*, 2016.

[102] S.-J. Wang and H. M. J. Hung. Adaptive enrichment with subpopulation selection at interim: methodologies, applications and design considerations. *Contemporary Clinical Trials*, 36(2):673–681, 2013.

[103] P. H. Westfall. *Resampling-based Multiple Testing: Examples and Methods for p-value Adjustment.* John Wiley & Sons, New York, 1993.

[104] P. H. Westfall and A. Krishen. Optimally weighted, fixed sequence and gatekeeper multiple testing procedures. *Journal of Statistical Planning and Inference*, 99(1):25–40, 2001.

[105] P. H. Westfall and R. D. Tobias. Multiple testing of general contrasts. *Journal of the American Statistical Association*, 102(478):487–494, 2007.

[106] P. H. Westfall, S. S. Young, and S. P. Wright. On adjusting p-values for multiplicity. *Biometrics*, 49(3):941–945, 1993.

[107] B. L. Wiens. A fixed sequence Bonferroni procedure for testing multiple endpoints. *Pharmaceutical Statistics*, 2(3):211–215, 2003.

[108] B. L. Wiens and A. Dmitrienko. The fallback procedure for evaluating a single family of hypotheses. *Journal of Biopharmaceutical Statistics*, 15(6):929–942, 2005.

[109] D. A. Williams. A test for differences between treatment means when several dose levels are compared with a zero dose control. *Biometrics*, 27(1):103–117, 1971.

[110] S. P. Wright. Adjusted p-values for simultaneous inference. *Biometrics*, 48:1005–1013, 1992.

[111] D. Xi and A. C. Tamhane. A general multistage procedure for k-out-of-n gatekeeping. *Statistics in Medicine*, 33(8):1321–1335, 2014.

[112] D. Xi and A. C. Tamhane. Allocating recycled significance levels in group sequential procedures for multiple endpoints. *Biometrical Journal*, 57(1):90–107, 2015.

4

Analysis of Safety Data

Steven Snapinn

Qi Jiang

CONTENTS

4.1 Introduction

In order to be of clinical value, any treatment must provide sufficient benefits to justify its use, and it must have a good safety profile relative to its benefits. In other words, the treatment must have a positive "benefit-risk" profile; that is, any harms caused by the treatment (also referred to here as adverse drug reactions or toxicities) must be of less clinical importance than the benefits it provides. Therefore, the assessment of the safety of any new drug is of critical importance [3, 22].

The critical role of the assessment of safety is true of any new drug, and there are a number of excellent references on the topic such as a recent paper by Xia and Jiang [57] and book by Jiang and Xia [31]. However, there are some unique aspects of the assessment of the safety of cancer treatments. This is noted, for example, in regulatory guidance documents such as one from the European Medicines Agency [20]. One difference between the development of a treatment for cancer and the development of a treatment for most other diseases is that cancer is a grievous illness, and the prognosis associated with many cancers is so poor that patients would accept a greater degree of toxicity in order to obtain an important benefit than they would for less grievous conditions. In fact, many cancer treatments, particularly older treatments, cause such severe adverse reactions that the challenge is often to identify a dose low enough to keep the adverse reactions at a manageable level but high enough to provide an important benefit.

This leads to a second important difference between the development of a treatment for cancer and the development of a treatment for most other diseases. Drug development proceeds in defined phases, and phase I clinical trials, where the treatment is given to human beings for the first time, are focused to a large extent on evaluating safety and tolerability. However, while phase I studies for most treatments are performed on normal volunteers, it is not ethical to subject normal volunteers to the kinds of adverse reactions caused by many treatments for cancer. Therefore, phase I clinical trials for cancer treatments are typically performed on patients with the disease for which the treatment is intended.

The remainder of this chapter is organized as follows. Section 4.2 discusses the assessment of safety and tolerability in phase I trials (see Chapter 6 for more detail on this topic), while the remainder of the chapter focuses on issues that arise later in the development of a cancer treatment. Section 4.3 discusses prospective plans for safety assessment in clinical development, including the Statistical Analysis Plan (SAP), which is written for individual clinical trials, and the Program Safety Analysis Plan (PSAP), which describes the plans for the program as a whole. Section 4.4 discusses safety signal detection, or the identification of new adverse drug reactions (i.e., harms caused by the treatment) from among the multitude of adverse effects that occur spontaneously during the course of clinical development. Section 4.5 provides some guidance for summarizing and graphically displaying safety data as an aid in the interpretation of safety information. Section 4.6 discusses meta-analysis, or the integration of safety information from multiple clinical trials. Section 4.7 presents some formal approaches for assessing whether the benefits of the treatment outweigh the harms it causes. Finally, Section 4.8 provides a summary.

4.2 Phase I Clinical Trials

All drugs have the potential to cause adverse reactions. In many cases, these adverse drug reactions are directly related to the mechanism of action of the drug. For example, the neutropenia commonly caused by cytotoxic drugs would be expected based on these drugs' mechanism of action [17]. In other cases, adverse drug reactions are unrelated to the mechanism of action. For example, the cardiotoxicity seen with some cancer treatments is a more surprising finding [23]. In addition, some side effects are so common that they would be expected to occur in many or most patients taking the drug, while others are so rare that they can only be detected after hundreds or thousands of patients are treated.

Phase I clinical trials are the first studies of a new treatment in human beings. As such, they proceed cautiously, starting with very low doses that have been shown to be safe in preclinical studies, with dose escalation as appropriate. These studies tend to be very small, and therefore are only able to detect the most frequent adverse drug reactions. In particular, phase I clinical trials for cancer treatments are designed to detect the kind of common toxicities that would be expected to occur with these treatments.

Drugs to treat cancer can be considered to belong to one of two broad categories: cytotoxic and cytostatic drugs. According to the European Medicines Agency [20], cytotoxic drugs are "anticancer compounds inducing irreversible lethal lesions through interference with DNA replication, mitosis, etc." Some examples of cytotoxic cancer treatments in common use are capecitabine, gemcitabine, pemetrexed, doxorubicin, epirubicin, docetaxel, irinotecan, paclitaxel, cisplatin, and oxaliplatin. Due to their lethal effects on cells, including both tumor cells and normal cells, cytotoxic drugs tend to have severe and dose-related toxicities. These include bone marrow suppression (anemia, neutropenia); effects on the cells lining the mouth (oral mucositis); damage to the stomach, intestine, and esophagus lining (nausea, vomiting, diarrhea); hair loss; and nervous system effects (fatigue, confusion). In many cases, these toxicities are so severe that they necessitate either a dose reduction or discontinuation of treatment; when this occurs in a patient, it is known as a dose-limiting toxicity (DLT).

Cytostatic drugs include biologic agents such as bevacizumab, panitumumab, gefitinib, and rituximab; and hormone or other treatments such as lenalidomide, letrozole, tamoxifen, and thalidomide. While these drugs typically cause fewer adverse reactions than cytotoxic drugs, they can also have important side effects.

Under the assumption that the higher the dose the greater the degree of efficacy, the initial evaluation of safety in phase I clinical trials of cytotoxic treatments involves finding the highest dose associated with an acceptable level of toxicity [1]. (Note that other potential objectives are possible, although less common [30]). In particular, phase I clinical trials of treatments for cancer have traditionally been designed to identify the highest dose such that the proportion of patients experiencing a DLT is at a reasonable level; this is known as the maximally tolerated dose (MTD).

As discussed above, while phase I clinical trials in most therapeutic areas are conducted on normal volunteers, phase I clinical trials for cancer treatments are conducted in cancer patients. This is both to avoid subjecting normal volunteers to the kinds of toxicities that are expected with these drugs and to provide these patients with a treatment that could possibly be beneficial. Therefore, there is a tension in phase I trials of cancer treatments between the caution that one needs to exercise when treating patients with an experimental treatment for the first time (i.e., begin with a subtherapeutic dose and escalate the dose slowly) and the desire to benefit patients with a grievous illness [46].

4.2.1 Phase I Designs

The simplest design for identifying the MTD, still in common use, is known as the 3+3 design. Using this design, a particular dose level is evaluated by treating an initial cohort of 3 patients, and, if necessary, a second cohort of 3 patients. If none of the initial cohort experiences a DLT, then the dose is considered to be safe. Similarly, if either two or three of the initial cohort experience a DLT, then the dose is considered unsafe. Only if exactly one of the initial cohort experiences a DLT is the second cohort considered necessary, and only if none of the second cohort experiences a DLT (i.e., exactly one of the total of six patients) is the dose considered to be safe.

One problem with the 3+3 design is that it can lead to a large number of patients being treated at subtherapeutic doses [33]. The continual reassessment method (CRM), a Bayesian dose escalation approach, was proposed by O'Quigley et al. [42] to address this problem. Unlike the 3+3 design, the CRM attempts to estimate the MTD from a continuous space of doses, it assumes a parametric model for the dose-response relationship, and it makes efficient use of all accumulating data in the study as well as prior information [24]. Yuan et al. [58] introduced an extension to the CRM that can account for the severity of toxicities.

Babb et al. [4] described a fully adaptive method that makes use of all the information available at the time of each dose assignment and attempts to control the probability of overdosing (i.e., treatment with a dose greater than the MTD). It is designed to approach the MTD as fast as possible subject to the constraint that the predicted proportion of patients who receive an overdose does not exceed a specified value. The authors found that this method leads to fewer overdoses than the CRM, while estimating the MTD with comparable accuracy.

The methods described above are all designed for the situation in which toxicities are expected to occur soon after the onset of treatment. Some authors have proposed designs for situations where toxicities may be delayed and, therefore, a time-to-event approach might be preferable. Cheung and Chappell [11] introduced a method for this situation, called the time-to-event continual reassessment method (TITE-CRM), and Bekele et al. [5] introduced a Bayesian dose-finding method similar to the TITE-CRM in which doses are chosen using time-to-toxicity data. However, the interpretability of the results from these methods can be limited unless the study is designed to collect complete information on delayed toxicities. If a substantial proportion of subjects exit the study at the time they discontinue treatment, and have no follow-up for adverse events, then there can be an issue of informative censoring, and the estimate of the treatment effect can be substantially biased.

Patients with cancer are often treated with multiple agents, and identification of an MTD in phase I trials is greatly complicated in this case. Conaway et al. [14] argued that when there are multiple agents, the dose-toxicity curve may not be monotonic, and they proposed a design for phase I trials in which the toxicity probabilities follow a partial order (i.e., there are pairs of treatments for which the ordering of the toxicity probabilities is not known at the start of the trial). Thall et al. [52] proposed an adaptive two-stage Bayesian design for finding one or more acceptable dose combinations of two cytotoxic agents used together.

Most phase I designs for cancer treatments were developed for cytotoxic treatments, where, due to their mechanism of action, toxicities are expected to be frequent. Some authors have suggested that designs for newer drugs, such as biologics targeted at specific gene mutations, should not follow the old paradigm. Korn [35] argued that, for a targeted, non-cytotoxic agent, toxicity and efficacy do not necessarily increase monotonically, and may plateau after reaching maximal toxicity or efficacy. He proposed that one might want to consider using a dose escalation design that is not based on occurrences of toxicity, but rather based on some other endpoint. Hoering et al. [27] also noted that toxicity and efficacy may not increase monotonically in this situation, and they proposed a phase I–II trial design for it. Messer et al. [39] argued that many newer agents hope to show efficacy without increasing the background rate of adverse events, and they proposed a new design, termed the phase I/II toxicity-evaluation design, for situations in which the therapeutic dose is expected to be well below the MTD.

4.3 Planning Safety Analyses

A key principle of any valid statistical analysis is that of prespecification. This is true both for efficacy analyses, where prespecification helps limit the probability of type I errors, and for safety analyses, where prespecification can aid in identifying true adverse drug reactions. In this section, we discuss some of the tools that can be used to prespecify safety analyses. Some of the information presented here is based on recommendations from the Safety Planning, Evaluation and Reporting Team (SPERT), a pharmaceutical industry group formed in 2006 by the Pharmaceutical Manufacturers of America [16]. In addition, detailed guidance on planning and prespecification of analyses of safety in the pre-market setting is provided by Xia and Jiang [57].

4.3.1 Events of Interest

One of the greatest difficulties in the evaluation of safety data is that patients can experience a multitude of adverse events, only some of which are true adverse drug reactions (i.e., caused by the treatment under investigation). Distinguishing between true adverse drug reactions and adverse events caused by other factors (e.g., by the underlying disease or by concomitant medications) is known as safety signal detection, and is discussed in detail in Section 4.4. In cancer clinical trials, patients tend to experience many adverse events, and a table of adverse events can be extremely long, with dozens or hundreds of distinct event types. In such cases, simply performing statistical tests on all adverse events can lead to many false positive results, while restricting hypothesis testing to a subset of events where there is some *a priori* reason to expect a relationship to the treatment under investigation can greatly reduce the frequency of false positives. This prespecified set of adverse events is known as adverse events of special interest (AESI) or simply as events of interest (EoI).

The set of AESI for an investigational treatment can change over the course of its development. The initial set of AESI will include events that are to be expected given the mechanism of action of the drug. This set can increase over time as clinical studies suggest that other events are possible adverse drug reactions. According to SPERT, some adverse events should always be considered AESI; these include QT prolongation, liver toxicity, immunogenicity, and bone marrow toxicity. (Note that the SPERT recommendations were not specific to oncology treatments.) AESI should always be clearly defined. Many adverse events can be coded in different ways in a given medical dictionary (see Section 4.4.1), and algorithms may need to be defined in order to determine which specific terms make up an AESI. In addition, data collection forms for clinical studies may need to be customized to capture more detailed information for the AESI than for standard adverse events.

4.3.2 The Statistical Analysis Plan (SAP)

All clinical trials have a protocol describing the rationale for the study, detailed procedures to be followed, and statistical design and analysis information. Many clinical trials also have a separate document, called a Statistical Analysis Plan, or SAP, that describes the statistical aspects of the study in much greater detail than the protocol. In particular, the SAP will provide the details of the safety analyses to be performed.

The safety analyses will always include an evaluation of adverse events, with special emphasis on AESI. In addition, it will include an evaluation of laboratory data, such as calculation of mean changes and calculation of percentages of patients whose laboratory values cross prespecified thresholds (e.g., a fold-increase in a liver enzyme that could indicate harm to liver, or a hemoglobin measurement low enough to indicate anemia). The SAP will provide details of these analyses and include a listing of the tables that will be produced, the prespecified thresholds for the laboratory analyses, a description of procedures for handling missing data and outliers, and definitions of the metrics that will be used to compare treatment groups.

4.3.3 The Program Safety Analysis Plan (PSAP)

One key recommendation by SPERT was the creation of a program safety analysis plan, or PSAP, which they described as a living document (amended as needed in response to the emerging safety profile) that will eventually form the basis for planning the summary safety information submitted to regulatory agencies to support a marketing application [15]. Used primarily by pharmaceutical industry sponsors, this document will contain information for the evaluation of safety for the program as a whole, but will not repeat the details of the planned analysis for specific studies contained in the individual SAPs.

The PSAP should have two main sections, one describing data collection and another describing the statistical analysis. The analytical section will describe a 3-tiered approach to the analysis of adverse events. The first tier focuses on the AESI, and includes hypothesis testing. The second tier is for adverse events that are not AESI, but are frequent enough for a meaningful analysis. Finally, the third tier is for events that are so infrequent that a simple tabulation is all that can be done. The PSAP will also describe how safety data from multiple studies should be combined, and the statistical and graphical methods that will be used. Similar to a SAP, the PSAP should address issues such as missing data, multiplicity, and analysis populations. It should also address the statistical power for the AESI in the analyses of the combined studies. SPERT also recommended that the PSAP be discussed with regulatory agencies at one of the regular meetings during the drug's development.

The PSAP should also describe the regular review of aggregate safety data across the program, as required by the US Food & Drug administration [55]. Some guiding issues to consider are which studies to be combined and presented (including how information from ongoing blinded studies will be handled), which data to include in the review, and which groups to compare (since different studies may use different dosages or have different control groups). They also provided the following main categories of analyses: a description of studies; a summary of subject exposure to treatment; demographic data; reasons for study and drug discontinuation; adverse events, including deaths, serious adverse events, AESI, and adverse events leading to study discontinuation. Finally, they provided some suggested analyses, such as a figure that simultaneously displays both incidence and risk estimates for adverse events; tables displaying subject-year-adjusted adverse event rates; bar graphs of the number of patients who experienced an adverse event in each system organ class; and a listing of unique combinations of system organ class, preferred term, and verbatim term.

4.3.4 Data Monitoring Committee (DMC)

While sponsors are responsible for the safety of their products, both marketed and in development, sponsors should remain blinded to the results of ongoing blinded clinical trials. For this reason, many clinical trials have a separate independent group, known as a Data Monitoring Committee (DMC), to monitor these trials. A DMC can have multiple responsibilities and objectives, but one objective common to all DMCs is to protect the safety of the participants in the clinical trial. DMC operations are described in detail in textbooks by Ellenberg, Fleming and DeMets [19] and Herson [26], and will be summarized briefly here.

Membership in a DMC consists of a number of clinical experts in the disease being studied as well as one or more biostatisticians; there may be additional members, such as an ethicist or a patient advocate. Members are typically chosen by the sponsor but are independent of the sponsor and have no substantial conflict of interest. The DMC's operations are governed by a charter that is reviewed and approved by the committee as well as by the sponsor. DMCs review the interim results of a clinical trial, or a set of trials, and assess whether or not patients in the trial are at undue risk. For example, if the DMC saw a substantial imbalance in an important adverse event (say, stroke) such that more patients taking the experimental treatment experienced a stroke than control patients, and there was no substantial benefit of the treatment that would balance the potential harm, the DMC might recommend to the sponsor that the trial terminate prematurely. The sponsor is ultimately responsible for deciding whether or not to accept the recommendation, and for implementing it.

In addition to recommending study termination, DMC recommendations could include pausing enrollment, discontinuing enrollment of a certain subset of subjects, reducing the dose, or modifying the protocol in some other way. While DMC charters sometime include specific statistical guidelines for making a recommendation, these guidelines typically apply to efficacy data only, and no such guidelines are provided for safety data. Therefore, the DMC must use their judgment to decide whether a safety finding represents a true adverse drug reaction or is likely due to play of chance, and whether a presumed adverse drug reaction is important enough to result in a somewhat drastic recommendation to modify or terminate an ongoing clinical trial.

In addition to recommending terminating the study due to a safety concern, some charters allow the DMC to recommend termination for overwhelming evidence of efficacy, while others allow the DMC to recommend termination for futility [48]. Futility is loosely defined as the inability of the trial to achieve its objectives, and includes both operational futility (e.g., slow enrollment) as well as a low probability of demonstrating a benefit. The latter deserves special attention in the context of late-stage cancer clinical trials, since it can be an important tool for protecting patient safety. Consider a phase III cancer clinical trial with an overall survival endpoint. While the hope is that the treatment under study will provide a benefit, there are many examples of cancer treatments that actually decrease survival, often due to a serious toxicity. In such a case, one would hope for the DMC to recommend termination as quickly as possible, and a futility rule allows this to happen. That is because the evidence to conclude that the treatment is unlikely to provide a benefit on the survival endpoint will typically appear well before the evidence to conclude that the treatment causes harm on the same endpoint.

4.4 Safety Signal Detection

As discussed in Section 4.3.1, it can be quite challenging to identify true adverse drug reactions from among the multitude of adverse events that may be reported during the course of a clinical trial. In this section we discuss the process of safety signal detection, focusing on issues such as the classification of events, multiplicity control, special considerations for single-arm and combination studies, and safety non-inferiority trials.

4.4.1 Classifying Adverse Events

The first challenge in safety signal detection is the accurate classification of adverse events. Whether an adverse event is identified by an investigator during a clinic visit, or reported directly by the patient, the same event can be described differently by different people. In order to do a statistical analysis of adverse event data, therefore, the events must first be coded according to some type of medical dictionary. This leads to a trade-off that must be carefully considered before beginning the analysis: The grouping of terms can be narrow, which can lead to an adverse drug reaction appearing separately with separate terms, and therefore can lead to low event counts and low statistical power; or the grouping of terms can be broad, which can lead to an adverse drug reaction being grouped with other events that are unaffected

TABLE 4.1: Common terminology criteria for adverse events (CTCAE) grades

Grade 1	Mild; asymptomatic or mild symptoms; clinical or diagnostic observations only; intervention not indicated.
Grade 2	Moderate; minimal, local, or noninvasive intervention indicated; limiting age-appropriate instrumental activities of daily living (ADL).
Grade 3	Severe or medically significant but not immediately life-threatening; hospitalization or prolongation of hospitalization indicated; disabling; limiting self-care ADL.
Grade 4	Life-threatening consequences; urgent intervention indicated.
Grade 5	Death related to AE.

by the treatment, leading to the addition of statistical noise and, again, low statistical power.

For example, if a treatment causes a broad set of cerebrovascular complications (say, ischemic stroke, hemorrhagic stroke, and transient ischemic attacks), an analysis that looks at each of the terms separately might miss detecting the adverse drug reaction due to small numbers within each category. On the other hand, if the cerebrovascular complications were grouped with other cardiovascular complications, such as myocardial infarction, the signal could be diluted. For this reason, it could be reasonable to do two or more separate analyses of adverse events, using different degrees of aggregation.

There are a number of different clinical dictionaries in common use for classifying adverse event terms. One that has been designed specifically for cancer treatments is the Common Terminology Criteria for Adverse Events. Developed by the National Institutes of Health, this dictionary undergoes regular revision, and version 4.0 was released in 2009 with 764 unique terms (http://evs.nci.nih.gov/ftp1/CTCAE/CTCAE_4.03_2010-06-14_QuickReference_5x7.pdf). For each term, the event is graded on a severity scale as shown in Table 4.1.

Another medical dictionary commonly used across many therapeutic areas is the Medical Dictionary for Regulatory Activities, or MedDRA (http://www.meddra.org). One key difference between MedDRA and CTCAE is the hierarchy of terms built into MedDRA. Version 12 of MedDRA contains 67,159 Lowest Level Terms; these are grouped into 18,483 Preferred Terms, which in turn are grouped into 1699 High Level Terms, then into 333 High Level Group Terms, and finally into 26 System Organ Classes. Since each term in version 4.0 of CTCAE corresponds to a Lowest Level Term in MedDRA, it is clear that the granularity of coding is far greater in MedDRA than in CTCAE.

Kübler et al. [36] discussed some of the limitations of MedDRA, including the fact that it was intended for assessment of individual cases, not analyses of clinical trials.

4.4.2 Statistical Methods for Late Phase Trials

The analysis of prespecified adverse events of special interest (AESI) is generally straightforward, but identifying other potential adverse drug reactions can be much more challenging. One problem is that the usual multiplicity paradigm is poorly suited to this task. For example, if there are 100 different adverse event terms reported by a sufficient number of patients during a clinical trial, and the goal were to control the overall significance level at 5%, a multiplicity correction approach such as Bonferroni would result in each term requiring a p-value of 0.0005, which could result in extremely low power and, therefore, a considerable type II error rate. On the other hand, avoiding a multiplicity correction altogether could lead to approximately 5 false positive results.

One approach that attempts to find a middle ground is an application of the false discovery rate [38], in which potential adverse drug reactions are flagged, and the expected proportion of flagged terms that represent false adverse drug reactions is controlled at a prespecified level. Note the subtle distinction between control of the false discovery rate and the type I error rate.

Berry and Berry [7] proposed a hierarchical mixture model to address this problem. This approach has three levels: the type of adverse event, the body system, and the collection of all body systems. This is a Bayesian approach that allows for borrowing of information across and within body systems. They argue that the probability that a drug caused a type of adverse event is greater if its rate is elevated for several types of adverse events within the same body system than if the adverse events with elevated rates are in different body systems.

Price et al. [44] discussed clinical trials focusing on safety endpoints, and the challenges associated with existing methods for their design and analysis. They proposed Bayesian methods for a variety of approaches, including sample size determination, frequent interim analyses, borrowing historical information, continuous monitoring of events, and hierarchical modeling.

Southworth and O'Connell [51] discussed a variety of approaches for the analysis of adverse event data from clinical trials. Their paper included an inside-out data mining method where the adverse events are used as exploratory variables to classify the treatments; a method that involves fitting separate regression models to each adverse event, with and without treatment; and a three-level hierarchical Bayesian mixture model.

Brewster et al. [9] described the safety signal process, known also as pharmacovigilance, followed by one large pharmaceutical company. They advocated a holistic approach to the review of safety data on an ongoing basis. In particular, with respect to statistical analysis, they recommended techniques such as time to event analysis, quantification of use, use of confidence intervals, and examination of adverse events in the context of the background incidence.

Chen et al. [10] compared the sensitivity and specificity of various methods for safety signal detection, and provided a set of recommendations.

4.4.3 Post-marketing Signal Detection

While a pre-marketing clinical program will identify many or most adverse drug reactions, it is inevitable that some adverse drug reactions will remain unidentified when the drug goes to the market. Ladewski et al. [37] examined this issue; in particular, they were interested in how frequently new adverse drug reactions were identified in the post-marketing setting for oncology drugs. They concluded that serious adverse drug reactions may be discovered as long as 36 years after a drug receives FDA approval, which suggests a need for continued vigilance and efficient strategies for dissemination of information.

However, the challenges in identifying these adverse drug reactions in the post-marketing setting are perhaps greater than in the pre-marketing setting. This is primarily related to the fact that adverse events occurring post-marketing do not occur in a carefully controlled experimental setting, which is designed for complete and accurate capture of all adverse events. Adverse event reports in the post-marketing setting are known as spontaneous reports, and it is well known that a large fraction of adverse events are never reported. Therefore, incidence rates based on spontaneous reports (i.e., the number of reports divided by the number of subjects who have been prescribed the treatment) are believed to be underestimates of the true incidence rates. Without a control group, the magnitude of the bias can be difficult to assess.

Identification of new adverse drug reactions in the post-marketing setting can be aided by a relatively new approach, known as disproportionality analysis [21]. Using this approach, it is not the incidence rate itself that is of interest, but rather the incidence for a particular adverse event relative to the incidence for all adverse events, or relative to the incidence of other specific adverse events. For example, if stroke and myocardial infarction occur at similar frequency with most treatments, but stroke is twice as frequent as myocardial infarction for the treatment under evaluation, this would suggest that stroke is an adverse drug reaction for that treatment.

Brewster et al. [9] discussed advances in post-marketing pharmacovigilance strategies and placed great emphasis on disproportionality analysis. They use a metric known as the relative reporting ratio, and calculate it for all possible drug-adverse event pairs in their database, relative to the background of all other drugs and adverse events in the database.

Huang et al. [28] examined statistical methods for post-market safety databases, such as the US Food and Drug Administration's adverse event reporting system (AERS). They proposed a likelihood ratio test for identifying drug-event combinations with disproportionately high frequencies; they found that this method has good power and can control both the type I error rate and the false discovery rate.

4.4.4 Single-arm Trials and Combination Studies

The ideal situation for identifying adverse drug reactions is a large clinical trial comparing a treatment used as monotherapy with a placebo. Unfortunately, not all situations are ideal, and in many cases a researcher will need to attempt to identify adverse drug reactions in single-arm trials, and in trials where the treatment is used in combination with other toxic treatments.

When capturing adverse event information, it is common to obtain the investigator's assessment of whether or not the event was drug-related. When there is a control group one could argue that this information is of little value, since the investigator may not be in a position to assess causality, and the comparison with the control group provides a more rigorous assessment. Causality determinations are particularly difficult for investigators in oncology studies because of the complex relationships between disease effects and drug effects. However, when there is no control group, the investigator's assessment may be better than nothing, and is often used as part of the statistical analysis.

Mukherjee et al. [41] conducted a study to understand the clinical reasoning used by the investigator when making the causality assessment. They conducted semi-structured interviews with medical oncologists and trial coordinators at six Canadian academic cancer centers. They concluded that attributing causality is a complex process, and that clinical trial researchers apply a logical system of reasoning, although they feel that the process could be improved.

In some cases there may be robust information on the background rate of an adverse event that can be used as a reference in the absence of a control group. However, such information is not always available, and Brewster et al. [9] recognized that it is difficult to evaluate adverse events from single-arm trials when there is little or no information on the expected background rate. They proposed using data from observational studies when possible, although they recognized the limitations. For example, data are often not recorded in a standardized and controlled manner, there is less patient-specific covariate information, and there is generally less information regarding the adverse events.

4.4.5 Safety Non-inferiority Trials

Non-inferiority trials have been the subject of multiple regulatory guidance documents and numerous publications (e.g., Snapinn [50]). Most non-inferiority trials focus on an efficacy endpoint, and attempt to demonstrate that one treatment has an effect that is either superior to that of another treatment, or similar to it. Non-inferiority trials can also focus on safety endpoints; the objective of such a trial is to determine whether or not the excess risk caused by the treatment exceeds some prespecified threshold. There are some similarities between efficacy and safety non-inferiority trials; most notably, both rely on the assumption of assay sensitivity, or the ability of the trial to detect differences between treatments. The concern is that a poorly designed or executed trial will fail to detect important differences. However, there are important distinctions between the two types of non-inferiority trials as well. The most important distinction is that efficacy non-inferiority trials inherently involve an indirect comparison between the experimental treatment and placebo, while safety non-inferiority trials are direct comparisons between the experimental treatment and the control, which is often a placebo. Snapinn and Jiang [49] provide additional details on safety non-inferiority trials.

4.5 Collecting, Summarizing, and Displaying Safety Data

The analysis of safety data has traditionally received much less attention from statisticians than the analysis of efficacy data. This is probably more a reflection of the inherent difficulties in the collection and analysis of safety data, such as the multitude of potential adverse events that are frequently reported as free text, than it is on the importance of the evaluation of safety. However, this is changing, as evidenced by the fact that the US Food and Drug Administration, as well as several pharmaceutical companies, have formed departments of safety biostatistics. In addition, there has been an increase in publications on this topic, such as the recent book by Jiang and Xia [31].

4.5.1 Data Collection

Safety data consist primarily of adverse event data, captured on a case report form at the investigator's site, and laboratory data, collected from the laboratories that analyze the samples. These two types of data often comprise a large fraction of the total study database. As with any clinical data, there is a natural tension between the desire to collect as much as possible, and the desire to minimize the cost and complexity of the study. Therefore, the goal is to find the balance that minimizes the data collection while including all necessary data to allow a clear presentation of the safety profile of the drug.

The US Food and Drug Administration has at least two guidance documents relevant to the collection of safety data in oncology trials: one is specific to safety data, but not oncology [54], and the other is specific to oncology, but not safety [53]. The former discusses the concept of targeted safety data collection, which could be accomplished by a separate case report form specific to prespecified adverse events of special interest (AESI), and safety data that could have abbreviated or no collection. The latter provides detailed information on the recommended data collection for toxicities, and provides a hypothetical example of data collection during the development of a cancer drug.

Kaiser et al. [32] addressed the optimal collection of adverse event information in oncology clinical trials, with an emphasis on studies conducted post-approval, when the adverse event profile of the drug is fairly well known. Their method involved reanalyzing data from eight completed prospective clinical trials and determining the new information obtained from these studies that was not already known about the drug. They reviewed 107,884 adverse events, and found four grade 1–2 events and nine grade 3–5 events they identified as true adverse drug reactions that were not included in the previously establish safety profiles of the drug. Their conclusion was that a much less rigorous approach to adverse event data capture could be used in this setting.

In a review of the paper by Kaiser et al. [32], Sargent and George [47] commented that the proposed more relaxed approach could potentially be used in some phase III clinical trials as well. They also commented on the attribution by the investigator of whether or not the adverse event was caused by the treatment. Given the lack of reliability of such information (they cited a study which demonstrated that 50% of adverse events on placebo arms were considered to be at least possibly related to the treatment), they felt that removing this information from the case report forms could simplify data collection with little consequence to the evaluation of the safety of the drug.

In multicenter trials, patient samples (blood, urine, etc.) can be assayed at local laboratories or at central laboratories. While using local laboratories may be simpler, central laboratories are often preferred, both because there can be wide variability in the assays used at different laboratories, and because the data formats prepared by different laboratories can differ; both of these issues can make it difficult to pool the information across all sites.

4.5.2 Reporting Safety Information

The simplest presentation of adverse event information involves estimation of a binomial proportion. For example, for a specific adverse event, if the event was experienced by e patients among n treated, the estimated proportion is $p = e/n$. Similarly, if there are two treatment arms, we can use subscripts to distinguish them (e.g., the subscript 0 for the control group and 1 for the treatment group). However, even in this simplest of situations, there is some disagreement with respect to the most valid metric for estimating the treatment effect. Three different metrics that could be used are the risk difference $(p_1 - p_0)$, the risk ratio (p_1/p_0), and the odds ratio $(\frac{p_1}{1-p_1}/\frac{p_0}{1-p_0})$.

These three metrics can lead to different rankings. For example, consider the three hypothetical situations in Table 4.2. The table gives three hypothetical adverse event results in the three columns, the three different metrics that could be used to estimate the treatment effect, and the rank of that metric from largest (1) to smallest (3) in that row. It is apparent that there is con-

TABLE 4.2: Hypothetical adverse event results and the corresponding metrics

Metric	Adverse Event Proportions		
	$p_0 = 0.10$ $p_1 = 0.20$	$p_0 = 0.65$ $p_1 = 0.40$	$p_0 = 0.85$ $p_1 = 0.65$
Risk Difference	0.10(3)	0.25(1)	0.20(2)
Risk Ratio	2.00(1)	1.63(2)	1.31(3)
Odds Ratio	2.25(3)	2.79(2)	3.05(1)

siderable disagreement among the three metrics with respect to the ranking. Therefore, when using a metric as a screening tool to identify "important" differences between treatment groups, care should be exercised in choosing the most appropriate metric.

The situation is more complicated when a simple proportion is not an adequate summary of the adverse event's occurrence. We consider here three different complications. In addition, these issues are discussed in more detail by Zhou et al. [59].

First, in a clinical trial with long-term follow-up, it may be important to account not only for whether or not the event occurred, but also when it occurred. One potential approach that can be used here is to sum the "at risk" time for each treatment group (s, or the sum of each patient's follow-up from enrollment through either occurrence of the event or discontinuation from follow-up), and calculate the event rate: $r = e/s$. Then the risk difference $(r_1 - r_0)$ and risk ratio (r_1/r_0) can be calculated. While these metrics can be useful, one limitation is their inherent assumption that the risk of the event is constant over time (i.e., a constant hazard rate). In the absence of constant hazards, these metrics may not be valid. In such situations, a full time-to-event analysis, including calculation of Kaplan-Meier curves and hazard ratios, may be appropriate. However, as mentioned above, such an analysis may not be interpretable if subjects discontinue from follow-up for reasons that are related to their likelihood of experiencing an adverse event.

A second complication is that some events may occur more than once during the course of follow-up. While an analysis of the first event alone is always valid, an analysis that takes into account the recurrent nature of the events may be more efficient.

Finally, not all events are of equal importance, and there can be a great difference between a CTCAE grade 1 (mild) event and a CTCAE grade 5 (fatal) event. Therefore, events are often captured and presented on such an ordinal scale. (When a patient experiences more than one event, it is customary to capture the most severe occurrence.) While the presentation of the proportion of patients in each category is common (where the sum of the proportions $= p$), the comparison of treatment groups based on such a presentation may not be appropriate. For example, consider the hypothetical results in Table 4.3. In this case, the total proportion who experience the event is somewhat higher

TABLE 4.3: Hypothetical toxicity grade distributions

Toxicity Grade	**Randomized Group**	
	Control	Treatment
1	0.15	0.10
2	0.10	0.15
3	0.10	0.05
4	0.00	0.05
5	0.00	0.05

in the treatment group (0.40) than in the control group (0.35). An evaluation by grade, however, might lead to the conclusion that the treatment reduces the incidence of grade 3 events, since the proportion in that group (0.05) is lower than in the control group (0.10). However, that would be a questionable conclusion, given that the sum of grade 3–5 events is higher in the treatment group (0.15) than in the control group (0.10).

As a general principle, it is inappropriate to compare treatment groups on the basis of the proportions in a middle category on an ordinal scale. As an illustration of that fact, consider that the comparison of proportions between two treatment groups is essentially equivalent to a comparison of the complement of those proportions; e.g., an analysis of the proportions of survivors is equivalent to an analysis of the proportions of deaths, etc. When considered in this way, an analysis of a middle category is equivalent to an analysis of the sum of the categories of greater and lesser severity than that category. For example, an analysis of the proportion of "good" on a scale of "excellent," "good," and "poor" is equivalent to an analysis of the combination of "excellent" and "poor," which seems illogical. For this reason, we recommend comparing treatment groups on the basis of cumulative categories, such as grade 1–5, grade 2–5, grade 3–5, etc.

The analysis of laboratory data generally takes one of two forms. First, there is an analysis of central tendency, such as the mean or median difference between groups with respect to the value obtained following treatment, or with respect to the change from baseline. Recognizing that small changes in some laboratory values, even changes that are consistent across patients, may not be clinically meaningful, another approach that is often used involves something called shift tables. With this approach, the possible distribution of the values of a laboratory parameter is divided into a set of r ranges (typically 3–5), and these ranges are arranged in a $r \times r$ grid comparing baseline and post-baseline results. The table is then populated with the proportions of patients who "shifted" from one category (represented by the rows) to another category (represented by the columns).

Representing the Consolidated Standards of Reporting Trials (CONSORT) group, Ioannidis et al. [29] provided a set of recommendations for reporting harms in publications. Among their ten recommendations are to clarify how safety information was collected, to describe the plans for presenting and analyzing safety information, to provide denominators for each analysis, and to present the absolute risk for each adverse event.

4.5.3 Graphical Approaches

Due to its complexity, a purely tabular display of safety information may not adequately convey the most important insights. While graphical presentation of both efficacy and safety information has long been used, the graphical display of safety data has received increasing attention [18]. Chuang-Stein et al. [13] and Amit et al. [2] provide some specific graphs. The 10 graphs by Amit et al. [2] include simple plots comparing distributions in the form of boxplots or cumulative plots; summaries comparing information over time (cumulative incidence, hazard, means with error bars); and multi-panel displays that include scatterplots, a trellis of individual profiles, and paired dotplots.

Brewster et al. [9] described the graphical displays that have been recommended for consideration during the routine analysis of safety data. They include graphs intended for regulatory submissions and for presentations and publications, and encompass all categories of safety data.

4.6 Meta-analysis of Safety Data

Many safety issues can be identified in individual clinical trials, even relatively small trials; in fact, as discussed above, phase I trials in oncology often attempt to identify safe doses with no more than six patients per dose. However, in some cases the safety issues, while important, are more subtle, and cannot be identified even in large individual clinical trials. In such cases, the use of meta-analysis, a technique for combining the results of multiple clinical trials, can be used to increase sensitivity. For example, Vansteenkiste et al. [56] attempted to determine whether or not the use of erythropoiesis-stimulating agents (ESAs) has an impact on various outcomes, including overall survival, in patients with lung cancer, and to do so they conducted a meta-analysis of nine clinical trials. The technique of meta-analysis has been well studied, and so we focus in this section on some current issues.

When conducting a meta-analysis, one must choose the metric to estimate the treatment effect in each study. For long-term outcomes studies, a natural metric would be the hazard ratio; however, meta-analyses are often conducted using published results, and hazard ratios are not always reported. Since publications will typically report the event proportions, which allow calculation of the odds ratio, meta-analyses will often use the odds ratio as the metric. And, in fact, when the event rates are relatively low, the odds ratio and hazard ratio are typically very close. However, when event rates are not low, the two metrics can be quite different, and the use of the odds ratio can be problematic.

Note that the meta-analysis by Vansteenkiste et al. [56] included one study, reported by Pirker et al. [43], in which there were 242 deaths among 299 patients (81%) in the darbepoetin alfa group and 251 deaths among 298 patients (84%) in the placebo group. The paper reported the hazard ratio and its 95% confidence interval as 0.93 (0.78, 1.11). The odds ratio can be calculated to be 0.795, and, using a common approximation to the variance of the log of the odds ratio (i.e., the sum of the four inverses of the numbers of deaths and the numbers of survivors in the two treatment groups), the 95% confidence interval for the odds ratio is (0.520, 1.216). Comparison of the hazard ratio and odds ratio for this study illustrates two facts that will occur in general when event rates are high: the odds ratio is farther from unity than the hazard ratio (i.e., the odds ratio exaggerates the magnitude of the effect as measured by the hazard ratio), and, perhaps more importantly, the confidence interval for the odds ratio is far wider than that for the hazard ratio. To avoid this problem, one might consider using the hazard ratio as the metric, using an approximation to the hazard ratio for those studies that don't report this metric directly. One simple approximation for the hazard ratio is $\ln(1 - p_1)/\ln(1 - p_0)$, and an approximation for the variance of the log of the hazard ratio is $(1/e_1) + (1/e_0)$. Note that using these approximations, the results of the study reported by Pirker et al. [43] would be a hazard ratio of 0.897, with a 95% confidence interval of (0.752, 1.071). While not perfect, this is certainly a far better approximation to the calculated hazard ratio than is the odds ratio.

One situation where individual clinical trials may not be sufficient to identify a safety issue is the opposite of the one just discussed; i.e., a rare but important adverse event, such that the event is expected to occur infrequently, if at all, in an individual trial. However, many meta-analysis techniques are based on large sample approximations, and so may not be valid in the case of a rare event. Bradburn et al. [8] evaluated the performance of various methods for pooling rare events, and found that most of the commonly used meta-analysis methods were biased. When using an odds ratio as the metric for pooling the studies, an issue arises when there are zero cases of the event in one of the treatment groups, since the odds ratio cannot be calculated in this case. One can apply a correction in this situation (e.g., addition of one-half case to each treatment group), but the results will be sensitive to the arbitrary choice of the correction. In fact, there is a current controversy over whether or not to include studies in the meta-analysis that have zero cases in the entire study.

Berlin et al. [6] addressed many issues arising in meta-analyses of safety data in the form of answers to frequently asked questions. This included the selection of studies to be included in the meta-analysis, adjustments for multiplicity (multiple endpoints and multiple analyses as studies are added), fixed-effects vs random-effects, and the use of individual patient data (IPD) meta-analyses. As discussed above, meta-analyses are typically based on published results, and, therefore, the analyst does not have access to the individual patient data. However, in those cases where the individual patient data are available, there are important advantages to doing an IPD meta-analysis. These include the ability to adjust for covariates at the patient level, the ability to map adverse event terms to a common dictionary, and the ability to conduct time-to-event analyses and construct Kaplan-Meier curves. As the pharmaceutical industry becomes more transparent with respect to sharing clinical trial databases with qualified researchers, the use of IPD meta-analysis should be expected to increase.

4.7 Benefit-risk Analysis

All treatments have the potential to cause harm, and in order to determine whether the treatment is valuable for use in patients those harms must be weighed against the benefits that the treatment provides. This is known as a benefit-risk assessment. In oncology, given the grievous nature of the illness, the benefits provided by effective treatments can be great, and therefore the harms that would be considered acceptable can be different from those in less serious diseases.

Benefit-risk analysis has typically been informal, but there has been recent emphasis on a more structured approach. There is a plethora of approaches for benefit-risk analysis, including both qualitative and quantitative approaches. In fact, at least 47 distinct approaches have been proposed, and various evaluations of these methods have been conducted [25, 40]. Most approaches involve some sort of structured presentation of both benefits and harms, while the quantitative approaches require the definition of utilities, or weights, that allow individual benefits and harms to be combined. Ke et al. [34] discussed some of the challenges with benefit-risk analysis. These include multifactoral sources of evidence, limited clinical data, and human judgment required to determine the utilities. Chuang-Stein et al. [12] reviewed quantitative measures that have been proposed in this context, including TWiST and Q-TWiST, benefit:risk ratio, global benefit:risk (GBR) score, ratio number needed to treat (NNT) for benefits and harms, benefit-less-risk measure, and benefit:risk index.

Quartey and Wang [45] argued that benefit-risk assessment should be a multi-disciplinary effort involving experts in clinical science, safety assessment, decision science, health economics, epidemiology, and biostatistics, and that biostatisticians should place greater emphasis on gaining expertise in this area.

4.8 Summary

The statistical evaluation of safety data from clinical trials has received increasing attention recently. The evaluation of safety in the oncology setting shares much in common with the corresponding evaluation in other therapeutic areas, but there are important distinctions as well. One such distinction is that phase I clinical trials, the first-in-human trials that attempt to gather information on drug safety, are conducted in patients in the oncology setting, but in normal volunteers in most other settings. In addition, one important medical dictionary, Common Terminology Criteria for Adverse Events, or CTCAE, was developed specifically for the cancer setting. While the grading of adverse events in this dictionary is helpful, comparisons between treatment groups should be based on cumulative categories of grades (e.g., grades 3–5 or grades 4–5), and not on individual grades from the middle of the scale. In general, safety analyses benefit from prespecification, including documentation of analysis plans and identification of adverse events of special interest (AESI). Data Monitoring Committees, or DMCs, play an important role in protecting the safety of patients in ongoing blinded trials, and implementation of futility rules by these committees can allow a trial to stop earlier than it otherwise would in the unlikely event that the treatment has a harmful effect on the study's primary endpoint. Safety signal detection presents many challenges regardless of therapeutic area; available statistical methods attempt to strike the right balance between sensitivity (ability to correctly identify new adverse drug reactions) and specificity (ability to keep false positives to a minimum). Meta-analysis can be a very useful tool when events are too rare to allow a signal to be detected in an individual clinical trial, but caution should be exercised when using the odds ratio as the treatment effect metric if the events are quite frequent. Structured approaches to the assessment of the benefit-risk balance are receiving considerable attention, although the large number of proposed approaches can make this area appear confusing to the novice.

Bibliography

[1] A. A. Adjei. What is the right dose? the elusive optimal biologic dose in phase I clinical trials. *Journal of Clinical Oncology*, 24:4054–4055, 2006.

[2] O. Amit, R. M. Heiberger, and P. W. Lane. Graphical approaches to the analysis of safety data from clinical trials. *Pharmaceutical Statistics*, 7:20–35, 2008.

[3] J. Avorn. Two centuries of assessing drug risks. *New England Journal of Medicine*, 367:193–197, 2012.

[4] J. Babb, A. Rogatko, and S. Zacks. Cancer phase I clinical trial: efficient dose escalation with overdose control. *Statistics in Medicine*, 17:1103–1120, 1998.

[5] B. N. Bekele, Y. Ji, Y. Shen, and P. F. Thall. Monitoring late-onset toxicities in phase I trials using predicted risks. *Biostatistics*, 9:442–457, 2008.

[6] J. A. Berlin, B. J. Crowe, E. Whalen, H. A. Xia, C. E. Koro, and J. Kuebler. Meta-analysis of clinical trial safety data in drug development program: answers to frequently asked questions. *Clinical Trials*, 10:20–31, 2012.

[7] S. M. Berry and D. A. Berry. Accounting for multiplicities in assessing drug safety: a three-level hierarchical mixture model. *Biometrics*, 60:418–426, 2004.

[8] M. J. Bradburn, J. J. Deeks, J. A. Berlin, and R. Localio. Much ado about nothing: a comparison of the performance of meta-analytic methods with rare events. *Statistics in Medicine*, 26:53–77, 2007.

[9] W. Brewster, T. Gibbs, K. LaCroix, A. Murray, M. Tydeman, and J. Almenoff. Evolving paradigms in pharmacovigilance. *Current Drug Safety*, 1:127–134, 2006.

[10] M. Chen, L. Zhu, P. Chiruvolu, and Q. Jiang. Evaluation of statistical methods for safety signal detection: a simulation study. *Pharmaceutical Statistics*, 14:11–19, 2015.

[11] Y. K. Cheung and R. Chappell. Sequential designs for phase I clinical trials with late-onset toxicities. *Biometrics*, 56:1177–1182, 2000.

[12] C. Chuang-Stein, R. Entsuah, and Y. Pritchett. Measures for conducting comparative benefit:risk assessment. *Drug Information Journal*, 42:223–233, 2008.

[13] C. Chuang-Stein, V. Le, and W. Chen. Recent advancements in the analysis and presentation of safety data. *Drug Information Journal*, 35:377–397, 2001.

[14] M. R. Conaway, S. Dunbar, and S. D. Peddada. Designs for single- or multiple-agent phase I trials. *Biometrics*, 60:661–669, 2004.

[15] B. Crowe, H. A. Xia, M. Nilsson, S. Shahin, W. Wang, and Q. Jiang. Program safety analysis plans: an implementation guide. In Q. Jiang and H. A. Xia, editors, *Quantitative Evaluation of Safety in Drug Development: Design, Analysis and Reporting*, pages 55–68. Chapman & Hall, London, 2014.

[16] B. J. Crowe, H. A. Xia, J. A. Berlin, D. J. Watson, H. Shi, S. L. Lin, J. Kuebler, R. C. Schriver, N. C. Santanello, G. Rochester, J. B. Porter, M. Oster, D. V. Mehrotra, Z. Li, E. C. King, E. S. Harpur, and D. B. Hall. Recommendations for safety planning, data collection, evaluation and reporting during drug, biologic, and vaccine development: a report of the safety planning, evaluation, and reporting team. *Clinical Trials*, 6:430–440, 2009.

[17] J. de Naurois, I. Novitzky-Basso, M. J. Gill, F. Marti Marti, M. H. Cullen, and F. Roila, on behalf of the ESMO Guidelines Working Group. Management of febrile neutropenia: ESMO clinical practice guidelines. *Annals of Oncology*, 21(suppl 5):v252–v256, 2010.

[18] S. P. Duke, Q. Jiang, L. Huang, M. Banach, and M. Cherny. Safety graphics. In Q. Jiang and H. A. Xia, editors, *Quantitative Evaluation of Safety in Drug Development: Design, Analysis and Reporting*, pages 195–224. Chapman & Hall, London, 2014.

[19] S. Ellenberg, T. Fleming, and D. DeMets. *Data Monitoring Committees in Clinical Trials: A Practical Perspective*. John Wiley & Sons, Hoboken, 2002.

[20] European Medicines Agency. Guideline on the evaluation of anticancer medicinal products in man, 2012. http://www.ema.europa.eu/docs/en_GB/document_library/Scientific_guideline/2013/01/WC500137128.pdf.

[21] S. J. Evans, P. C. Waller, and S. Davis. Use of proportional reporting ratios (PRRs) for signal generation from spontaneous drug reaction reports. *Pharmacoepidemiology and Drug Safety*, 10:483–486, 2001.

[22] T. R. Fleming. Identifying and addressing safety signals in clinical trials. *New England Journal of Medicine*, 359:1400–1402, 2008.

[23] J. D. Floyd, D. T. Nguyen, R. L. Lobins, Q. Bashir, D. C. Doll, and M. C. Perry. Cardiotoxicity of cancer therapy. *Journal of Clinical Oncology*, 23:7685–7696, 2005.

[24] S. Guan. Statistical designs for early phases of cancer clinical trials. *Journal of Biopharmaceutical Statistics*, 22:1109–1126, 2012.

[25] J. J. Guo, S. Pandey, J. Doyle, B. Bian, Y. Lis, and D. W. Raisch. A review of quantitative risk-benefit methodologies for assessing drug safety and efficacy - report of the ISPOR risk-benefit management working group. *Value Health*, 13:657–666, 2010.

[26] J. Herson. *Data and Safety Monitoring Committees in Clinical Trials*. Chapman & Hall, London, 2009.

[27] A. Hoering, M. LeBlanc, and J. Crowley. Seamless phase I-II design for assessing toxicity and efficacy for targeted agents. *Clinical Cancer Research*, 17:640–646, 2011.

[28] L. Huang, J. Zalkikar, and R. Tiwari. A likelihood ratio test based method for signal detection with application to FDA's safety data. *Journal of the American Statistical Association*, 106:1230–1241, 2011.

[29] J. P. A. Ioannidis, S. J. W. Evans, P. C. Gotzsche, R. T. O'Neill, D. G. Altman, K. Schulz, and D. Moher, for the CONSORT Group. Better reporting of harms in randomized trials: an extension of the CONSORT statement. *Annals of Internal Medicine*, 141:781–788, 2004.

[30] A. Ivanova and S. H. Kim. Dose finding for continuous and ordinal outcomes with a monotone objective function: a unified approach. *Biometrics*, 65:307–315, 2009.

[31] Q. Jiang and H. A. Xia. *Quantitative Evaluation of Safety in Drug Development: Design, Analysis and Reporting*. Chapman & Hall, London, 2014.

[32] L. D. Kaiser, A. S. Melemed, A. J. Preston, H. A. Chaudri Ross, D. Niedzwiecki, G. A. Fyfe, J. M. Gough, W. D. Bushnell, C. L. Stephens, M. K. Mace, J. S. Abrams, and R. L. Schilsky. Optimizing collection of adverse event data in cancer clinical trials supporting supplemental indications. *Journal of Clinical Oncology*, 28:5046–5053, 2010.

[33] S.-H. Kang and C. Ahn. Phase I cancer clinical trials. In S.-C. Chow, editor, *Encyclopedia of Biopharmaceutical Statistics, 3rd Ed*, pages 1011–1015. Informa Health, New York, London, 2010.

[34] C. Ke, Q. Jiang, and S. Snapinn. Benefit-risk assessment approaches. In Q. Jiang and H. A. Xia, editors, *Quantitative Evaluation of Safety in Drug Development: Design, Analysis and Reporting*, pages 267–288. Chapman & Hall, London, 2014.

[35] E. L. Korn. Nontoxicity endpoints in phase I trial designs for targeted, non-cytotoxic agents. *Journal of the National Cancer Institute*, 96:977–978, 2004.

[36] J. Kübler, R. Vonk, S. Beimel, W. Gunselmann, M. Homering, D. Nehrdich, J. Köster, K. Theobald, and P. Voleske. Adverse event analysis and MedDRA: business as usual or challenge? *Drug Information Journal*, 39:63–72, 2005.

[37] L. A. Ladewski, S. M. Belknap, J. R. Nebeker, O. Sartor, E. A. Lyons, T. C. Kuzel, M. S. Tallman, D. W. Raisch, A. R. Auerbach, G. T. Schumock, H. C. Kwaan, and C. L. Bennett. Dissemination of information on potentially fatal adverse drug reactions for cancer drugs from 2000 to

2002: first results from the Research on Adverse Drug Events and Reports project. *Journal of Clinical Oncology*, 21:3859–3866, 2003.

[38] D. V. Mehrotra and J. F. Heyse. Use of the false discover rate for evaluating clinical safety data. *Statistical Methods in Medical Research*, 13:227–238, 2004.

[39] K. Messer, L. Natarajan, E. D. Ball, and T. A. Lane. Toxicity-evaluation designs for phase I/II cancer immunotherapy trials. *Statistics in Medicine*, 29:712–720, 2010.

[40] S. Mt-Isa, N. Wang, C. E. Hallgreen, T. Callreus, G. Genov, I. Hirsch, S. Hobbiger, K. S. Hockley, D. Luciani, L. D. Phillips, G. Quartey, S. B. Sarac, I. Stoeckert, A. Micaleff, D. Ashby, and I. Tzoulake. Review of methodologies for benefit and risk assessment of medication, 2012. http://www.imi-protect.eu/benefit-risk.html.

[41] S. D. Mukherjee, M. E. Coombes, M. Levine, J. Cosby, B. Kowaleski, and A. Arnold. A qualitative study evaluating causality attribution for serious adverse events during early phase oncology clinical trials. *Investigational New Drugs*, 29:1013–1020, 2011.

[42] J. O'Quigley, M. Pepe, and L. Fisher. Continual reassessment method: a practical design for phase I clinical trials in cancer. *Biometrics*, 46:33–48, 1990.

[43] R. Pirker, R. A. Ramlau, W. Schuette, P. Zatloukal, I. Ferreira, T. Lillie, and J. F. Vansteenkiste. Safety and efficacy of darbepoetin alfa in previously untreated extensive-stage small cell lung cancer treated with platinum plus etoposide. *Journal of Clinical Oncology*, 26:2342–2349, 2008.

[44] K. L. Price, H. A. Xia, M. Lakshminarayanan, D. Madigan, D. Manner, J. Scott, J. D. Stamey, and L. Thompson. Bayesian methods for design and analysis of safety trials. model choice via Markov chain Monte Carlo methods. *Pharmaceutical Statistics*, 13:13–24, 2014.

[45] G. Quartey and J. Wang. Statistical aspects in comparative benefit-risk assessment: challenges and opportunities for pharmaceutical statisticians. *Pharmaceutical Statistics*, 11:82–85, 2012.

[46] M. J. Ratain, D. Collyar, B. A. Kamen, E. Eisenhauer, T. S. Lawrence, C. Runowicz, S. Turner, and J. L. Wade III. Critical role of phase I clinical trials in cancer treatment. *Journal of Clinical Oncology*, 15:853–859, 1997.

[47] D. J. Sargent and S. L. George. Clinical trial data collection: when less is more. *Journal of Clinical Oncology*, 28:5019–5021, 2010.

[48] S. Snapinn, M.-G. Chen, Q. Jiang, and T. Koutsoukos. Assessment of futility in clinical trials. *Pharmaceutical Statistics*, 5:273–281, 2006.

[49] S. Snapinn and Q. Jiang. Non-inferiority study design and analysis for safety endpoints. In Q. Jiang and H. A. Xia, editors, *Quantitative Evaluation of Safety in Drug Development: Design, Analysis and Reporting*, pages 39–54. Chapman & Hall, London, 2014.

[50] S. M. Snapinn. Non-inferiority trials. *Current Controlled Trials in Cardiovascular Medicine*, 1:19–21, 2000.

[51] H. Southworth and M. O'Connell. Data mining and statistically guided clinical review of adverse event data in clinical trials. *Journal of Biopharmaceutical Statistics*, 19:803–817, 2009.

[52] P. F. Thall, R. E. Millikan, P. Mueller, and S.-J. Lee. Dose-finding with two agents in phase I oncology trials. *Biometrics*, 59:487–496, 2003.

[53] U.S. Food & Drug Administration. Guidance for Industry: Cancer Drug and Biological Products - clinical data in marketing applications, 2001. http://www.fda.gov/downloads/Drugs/GuidanceCompliance/RegulatoryInformation/Guidances/ucm071323.pdf.

[54] U.S. Food & Drug Administration. Draft Guidance for Industry: determining the extent of safety data collection needed in late stage premarket and postapproval clinical investigations, 2012. http://www.fda.gov/downloads/Drugs/GuidanceCompliance/RegulatoryInformation/Guidances/UCM291158.pdf.

[55] U.S. Food & Drug Administration. Guidance for Industry and Investigators: safety reporting requirements for INDs and BA/BE studies, 2012. http://www.fda.gov/downloads/Drugs/GuidanceCompliance/RegulatoryInformation/Guidances/UCM227351.pdf.

[56] J. Vansteenkiste, J. Glaspy, D. Henry, H. Ludwig, R. Pirker, D. Tomita, H. Collins, and J. Crawford. Benefits and risks of using erythropoiesis-stimulating agents (ESAs) in lung cancer patients: study-level and patient-level meta-analyses. *Biometrics*, 76:478–485, 2012.

[57] H. A. Xia and Q. Jiang. Statistical evaluation of drug safety data. *Therapeutic Innovation & Regulatory Science*, 48:109–120, 2014.

[58] Z. Yuan, R. Chappell, and H. Bailey. The continual reassessment method for multiple toxicity grades: a Bayesian quasi-likelihood approach. *Biometrics*, 63:173–179, 2007.

[59] Y. Zhou, C. Ke, Q. Jiang, S. Shahin, and S. Snapinn. 49(3), 2015.

Part II

Early Phase Clinical Trials

5

Development and Validation of Predictive Signatures

Michael C. Sachs

Lisa M. McShane

CONTENTS

5.1 Introduction

A biological signature is a discernible pattern of measurements that is of interest for its ability to distinguish subgroups with distinct biological or clinical phenotypes, or behaviors. The increasing availability of omics assays, defined as assays permitting the comprehensive evaluation of related sets of biological molecules [57] such as DNAs, RNAs, or proteins, has fueled much research directed at identification of signatures in cancer which can aid in clinical management decisions for patients. Historically in oncology, signatures have usually been derived from a single high-throughput assay platform, for example a gene expression microarray which can simultaneously measure expression levels of thousands of genes in one biological sample. Restriction to a single assay platform is not essential, however, to the concept of a signature; nor must a signature be composed of a large number of measurements even if the underlying assay platform generates high-dimensional biomarker data. Due to the widespread use of high-throughput omics assays for signature development and the diverse set of issues that arise in their use, omics-based signatures and the clinical tests based on them will be the focus of discussions here.

High quality evidence must be generated to support incorporation of an omics-based signature into decision making for routine clinical practice. Omics assays generate high-dimensional data, often hundreds or thousands of measurements. In order to translate these data into reliable and interpretable clinical decision tools that can be applied to individual cases, specialized statistical methods that are appropriate for use in high-dimensional data settings must be used. An omics signature is operationalized by development of an omics-based test that has the ability to calculate or detect the signature. The test may incorporate the omics data into a continuous measure, such as a risk score developed from a statistical model, or the omics data may be processed through an algorithm that classifies each case into two or more signature categories. Statistical approaches to develop these models or algorithms must be chosen with care to avoid common pitfalls such as model over-fitting and biased assessment of model or algorithm performance. A series of studies must be performed to develop and validate the omics test, culminating in specification of a final test which is established to be reliable and clinically useful. Decisions concerning when an omics test is ready for incorporation into a clinical trial or use in clinical care require careful examination of the quality and reliability of evidence generated along with potential benefits and risks of use.

A general approach to development of a predictive omics-based test to guide treatment decisions can be summarized as follows: (i) Development of a model or classifier for the signature using preclinical and early phase studies based on research-grade omics assays; (ii) Development of a clinical-grade assay and test procedure; (iii) Establishment of the analytical performance and evaluation of the preliminary clinical performance of the test using stored specimen sets with associated clinical data; (iv) Assessment of the clinical utility of the locked down omics test either in a prospective clinical trial, or using specimens stored from a completed prospective trial. Preliminary evaluation of the predictive signature may indicate a need to refine the assay and, likewise, refinements to the assay procedures may trigger further refinement of the signature. Several iterations through steps (i)–(iii) may be needed before sufficiently compelling evidence is generated to advance to step (iv). A switch from a high-throughput omics assay to another assay more feasible to use in clinical settings may be required.

Critical elements that must be established by the end of the development and validation process are that the signature has analytic validity, clinical validity, and clinical utility. Analytic validity means that the signature measurement can be done reliably, reproducibly, and accurately in the clinical context (i.e., stage of disease, specimen type). Clinical validity means that there is a strong and statistically significant association between the signature and the clinical outcome of interest. Clinical utility means that the use of the signature in clinical practice leads to an overall benefit to the patient. These definitions are adapted from Teutsch et al. [83] and we expand on their meaning later. Each of these steps in the development and validation process will now be discussed in the sections that follow. For simplicity, the various topics will be discussed as though the process occurs in an orderly linear fashion, but as already noted there can be many iterations of the process.

5.1.1 Prognostic and Predictive Omics Signatures

An early focus on the intended clinical use for a signature is strongly advised so that developmental studies can be planned with the context in mind in order to maximize their relevance. Investigators should specify the type of clinical decision that the omics test is intended to inform as well as the patient population for which use of the signature would be recommended. Omics-based signatures in oncology clinical trials are most often used for one of two purposes: prognosis or prediction of treatment benefit. A prognostic signature is used to predict patient outcome in the absence of therapy or in the context of a standard therapy all patients are likely to receive. A prognostic signature should exhibit a statistically strong association with a meaningful clinical outcome such as overall survival or quality of life. To be clinically useful, the association must be strong enough that the expected clinical course in different subgroups defined by the signature would warrant different clinical management. For instance, a patient with a very good prognosis after surgical resection of his or her tumor may opt not to receive any adjuvant chemotherapy, while a patient with a poor prognosis may opt for more aggressive treatment which may carry additional risks and side effects.

Predictive, also known as treatment-selection or therapy guiding, signatures are intended for selecting patient sub-populations for specific treatments, usually molecularly targeted therapies. Many new treatment regimens target multiple pathways in ways that are not well understood [23]; therefore there is much potential for omics-based signatures to perform better than single biomarkers in identifying patients who are likely to benefit from these treatments [8, 30]. Predictive signatures may also identify a subgroup that is more prone to treatment-related toxicity and thus should be spared that treatment. A predictive signature should exhibit a statistical interaction with a therapy such that the therapy is beneficial in one signature subgroup and is harmful or not beneficial in another subgroup, called a qualitative interaction [68]. A predictive signature having this property will also demonstrate different prognostic ability with different treatments, but the converse is not necessarily true. It is a common misconception that if a signature is prognostic in the treated population and not prognostic in the untreated population, then it

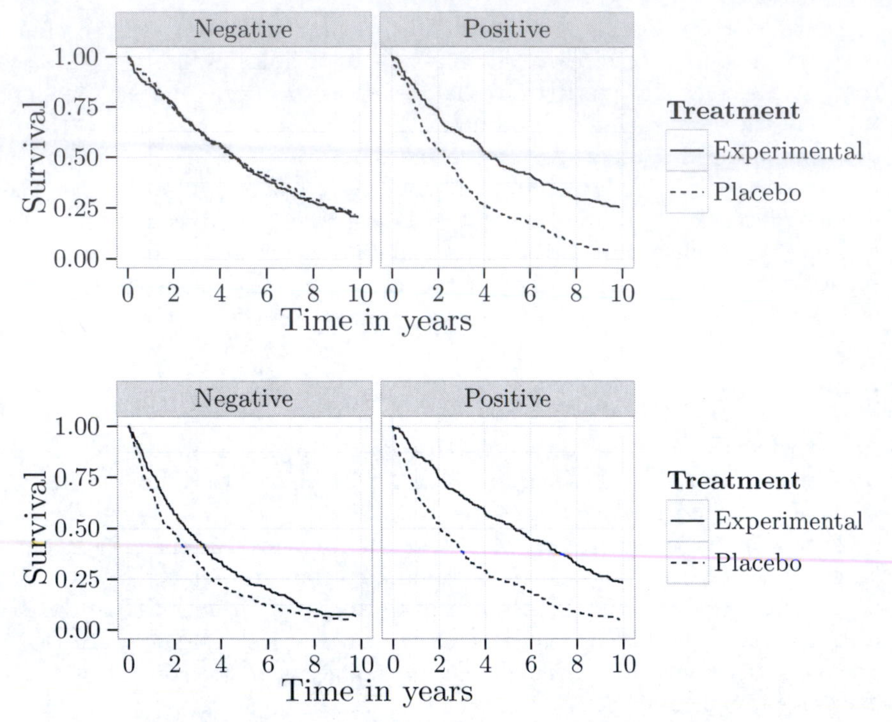

FIGURE 5.1: The top panel shows an example of a predictive signature that is useful for therapy selection. The signature positive group shows good treatment efficacy, while the negative group does not. The bottom panel shows an example of a predictive signature that may not be useful for therapy selection. Both signature groups show treatment efficacy, but to different degrees.

must be suitable for therapy selection. It is possible that there is a therapy benefit in both signature positive and negative groups but the magnitude of benefit in the positive subgroup is greater than in the negative subgroup. This is called a quantitative interaction. If the treatment benefit in the negative subgroup is still large enough to be clinically meaningful, then it may be reasonable to provide the new therapy to all patients and no signature would be needed. Figure 5.1 illustrates this concept and shows an example of a predictive signature that is useful for therapy selection compared to a predictive signature that is not useful for therapy selection.

5.2 Signature Development

The process of developing an omics signature to the point where it is ready for use in a phase II or III clinical trial can be challenging. Unlike in therapeutic trials, there has not been wide adoption of a well-structured, phased approach to developing and translating omics-based signatures into clinical practice. Many omics signatures stall in the exploratory phase. Frequently, studies are conducted using convenience sets of specimens not representative of any particular clinical setting and without much thought given to an eventual clinical use. An interesting biological or clinical signature may be identified, but translation of the signature into a clinical tool often never occurs. There have been some proposals for structured approaches to the development of biomarkers for diagnosis [66] and for prediction and prognosis [31, 74]. These proposals were not intended to address the complexities inherent in the development of signatures from high-dimensional omics data, but once an omics signature has been developed to the point of being represented by a single score or classification system, these existing structured approaches offer helpful guidance. McShane et al. [54, 55] bring together principles of signature development and these structured approaches to general biomarker development to propose a set of criteria for determination of the readiness of an omics signature to be used in a clinical trial.

As in development of therapeutics, preliminary data for omics-based signatures for prognosis or prediction are often gathered *in vitro* or in animal studies. Experiments on human cancer cell lines can be used to provide evidence supporting a biological rationale and help focus further study. Mouse xenograft models, in which human tumor cells are transplanted into mice, are often used in drug development and may also provide preliminary evidence of predictive molecular features [48, 82, 88]. Preclinical models may permit measurement of a variety of molecular characteristics using omics assays, including DNA, RNA, and protein. These data can be interrogated to identify preliminary sets of molecular features such as mutations or expression levels (RNA or protein) of particular genes that appear promising due to their observed association with the phenotype that the signature is intended to predict.

5.2.1 Assay Development and Validation

Although useful information can be obtained from preclinical studies, definitive evaluation to determine readiness for clinical use eventually requires an independent validation study in human samples. This may require multiple steps to establish that the biologic signals persist in human samples and to establish a measurement process that is robust enough for use with specimens collected under routine clinical conditions. The development of detailed standard operating procedures is critical to enable reliable and accurate measurements. Assay development also includes evaluation of the impact of technical factors on the assay results. Multiple factors may influence the results obtained from the measurement process, including tissue processing and storage methods [79, 80, 87] and technical aspects of the assay itself, such as reagents and imaging settings. It is important for all of these aspects to be fully specified and locked down prior to final validation. In addition, most assays are subject to influence by nuisance factors such as batch effects or specimen quality deficits that can have substantial effects yet are often ignored [45]. Standard operating procedures should include quality control criteria to qualify specimens and omics assay results. Criteria for screening out poor quality specimens prior to running the assay should be developed. Generally, these criteria are based on specimen characteristics such as sample amount, purity, percent tumor, percent necrosis, or some other metrics of sample quantity or quality.

An omics assay is considered to have analytic validity when it is empirically demonstrated that the assay measures its intended target accurately, reliably, and reproducibly. For signatures that depend on a multitude of omics features, there are differing opinions on whether only the final signature output needs to be analytically validated, or if each of the features going into the signature needs to be individually analytically validated. If the signature incorporates hundreds or thousands of features, then it is generally not feasible to separately evaluate analytical performance of each feature. Moreover, it can be difficult to predict how even a small amount of random or systematic error in each feature measurement will translate into errors in the final signature. The impact of feature-specific errors will depend on their correlation with other feature measurements and how influential the most error-prone features are in the signature. This suggests that a reasonable compromise when evaluating the analytical performance of an omics assay composed of a very large number of features is to use clinical specimens that are representative of the population in which the signature is intended to be used, thereby covering a representative range of possible combinations of features that are likely to be encountered in practice. Different combinations of features may map to the same final signature result, but it is of interest to determine whether performance in a given range of final signature result varies depending on feature value inputs.

A number of helpful review articles provide general guidance on approaches for assessment of analytic performance of standard types of molecular assays [43, 65]. Additionally, several guidance documents are available which describe standards for assessing and reporting the analytical performance of omics assays [52, 69, 73]. A few of the basic performance metrics will be described here, with the reader referred to the cited references for more in-depth discussion of additional metrics. Some examples of well-conducted and reported analytical validation studies are those for the Oncotype DX signature [20] and for the PAM50-ROR signature [60] which are used in practice to estimate the probability of recurrence of node-negative hormone-receptor positive breast cancer.

Accuracy and precision are two analytical performance metrics for continuous biomarker or signature values that are typically examined. Precision is defined as the closeness of values obtained by repeated measurement of the same specimen under the same conditions. Precision is typically quantified as a standard deviation or in a relative sense as the coefficient of variation, which is defined as the standard deviation divided by the mean. Measurement accuracy refers to how close individual repeated measurements on the same sample or same individual are to an accepted true value; it reflects both bias and precision. Bias refers to the average difference between a measurement result and a known value or an accepted reference value. For many omics platforms, there are not accepted true values for every single feature and analytical bias cannot be evaluated. For omics platforms that generate binary features, such as the presence or absence of mutations, accuracy can be evaluated by estimating the sensitivity and specificity of the assay. Some binary assay results may have continuous measurements underlying them, such as next generation sequencing which counts alleles to determine the presence or absence of mutations.

Assay limits of detection and the related issue of handling of missing feature measurements deserve special mention. For any omics signature comprising more than one feature measurement, a single indeterminate or missing value precludes direct computation of the signature. Missing values often occur because a feature value associated with a specimen falls below or above the range of signals that the assay system is capable of detecting (limits of detection) and either no signal is recorded (below limit of detection) or the recorded value is saturated at the maximum detectable value (above limit of detection). Missing values require one to either declare that the signature cannot be calculated or to impute a value for the missing observations. Failure to impute missing values means that it might not be possible to reach a clinical decision using the signature and the assay will have been performed on the patient's specimen for naught. During the analytical validation assessments it is important to assess the expected rate of assay failures as it will have a bearing on the clinical practicality of the signature. In many cases it will be reasonable to impute values for the missing feature measurements. Simple imputation methods include substitution of the lower limit of detection, or half that value, for any feature value below the lower limit of detection, and substitution of the upper limit of detection for any saturated value. Values missing for other reasons can be imputed by a variety of methods including substitution of a mean or a value predicted from a model based on non-missing values [47]. When the clinical performance of the signature is assessed, it will be particularly important to examine the impact of missing values and their imputations.

Omics assays can be run on a variety of specimen types, but the results may be affected by factors encountered in specimen collection, processing, and storage. Different tissue collection methods may result in varying levels of quality of the specimen (for example surgical excision versus core needle biopsy). The condition of the specimen once removed from the host can quickly degrade. Molecular assays can successfully be run on decades old formalin-fixed, paraffin-embedded (FFPE) tissue [15, 39] but storage method and delays to fixation can have an impact on the results [79, 80, 87]. In clinical settings, collection, processing, and storage may occur under a range of conditions. An analytical performance assessment should include verification that the omics assay performs satisfactorily in that anticipated range. If it does not, then restrictive requirements for specimen collection and processing should be clearly specified; however, severe restrictions may limit the future clinical utility of a signature.

A guiding principle regarding how good the analytical performance must be is that it must be good enough to not have a significant detrimental impact on the clinical performance of the signature. The acceptable level of clinical performance will depend on the intended use. We discuss this issue further in Section 5.3.

5.2.2 Statistical Development

Development of a mathematical model or classifier that translates the omics features into a clinically useful quantity is a multi-step process. Selection of features to include in the model or classifier is typically a first step, although as will be discussed later, there are several modeling approaches that permit simultaneous feature selection and model parameter estimation. For purposes of providing an overview we discuss first the conceptually simple approach of performing feature selections separately from model building. If the goal is to develop a prognostic omics test, then feature selection aims to identify a subset of features that either alone or in combination with other features demonstrate an association with the clinical outcome of interest. The vast majority of omics signatures published to date are prognostic signatures. To select features for a predictive omics test for use in deciding between two treatments (A and B, say), the goal is to identify features that, either alone or in combination with other features, identify subgroups of patients such that one subgroup has a better outcome on treatment A than on B, while the other subgroup has similar or worse outcome on treatment A compared to treatment B. This kind of relationship that is desired for predictive features is referred to as a qualitative interaction, as defined earlier. The selected features are then combined into a multivariable prediction model or algorithm, possibly along with established prognostic or predictive variables. If the clinical distinction of interest is binary, for example respond or not respond to a particular therapy, and the output of the statistical model is a continuous score, then a cutpoint to dichotomize the score may be suggested for clinical decision making. The clinical test Oncotype DX, for example, is reported as a continuous risk score along with a plot showing the score's relationship to

10-year distant recurrence free survival and recommended cutpoints of 18% and 31% to define low, intermediate, and high risk categories (an example is shown in Figure 5.2). It has been demonstrated that the low risk subgroup has sufficiently low risk that patients in that subgroup are not likely to benefit from chemotherapy [78]. It is advisable to maintain the continuous score as far into the model development process as possible as any dichotomization causes a loss of information [77].

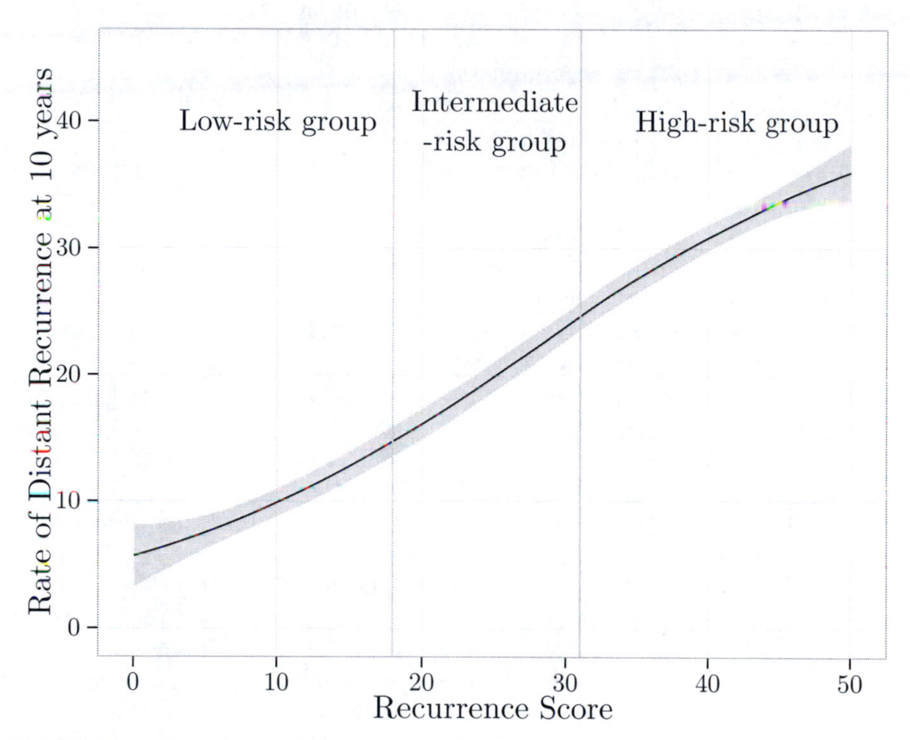

FIGURE 5.2: Sample graph illustrating the association between the Oncotype DX test for distant recurrence of ER positive, node negative breast cancer, and the rate of distant recurrence in a sample at 10 years. Figure is Figure 2B from Sparano and Paik [78]. Reprinted with permission.

The signature development process is iterative. During development and before the model or classifier is established and locked down, it is possible to go back to optimize things like the assay measurement procedures, quality control criteria, model features and parameter estimates, or algorithmic rules used to identify signature-driven subgroups. Preliminary evidence supporting the usefulness of the signature should be established, typically employing some form of internal validation, during the course of model or algorithm development. In the discussions that follow we elaborate on each of these steps in the development process.

Criteria for selection of features for inclusion into a model or algorithm may depend on more than their observed associations with outcomes or phenotypes. Individual features (e.g., genes, proteins, transcripts) may be rejected for other technical or biological reasons. As a concrete example, in the development of the gene expression-based prognostic signature EndoPredict, investigators chose to exclude probes that exhibited narrow measurement dynamic range, low detection rates, or poor correlation between measurements for the same gene generated by different omics assay platforms (gene expression microarrays versus RT-qPCR in this example)[24]. Quality criteria of these types can enhance the robustness and reliability of the test; however, criteria such as these are generally applied *ad hoc* and we are not aware of formal comparisons or evaluations of different approaches.

In recent years there has been an increase in the number of computational approaches to classification and prediction described in the statistical literature. In practice, *ad hoc* approaches to selection and estimation are commonly used with varying degrees of success. To name a few, there are centroid-based approaches like K nearest neighbors [4] and shrunken centroids [85], tree-based approaches like classification and regression trees [14] and random forests [13], and regression-based approaches such as subset selection, shrinkage, linear discriminant analysis, support vector machines [19], and supervised principal components [7]. Hastie et al. [33] is an excellent reference for many modern statistical methods for prediction. Instead of attempting to comprehensively review these methods, we aim to frame the critical statistical challenges inherent in the development of a predictive signature from high dimensional omics-based data.

The defining statistical challenge in the development of omics based signatures is the vast number of features or variables measured relative to the number of independent specimens (or study participants). Having many more features (p) than specimens (n), the $p > n$ problem causes difficulties for standard statistical approaches for combining features such as regression or linear discriminant analysis. To illustrate this problem, consider simple linear regression with a n by p design matrix X and response vector Y. The least squares solution for the regression coefficient β solves the equation $X^T X\beta = X^T Y$. When $p > n$, this equation does not have a unique solution for β because $X^T X$ is not invertible.

There are two broad approaches to overcome this $p > n$ estimation problem: (1) Reduce the number of candidate features by screening them or combining them (filtering or data-reduction); (2) Modify the estimation algorithm with a penalty term (regularization). With filtering, univariate methods are applied to each of the many omics features in turn where the univariate method involves estimating the association of the feature with the clinical outcome. Then, some criterion, which is chosen in advance or selected using cross-validation, is applied to the statistic to select a subset of p^* features such that $p^* < n$. With regularization, the optimization involved in estimating regression coefficients is constrained in a special way, which leads to a unique solution that can have desirable properties.

To illustrate the mechanics of feature selection (filtering), consider using a large set of continuous gene expression values $X_j, j = 1, \ldots, p$ to develop a prognostic signature for a binary treatment outcome $Y \in \{0, 1\}$ (e.g., alive at 5 years or deceased prior to 5 years). The number of features, p, is too large to incorporate all of the X_j values into a multivariable prognostic model, so we will select only those genes with a promising univariate association with Y. As a first step, for each $j = 1, \ldots, p$, we calculate the two-sample t-statistic comparing values of X_j by levels of Y. Then, we filter out the genes that have weak associations with Y by selecting only the top 5% of t-statistics in absolute value. In the second step, those top 5% are then included in a multivariable logistic regression model to predict Y. This general procedure allows for many different modeling approaches. Instead of selecting the top 5%, an investigator could select only those genes whose t-statistics exceed some threshold θ in absolute value. The threshold can be determined by cross-validation as part of the model building process (to be discussed later). Many other criteria or test statistics could also be used. Any type of statistical model can be used in the second step, for example, Bair et al. [6] filter genes based on regression coefficients and then use principal components analysis to identify linear combinations of variables for inclusion in a multivariable regression model. Proportional-hazards regression or other time-to-event models incorporating treatment by gene interactions would be suitable for developing predictive signatures in settings where the primary outcome is time to an event such as recurrence or death. The main criticism of the filtering strategy just described is that the univariate models in step one fail to account for complex multivariable relationships, such as confounding and interactions. [81] shows empirically that when a true relationship between an X_j and Y is confounded by a third variable, that relationship could be inappropriately rejected or included based on univariate filtering, depending on whether or not the confounder attenuates or accentuates the association.

Regularization approaches directly model the multivariable relationships of all the features. To overcome the $p > n$ optimization problem described above, constraints on the regression coefficients are incorporated into the model. To illustrate the concept, consider again, for each of $i = 1, \ldots, n$ subjects, a large set of continuous gene expression values $X_{ij}, j = 1, \ldots, p$ and a continuous outcome Y_i. Let Y denote the column vector of Y_i values, and X the design matrix with n rows and p columns. The goal is to fit the linear regression model $E[Y|X] = X^T\beta$ by finding an estimate of β. The least squares estimate is the value of β that minimizes the expression

$$\sum_{i=1}^{n}(Y_i - X_i^T\beta)^2.$$

The solution to the problem of non-uniqueness of the estimate when $p > n$ is to incorporate a penalty function on β and instead minimize

$$\sum_{i=1}^{n}(Y_i - X_i^T\beta)^2 + f(\beta, \lambda),$$

where λ is a vector of tuning parameters. The tuning parameters λ cannot be estimated using standard techniques and instead must be specified prior to estimating β. The nature of the penalty function f determines the properties of the resulting estimate of β. The earliest form suggested was ridge regression [34], wherein $f(\beta, \lambda) = \lambda \sum_{j=1}^{p} \beta_j^2$ for $\lambda > 0$. In this case the solution for β is

$$\hat{\beta} = (X^TX + \lambda I)^{-1}X^TY,$$

where I is the identity matrix. Compared to the standard least squares estimate (if it is unique), it can be seen that the ridge estimate of β is shrunken towards 0. When $\lambda = 0$ there is no shrinkage and the degree of shrinkage increases as λ increases. The specific value of λ used in practice must be selected, either by cross-validation or by prespecifying it. The prediction performance of the model will vary as a function of λ and it is tempting to select the value of λ that yields the best in-sample performance. To avoid substitution bias in doing so, one can use cross-validation to obtain valid estimates of the out-of-sample prediction performance while simultaneously selecting the optimal value for λ. Cross-validation is described in Section 5.2.5.

This shrinkage is a way to reduce model complexity and allow for an estimate when $p > n$. There are a multitude of penalty functions that have been studied in the statistical literature, each with different properties. An important type of regularization in omics-based signature development is the lasso [84]. The lasso uses the penalty function $f(\beta, \lambda) = \lambda \sum_{j=1}^{p} |\beta_j|$. A desirable property of the lasso penalty is that it encourages non-important components of β to be set exactly to 0, effectively performing simultaneous variable selection and multivariable estimation. Another type of penalty is called the elastic net [95], which is designed to be better suited to problems in which there is large amount of correlation among the features. The elastic net penalty function is $f(\beta, \lambda_1, \lambda_2) = \lambda_1 \sum_{j=1}^{p} |\beta_j| + \lambda_2 \sum_{j=1}^{p}(\beta_j)^2$. Penalty functions can be incorporated into the relevant optimization criteria for estimation of a variety of regression models. For instance, in logistic regression the binomial log-likelihood would be penalized, and in Cox regression the partial log-likelihood would be penalized.

Feature selection for building predictive (treatment-selection) signatures relies on criteria different than those for prognostic signatures. In order to effectively guide therapy, an omics-based signature must have a strong and qualitative interaction effect with the treatment in question; hence features should be selected according to this same principle. The naïve approach to this in our examples would be to expand the design matrix by including all possible treatment by gene interactions and then proceed with filtering or regularization. This might have the undesirable side effect of including an interaction term without including the main effect. To get around this problem, Bien et al. [10] propose to use the hierarchical grouped-lasso, which is an extension of the lasso penalty that forces main effects to be included if the interaction effects are non-zero. Lim and Hastie [46] offer an alternative solution to the same problem. In a filtering approach, the main effects can be forced into the resulting models at the second stage.

Clustering is another approach to feature selection and data-reduction that is commonly used in omics-based signature development. Unlike filtering or regularization, clustering is performed in an unsupervised manner, that is, without regard to the clinical outcome. Clustering methods use only the omics features themselves in an attempt to identify biologically distinct subgroups. Proponents of clustering methods for prediction argue that the resulting groups are easy to interpret and important biological features of the groups can be identified. Furthermore, if truly distinct biological processes are uncovered, then they are likely to correlate with clinical outcome or response to treatment or provide targets for future drug development. Opponents of using clustering methods for prediction argue that if the omics features contain sufficient information to successfully predict outcome, then methods designed for that task will perform better [75]. Likewise, biological discoveries based on clustering are identified *post hoc*, using visual inspection and subjective interpretation of the data, and therefore may not be valid or reproducible. Despite the controversies, omics-based signatures have been discovered using clustering methods such as hierarchical clustering [1] and non-negative matrix factorization [44].

Investigators need not wed themselves to a particular statistical method or even class of methods. Indeed, in high dimensional settings, it is quite common to combine filtering, regularization, and even data reduction steps by clustering. For example Bair et al. [7] filter genes with univariate regression models before entering the selected ones into a principal components analysis. Witten and Tibshirani [90] reduce the dimension of genetic data with principal components analysis prior to fitting a lasso-like model. The use of a variety of different methods in a particular setting can result in a multitude of potential statistical models that may contain distinct parameters and subsets of features. Bayesian model averaging [35] is a formal approach to combining results from multiple models that accounts for uncertainty about the optimal subset of features to include in the signature. Bayesian model averaging has been used to build a classification tool based on gene expression microarrays [93].

5.2.3 Iteration and Refinement

The results of a preliminary validation may indicate a need to go back and refine certain aspects of the signature. If problems with the assay itself are indicated, adjustments to the assay protocol may be needed. Other aspects such as the data pre-processing steps, overall data quality assessments, exclusion of unreliable measurements, data normalization, or calculation of intermediate summary statistics (for example, calculation of gene-level summary expression levels from probe intensity values in microarray data) may need to be refined. Aspects of the statistical approach may also need to be refined; these aspects may include decisions about constraints on the number of variables in the model, constraints on the weight given to any single variable, how to handle unusual measurements, how to summarize redundant variables, and where to set cutpoints on risk scores for therapy selection. Unlike the linear phased approach of therapy development, omics-based signature development can be much more iterative and therefore resource-intensive. Thus it is important to have a clear development plan in place, with a focus on the clinical need addressed by the predictive signature. If any changes are made along the way, it may be necessary to re-validate the signature. Once an acceptable level of performance is demonstrated and the assay and signature is shown to be standardized and reproducible, the omics signature can be considered to have clinical validity. Clinical validity means that the signature has demonstrated a statistically convincing association with a clinical outcome. The sections that follow elaborate on the process of establishing clinical validity of a predictive signature.

5.2.4 Performance Metrics

As noted by Pepe et al. [67], assessing the performance of a signature for predicting response to treatment in individual patients requires more than just an odds ratio or hazard ratio. Polley et al. [68] advocate presenting survival curves and hazard ratios with confidence intervals for each subgroup defined by the signature (i.e., predicted benefit and predicted no benefit). This allows researchers to evaluate the efficacy of treatment in each of the potential treatment selection subgroups in a familiar way. It is important to present comprehensive results of the inference, including survival curves, point estimates, confidence intervals, in addition to p-values. Reduction of the results to p-values alone will often inhibit clear interpretation of the results. When there is a significant p-value in one signature group, but a nonsignificant p-value in the other, researchers may incorrectly conclude that the treatment effects are significantly different from each other. The significance of a p-value can depend on many things, only one of which is the situation where the true treatment effects differ. This is a common statistical fallacy that should be avoided by directly testing whether the treatment effects differ [29].

Survival curves calculated for subgroups defined by a signature may show a strong separation as reflected in a large hazard ratio, but the distributions of actual survival times for the two subgroups can overlap substantially, resulting in dependency of the accuracy estimate on the particular timepoint. Accuracy of prediction will be poor at timepoints where there is heaviest overlap of the survival time distributions, but good at timepoints where the distributions do not overlap much [70, 91]. This is potentially also a limitation of the Janes et al. [40] method, that we summarize below, if naïvely applied using a single, arbitrarily selected time point for dichotomizing a time-to-event outcome.

Performance of a model or classifier that evaluates a predictive signature can be quantified by several different metrics that address the associations between the signature, the treatment, and a clinical outcome. The most common clinical outcome in oncology is a time-to-event outcome such as progression-free survival or overall survival. Choodari-Oskooei et al. [16, 17] provide thorough evaluations of the variety of metrics to assess performance of a prognostic model with censored time-to-event outcomes. They conclude that measures of explained variation, that is the ratio of the variance in the survival outcome explained by the signature to the overall variance, are preferred. Interested readers can refer to those papers for the details of the estimation methods. Evaluation of performance of predictive (therapy-selection) models is trickier because it is the magnitude of the interaction effect and whether the interaction is qualitative (preferred) or quantitative that is relevant to model performance. It is not sufficient to establish that a putatively predictive signature for a new drug separates patients who receive the new drug into groups with different survival outcomes, because the separation could be driven by an underlying prognostic ability of the signature. Showing, in addition, that the signature does not separate patients who received control therapy still does not establish the desired qualitative interaction. The limitation of that approach is that it is possible for such scenarios to result purely from quantitative treatment-by-signature interactions with all subgroups benefiting from the new therapy but by different amounts. Janes et al. [42] describe several standard approaches and their limitations. Janes et al. [40] is a comprehensive approach to evaluating predictive performance that we will summarize and illustrate in the next section.

5.2.5 Estimation of Performance Metrics

Regardless of the metric used to evaluate a signature's performance, it is important to avoid biases that can creep into performance estimates when data used to build the signature are also used to evaluate its performance. Although the ideal situation is to have multiple independent data sets on which to develop, refine, and test a model, these are often not available. Then one must use various strategies to split an existing data set into portions used for model development and portions for model testing. It is advisable to obtain preliminary model performance estimates periodically throughout the model development process to increase the chances that the final model will perform well on an independent data set. Investigators may use data-driven approaches to choose from among multiple models developed using different methods, and within a particular modeling method data are used to estimate precise characteristics of a model, such as regression coefficients or cutpoints for classification. Thus, there are multiple opportunities to tune the model to the data used to build it. Model overfitting occurs when a fitted model is overly complex or when there are very large numbers of features relative to number of independent observations, and the model is fit to noise in the data [75]. An overfit model usually performs poorly on an independent data set. Careful planning of the signature development studies is needed to not be misled about a model's or classifier's performance.

It is well established that using the same data that were used to select and estimate the model to evaluate the model results in optimistic bias in estimates of model performance. The most egregious practice of assessing model performance by inserting into the model exactly the same full data set used to build it is known as resubstitution; this can lead to extremely biased performance estimates, particularly when there are very large numbers of features available for potential inclusion in the model during development. Partial resubstitution is also problematic; this refers to using the full data set for initial selection of features based on their associations with clinical outcome, but using only a portion of the data set to fit model parameters and the remaining portion to test model performance. Surprisingly, the initial use of the full data for feature selection only can still introduce substantial bias in model performance estimates.

The primary way to guard against resubstitution bias in preliminary model performance estimates is to strictly separate the data used to select and estimate the model from that used to evaluate it. This can be done directly, by using one sample to select and estimate a model, and then evaluating that model on a statistically independent sample. If an independent sample is not available, then one can randomly split a single sample into separate training and validation subsets. Common split-sample approaches use 1/2 or 2/3 of the sample for training and the rest for validation. Dobbin and Simon [22] investigate and propose strategies for allocating samples into training and test sets. They conclude that the optimal allocation depends on the number of available subjects and the signal-to-noise ratio of the omics features.

Cross-validation is another approach that can provide unbiased estimates of the expected out-of-sample prediction performance. With cross-validation, the concept of split-sample training and validation is combined with resampling methods. To perform cross-validation we partition the sample into K subsets of approximately size $n/K = k$ where n is the size of the full data set. Then, for $i \in 1, \dots, K$, the ith subset is excluded while the remaining data are used to select and estimate the model. The performance of that model is evaluated on the left-out ith subset. This process is repeated K times to yield K estimates of model performance, which allows for both a point estimate and a standard error for the model performance. This is referred to as "K-fold" or "leave-k-out" cross-validation. The choice of K to use in practice depends on the trade-off between bias and variance of the modeling approach used for the prediction task. If the size of the subsets k is small relative to n (even sets of size 1 can be used, known as "leave-one-out cross-validation"), then the performance estimates will be approximately unbiased but may have high variance because the training sets would be substantially overlapping. If the size of the subsets k is large relative to n, then the training sets would be smaller, potentially increasing the variability in the fitted model and potentially biasing each performance estimate. At each fold of the procedure, it is critical that all of the model selection and estimation steps are repeated, including selection of any tuning parameters involved in the statistical model. Failing to do so would be a variation on partial resubstitution, causing optimistically biased estimates of performance. If the modeling approach is not entirely algorithmic, e.g., if it involves some sort of subjective assessment, then cross-validation could be very difficult to implement properly. Hastie et al. [33], Chapter 7, gives a nice overview of these and related model assessment issues. Pang and Jung [63] compare the properties of the split sample approach to cross-validation and provide some useful considerations for sample size planning of signature development studies.

Bonetti and Gelber [12] describe a graphical approach to determining treatment by signature interactions in the time-to-event setting with a signature that yields a continuous value. They suggest a simple smoothing approach to estimate treatment hazard ratios in subgroups defined by the signature value and then plot the hazard ratios as a function of the signature value. This can be useful for determining whether there is a treatment-by-signature interaction, and, if so, can offer some guidance as to where to set a clinically relevant cutpoint for determination of predicted benefit *versus* predicted no-benefit. Another common approach to cutpoint selection is to simply use the observed median of the signature in the training sample, but this is less desirable because the choice is arbitrary and does not take into account the magnitude or direction of the hazard ratios. It should be appreciated that clinical decisions based on a continuous score near a decision cutpoint are more vulnerable to errors or noise in the omics score contributed by the assay system. For this reason, we advise that continuous signature values be maintained throughout the signature development process and even be included in diagnostic reports, if the signature is eventually used in clinical practice.

5.2.6 Computational Reproducibility

If an omics signature appears to work well, then others will want to evaluate and use it. To facilitate that, the methodology must be reported accurately and with sufficient detail for others to calculate the signature. In addition to supplying protocols for specimen collection and laboratory procedures, it is critical that the computational aspects of the signature calculation are reproducible and well documented. Software is written and used at every stage of the development and evaluation of omics signatures. Statistical software is used to develop the signature, with specialized packages for omics data, and to analyze the results. This aspect of reproducibility is often overlooked but is gaining attention in many scientific fields. The biggest barriers to reproducibility of an omics signature are poor reporting of the methodology [18] and a lack of well-documented code [64]. Wilson et al. [89] outlines some guidelines for scientific computing that are relevant for developing and implementing omics signatures such as using version control, developing automated tests, collaborating, and developing documentation.

Analyses involving omics data involve complex software for processing, normalization, and signature calculation. Some of this software may be custom, require in-depth knowledge of the biology, and may be developed specifically for a given application. Many scientists, however, are self-taught with regard to software development and thus the accuracy, reliability, and transportability of the computational procedures are often left unevaluated [32]. Some computational methods such as determination of starting values or Monte Carlo methods may involve random number generation, which leaves the possibility that identical inputs to the signature calculation may give different results. This can be considered a component of the assay variability, but it is better avoided by specifying random number generator seeds.

Scientific software builds upon existing resources, such as operating systems, standard statistical packages such as `R` [25], and other open-source resources. It is important to clearly document such dependencies, but documentation is not enough. Since cancer clinical trials often take years to complete, dependencies can be updated over that course, fixing bugs, adding features, and removing old features. Any of these changes can potentially alter the results of omics analyses.

Recently, several approaches to managing dependencies have gained attention in the statistical computing literature, mainly in the context of using `R`. Packrat [38] and the Reproducible `R` Toolkit [5] are both `R` packages that create archives of all dependencies used in an analysis. These dependencies can be combined with the resulting analysis to ensure future replication, even if the dependencies change downstream. A more comprehensive approach is Docker [37] which is a general-purpose application that archives a complete computing environment, from the operating system down to the software dependencies. Boettiger [11] gives an overview of using Docker for reproducible science, with again a focus on `R`.

Software-development efforts have been made to encourage researchers to document their entire scientific workflow, from the lab bench to the bedside. Kepler [2] and Taverna [36] are two software packages with graphical user interfaces for documenting workflows. They are flexible tools that enable researchers to document and track data inputs, versioning, processing steps, analysis tools, and outputs in a graphical way.

5.2.7 Practical Considerations

A potentially valuable and useful omics signature can be difficult to implement clinically if there are too many practical barriers. A predictive or prognostic test must be completed in a timely manner in order for it to benefit the patient. Specimen collection, processing, shipping, assay completion, data generation, and computation of the signature must be completed in an acceptable time frame without significantly delaying treatment decisions or causing undue burden on the patient. Signatures that integrate information from multiple platforms can magnify potential delays and costs. Reduction of the number of features going into a signature may be desirable if moving to another assay platform, for example, from gene-expression microarray to multiplex qRT-PCR. This can reduce the cost and the time to run the assay and offer more reliable performance on typical clinical specimens. This practical aspect should also be considered in the model development process when choosing a feature reduction method as data reduction by clustering does not necessarily allow one to reduce the number of features measured.

To meet the clinical requirements in real time, it must be possible and feasible to estimate the signature on a case-by-case basis. Many omics signature calculation methods contain data normalization or pre-processing steps, such as centering features by their sample means, that depend on other specimens run in the same batch. The statistical algorithm may also use information from other specimens in the sample, for example, many clustering algorithms require a group of specimens [85]. Such normalization steps are not acceptable in clinical practice, as assays must be run in real time for a single case in order to avoid lengthy treatment delays. It is possible, however, to have a fixed reference sample in place to be used for these types of pre-processing steps [53, 61].

The expected distribution of the signature groups is an important consideration in planning a definitive validation study. It may be that a signature is highly predictive, but the subgroup expected to benefit from therapy is very rare. In that case, it may be impractical to accrue a sufficient number of study subjects to demonstrate benefit in that subgroup.

5.3 Clinical Utility Assessment

After developing and refining the predictive omics signature and demonstrating preliminary evidence of promising performance by establishing analytic and clinical validity, a final step is to establish clinical utility. Demonstrating clinical utility requires evidence that the use of the signature to guide patient care results in measurable improved clinical outcomes as compared to non-use of the signature [56]. No further refinement to the signature evaluation process is allowed at this phase. Rather, the goal is to obtain an unbiased and sufficiently precise estimate of the performance of the signature in the context of a phase II or III randomized controlled trial. Interpretation and final assessment of whether the signature will be adopted for clinical use is context-dependent and requires expert judgment. We consider mainly the situation in which the intended clinical use of a signature is as a companion diagnostic: to identify a subpopulation that will be treated with a therapy (predicted benefit/test positive) while the remaining subpopulation will receive the standard of care (predicted no benefit/test negative). Signatures that are extremely prognostic may also be clinically useful for guiding therapy, even though they would not be considered a companion diagnostic to any particular treatment.

A variety of study designs exist to evaluate a prognostic or predictive signature [26, 27, 51, 72]. The type of study used to evaluate a particular signature will depend on the level and quality of prior evidence, both empirical and theoretical, supporting its utility. The study should have a clear and comprehensive protocol prespecified, including specimen handling procedures, assay procedures, and statistical analysis plans. Investigators should prespecify a statistic or set of statistics that address the intended clinical use of the signature and conduct a power and sample size analysis to ensure that the study has a high probability of definitively assessing the clinical utility of the signature.

A prognostic signature does not require a randomized controlled trial in order to demonstrate its clinical utility. An observational study in which all subjects receive a standard therapy can be used to demonstrate that a prognostic signature has a strong association with a clinical outcome. However, a strong association with clinical outcome alone does not demonstrate the clinical utility of a prognostic signature. Prognosis can be obtained using standard clinical, pathological, and other existing features, and in order to be useful, a prognostic signature must contain information above and beyond the standard prognostic tools. This is often referred to as the incremental value. Moons et al. [58, 59] provide excellent reviews of the steps in developing and validating a prognostic marker, including assessing the incremental value.

For the evaluation of a potentially predictive signature, the choice of study design depends on the prior evidence supporting the signature in the context of the study population and the treatment options. Each signature will have associated with it a different level of biological understanding, preclinical data, and preliminary clinical evidence. Strong biological and preclinical data may support the use of a signature for guiding a well-understood targeted agent. In settings lacking a strong biological understanding, a large amount of high-quality preliminary clinical data may be needed to support further study. In assessing the prior evidence, it is important to be aware of the quality of the background studies and the validity of the analyses. When evaluating the credentials of a potentially predictive omics-based signature for use in a clinical trial, it is important to carefully consider the pitfalls described in the previous section and elsewhere [18, 75, 92].

5.3.1 How Omics Signatures Are Used in Clinical Trials

Predictive or potentially predictive omics signatures are evaluated by measuring them as pre-treatment baseline variables in randomized controlled trials.

How a signature is precisely evaluated in a trial depends on the level of prior evidence supporting the predictive value of the signature weighted against practical concerns. A signature can be used as an eligibility criterion, wherein patients are screened and have the omics signature measured prior to enrollment. Then only those patients who meet the prespecified definition for predicted benefit would be enrolled in the trial. This is called an **enrichment design** and while it can be more efficient than a non-enrichment design, it does not generate any evidence for the efficacy of treatment in any other subpopulation [26].

A omics-based signature lacking very strong credentials may instead be used as a stratification factor in a clinical trial conducted in a broad patient population, with the intent to determine whether the treatment effect differs across signature subgroups. Stratification ensures that the distribution of the signature subgroups is balanced over the treatment arms, which prevents a loss of efficiency if the signature turns out to be highly predictive of treatment response [94]. For large trials, there is little risk of a loss of efficiency due to imbalance. The rule of thumb is several hundred participants or more, although that depends on the number and size of the strata [62].

The stratified design requires that the specimen needed for the omics assay be gathered from a patient prior to enrollment, the assay run, the signature calculated, and then the patient randomized conditionally on their omics signature value. This adds risk to the patients if treatment is delayed due to the extra time needed to perform these steps, and costs to running the trial. For larger trials in which there is little risk of imbalance over treatment arms and where it is elected to perform the omics assay after randomization, the omics signature may simply be a baseline measurement that does not affect the conduct of the trial. Again, the intent of the analysis at the end of the trial is to determine whether the treatment effect differs by the omics signature. The practical difference is that the omics signature may be calculated at any time prior to the analysis, as long as the tissue that goes into the assay is collected at baseline prior to treatment and comparable assay results are obtained whether the specimen is fresh or has been stored. Note, however, that in order to be implemented in clinical use, it must be feasible to evaluate the signature (including running the assay) in real time.

The omics analysis may even be conducted retrospectively on stored specimens, even if the omics signature evaluation was not pre-planned at the start of the trial. If a rigorous protocol for signature evaluation is prespecified and followed then a high level of evidence supporting the signature can be generated [76]. This is not license to conduct a multitude of exploratory analyses and call a positive result confirmatory.

Regardless of whether the omics signature is used as a trial enrichment criteria, stratification factor, or baseline measurement, the end goal is to examine the associations among the treatment, the signature, and clinical outcome. There are many analytic approaches that one can take, including simple stratified analyses, group sequential designs, and adaptive approaches. The choice of specific study design depends on the clinical question of interest and the biological and empirical evidence regarding the omics signature. For details on the specific study designs, we refer readers to Chapter 13.

5.3.2 Evaluating Clinical Utility

A signature is predictive if the effect of a therapy depends on the signature value. The degree to which the treatment effect differs determines the clinical utility of the signature. How do we quantify this? Generally speaking, most phase III clinical trials in oncology have some survival outcome (e.g., overall survival, disease-free survival) as the primary outcome. The most direct way to visualize the predictive value of a signature, and the one advocated by Polley et al. [68], is to plot survival curves by treatment arm and by signature subgroups (i.e., predicted benefit *versus* predicted no benefit or harm). Since the goal is to compare the treatment effect across signature groups, it is best to have panels separately by signature group, keeping the comparison by treatment arm within panel. An example of this is depicted in the top plot of Figure 5.3. The viewer can assess the treatment effect in a familiar way to determine whether the difference in treatment effect by signature group is sufficient for clinical use. Along with such a plot, hazard ratios for treatment (with confidence intervals) within each of the signature strata should be presented. In an appropriate context, the plot provides sufficient information to determine whether the use of the signature would lead to different treatment decisions. These plots do assume an existing dichomization of the signature. Altering the signature cutpoints could change the impression of the predictive value of the signature.

Survival outcomes can be dichotomized, as we show in the middle plot of Figure 5.3, to highlight the differences in treatment effect for a clinical outcome such as death or recurrence within a specified time period, 5 years or 10 years, for example. The impression of the predictive value of the signature may change depending on the choice of time cutpoint. In the case where the signature is continuous-valued, such as a risk score for treatment benefit, Janes et al. [40] describe several ways to assess the differences in treatment effect by signature value. One example is shown in the bottom panel of Figure 5.3, which shows the estimated risk along the y-axis versus the signature percentile on the x-axis, by treatment group. The crossing curves show a gradient of treatment effect differences, with the new treatment being less effective than standard below the 25-th signature percentile, and beneficial above the 25-th percentile. Plots showing treatment effect differences paired with inference and appropriate context are the best way to make a judgment about clinical utility. The complexity of predictive signatures makes it difficult to capture the results in a single metric in a clinically meaningful way.

Many investigators choose to perform statistical tests of the treatment by signature interaction in a Cox regression model. A p-value that is less than 0.05 is then incorrectly used as evidence of the predictive value and thus clin-

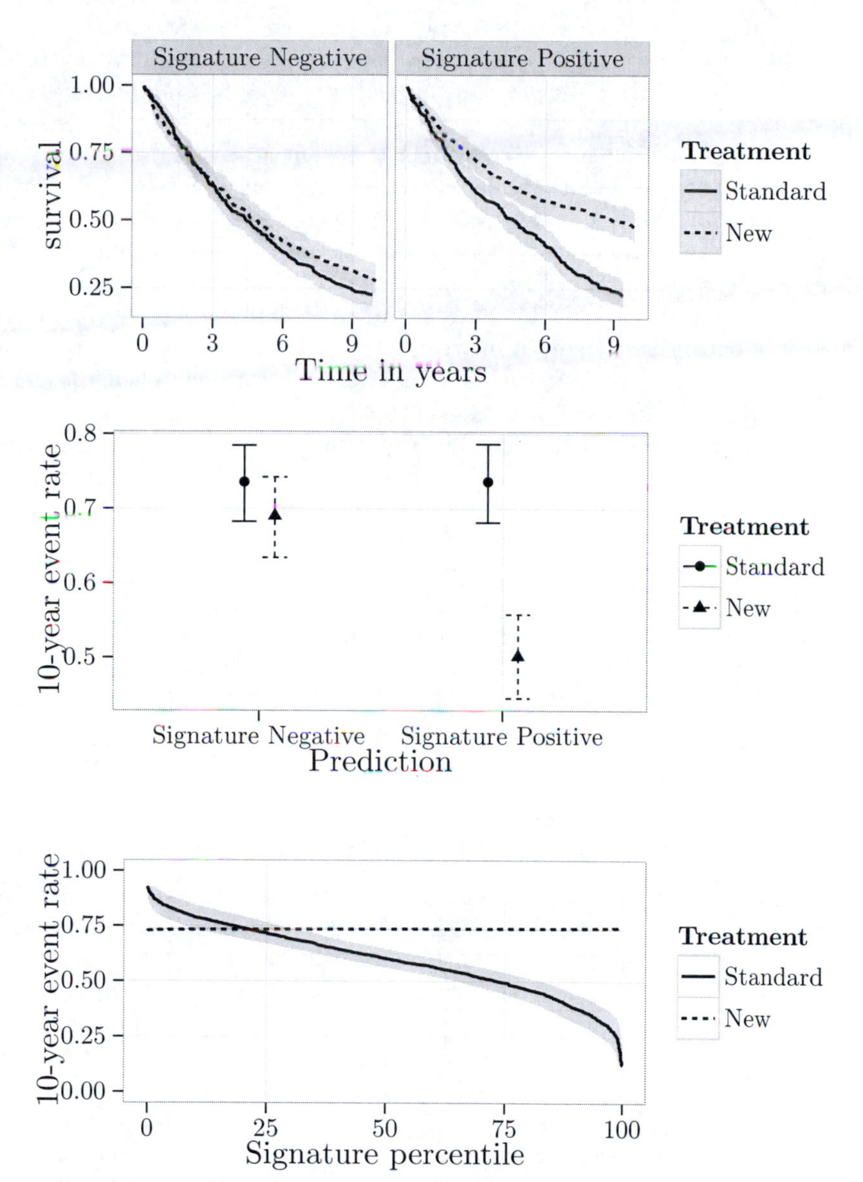

FIGURE 5.3: Three ways to visualize clinical utility of a predictive signature. The top plot shows survival curves by treatment group and by signature group (predicted no benefit vs predicted benefit). The middle plot shows the estimated 10-year event probabilities by the same strata. The bottom plot shows the predicted 10-year risk by percentiles of a continuous valued signature, by treatment group.

ical utility of the signature for therapy selection. The existence of a treatment by signature interaction is necessary but not sufficient for the signature to be clinically useful in guiding therapy [68]. However it may be difficult to detect such an interaction because clinical trials designed to evaluate treatment differences are generally not powered sufficiently to detect interactions with treatment. It is possible for the treatment to be efficacious in both groups but to a different degree. For example, a randomized study of pazopanib versus placebo on progression-free survival in renal cell carcinoma patients looked at the difference in treatment effect by serum concentration of interleukin 6 (IL-6) [86]. Pazopanib was clearly beneficial, with a hazard ratio of 0.31 (0.31 to 0.58) in the high IL-6 group and a hazard ratio of 0.55 (0.28 to 0.71) in the low IL-6 group. This difference in treatment effect (interaction) was statistically significant ($p = 0.009$), yet it is clear that the treatment choice would be for pazopanib regardless of IL-6 concentration. This is called a quantitative interaction because the effect goes in the same direction, but has different magnitudes. Quantitative interactions may still be clinically useful for therapy selection if there are concerns about significant toxicity of the agent. The clinical interpretation is much more clear with qualitative interactions, in which the new treatment is beneficial in one group and inferior or similar to new treatment in the other group. If the treatment is sufficiently beneficial in a signature-determined subgroup (which may depend on the context), then the clinical use for therapy selection is clear: treat those in the signature subgroup predicted to benefit. Critical examination of the distribution of the treatment effects in all signature-defined subgroups and context-appropriate clinical judgment are essential for proper evaluation of clinical utility.

5.3.3 Power and Sample Size Considerations

For enrichment designs, the primary hypothesis test is concerned with estimating the treatment effect in the eligible subgroup. Therefore, if the expected proportion of the population eligible for the trial is known, then standard approaches to estimating power and sample size in clinical trials apply in that case. Maitournam and Simon [50] studied the efficiency of enrichment designs relative to stratified or all-comers designs. They found that the relative efficiency depends on the prevalence of the eligible population and the treatment effect in the ineligible population. Successfully enrolling the target number of eligible patients requires screening more subjects by gathering specimens, running assays, and computing results in order to identify the eligible subgroup. These additional costs must be considered in the planning of a prospective trial. While the total number of subjects required may be smaller, the time it takes to screen and enroll subjects means that it might require more resources compared to an all-comers design.

For stratified or all-comers designs, it is slightly more complicated to determine power and sample size because addressing the question of predictiveness requires multiple tests and/or non-standard methods. Many phase III all-comers designs incorporating predictive signatures are designed to power the test of a treatment by signature interaction effect [71]. As we described above, an interaction can be qualitative or quantitative, therefore this approach of sizing a study for any interaction effect does not directly address the question of clinical utility. Polley et al. [68] show examples of biomarkers that have significant interactions with treatment but would not be considered clinically useful because the treatment is still sufficiently useful in every subgroup. Statistical methods exist to test for qualitative interaction and have a fairly long history in subgroup analysis [9, 21, 28]. Therefore, if an investigator is able to specify a threshold for the treatment effect, under which it would not be considered useful to apply the therapy, then these methods can be used to size a study to address the clinical aim. Mackey and Bengtsson [49] suggest an alternative, sequential testing approach of the three questions: (i) Do any patients benefit from the treatment?; (ii) Do any patients not benefit from the treatment?; and (iii) What is the biomarker threshold (if applicable)? These questions clearly address the clinical aim; however, this approach has not formally been compared to other strategies. Janes et al. [41] discuss the different study designs and sample size requirements for evaluating treatment selection biomarkers using different criteria.

5.4 Summary

Predictive signatures are used in oncology for investigating treatment benefits in relation to the signature value with the ultimate goal of using the signature to guide therapy, thereby improving patient outcome. Signatures do not always work well in practice; thus they must be properly validated. As illustrated by the discussions in this chapter, there are many aspects to validation, including analytic validity, clinical validity, and clinical utility. Achieving all three may require a lengthy iterative process. Altman and Royston [3] provide an excellent discussion of similar issues in the context of prognostic models. A quote from Altman and Royston [3] is apt in the predictive setting as well (p. 463): "Focus on clinically relevant measures that quantify the performance of a model and accept that the final assessment requires clinical judgment and is context-dependent." The development of a signature for treatment selection requires a thoughtful development plan, careful execution to avoid pitfalls, and a strong interdisciplinary team involved in every step to ensure that the final signature is fit for the intended clinical use.

Bibliography

[1] A. A. Alizadeh, M. B. Eisen, R. E. Davis, C. Ma, I. S. Lossos, A. Rosenwald, J. C. Boldrick, H. Sabet, T. Tran, X. Yu, et al. Distinct types of diffuse large b-cell lymphoma identified by gene expression profiling. *Nature*, 403(6769):503–511, 2000.

[2] I. Altintas, C. Berkley, E. Jaeger, M. Jones, B. Ludascher, and S. Mock. Kepler: an extensible system for design and execution of scientific workflows. In *Proceedings. 16th International Conference on Scientific and Statistical Database Management 2004*, pages 423–424. IEEE, 2004.

[3] D. G. Altman and P. Royston. What do we mean by validating a prognostic model? *Statistics in Medicine*, 19(4):453–473, 2000.

[4] N. S. Altman. An introduction to kernel and nearest-neighbor nonparametric regression. *American Statistician*, 46(3):175–185, 1992.

[5] Revolution Analytics. Reproducible R Toolkit, 2014. http://projects.revolutionanalytics.com/documents/rrt/rrtpkgs/.

[6] E. Bair, T. Hastie, D. Paul, and R. Tibshirani. Prediction by supervised principal components. *Journal of the American Statistical Association*, 101(473):119–137, 2006.

[7] E. Bair and R. Tibshirani. Semi-supervised methods to predict patient survival from gene expression data. *PLoS Biology*, 2(4):e108, 2004.

[8] T. T. Batchelor, D. A. Reardon, W. Wick, and M. Weller. Antiangiogenic therapy for glioblastoma: current status and future prospects. *Clinical Cancer Research*, 20(22):5612–5619, 2014.

[9] E. O. Bayman, K. Chaloner, and M. K. Cowles. Detecting qualitative interaction: A Bayesian approach. *Statistics in Medicine*, 29(4):455–463, 2010.

[10] J. Bien, J. Taylor, and R. Tibshirani. A lasso for hierarchical interactions. *Annals of Statistics*, 41(3):1111–1141, 2013.

[11] C. Boettiger. An introduction to Docker for reproducible research, with examples from the R environment, 2014. http://arxiv.org/abs/1410.0846.

[12] M. Bonetti and R. D. Gelber. A graphical method to assess treatment-covariate interactions using the Cox model on subsets of the data. *Statistics in Medicine*, 19(19):2595–2609, 2000.

[13] L. Breiman. Random forests. *Machine learning*, 45(1):5–32, 2001.

[14] L. Breiman, J. Friedman, C. J. Stone, and R. A. Olshen. *Classification and Regression Trees.* CRC Press, 1984.

[15] D. M. Carrick, M. G. Mehaffey, M. C. Sachs, S. Altekruse, C. Camalier, R. Chuaqui, W. Cozen, B. Das, B. Y. Hernandez, C-J. Lih, et al. Robustness of next generation sequencing on older formalin-fixed paraffin-embedded tissue. *PloS One*, 10(7), 2015.

[16] B. Choodari-Oskooei, P. Royston, and M. K. B. Parmar. A simulation study of predictive ability measures in a survival model I: explained variation measures. *Statistics in Medicine*, 31(23):2627–2643, 2012.

[17] B. Choodari-Oskooei, P. Royston, and M. K. B. Parmar. A simulation study of predictive ability measures in a survival model II: explained randomness and predictive accuracy. *Statistics in Medicine*, 31(23):2644–2659, 2012.

[18] G. S. Collins, S. Dutton, O. Omar, M. Shanyinde, A. Tajar, M. Voysey, R. Wharton, L. Yu, K. G. Moons, et al. External validation of multivariable prediction models: a systematic review of methodological conduct and reporting. *BMC Medical Research Methodology*, 14(1):40, 2014.

[19] C. Cortes and V. Vapnik. Support-vector networks. *Machine Learning*, 20(3):273–297, 1995.

[20] M. Cronin, C. Sangli, M. Liu, M. Pho, D. Dutta, A. Nguyen, J. Jeong, J. Wu, K. C. Langone, and D. Watson. Analytical validation of the oncotype dx genomic diagnostic test for recurrence prognosis and therapeutic response prediction in node-negative, estrogen receptor-positive breast cancer. *Clinical Chemistry*, 53(6):1084–1091, 2007.

[21] D. O. Dixon and R. Simon. Bayesian subset analysis. *Biometrics*, 47(3):871–881, 1991.

[22] K. K. Dobbin and R. M. Simon. Optimally splitting cases for training and testing high dimensional classifiers. *BMC Medical Genomics*, 4(1):31, 2011.

[23] S. Faivre, S. Djelloul, and E. Raymond. New paradigms in anticancer therapy: targeting multiple signaling pathways with kinase inhibitors. *Seminars in Oncology*, 33(4):407–420, 2006.

[24] M. Filipits, M. Rudas, R. Jakesz, P. Dubsky, F. Fitzal, C. F. Singer, O. Dietze, R. Greil, A. Jelen, P. Sevelda, et al. A new molecular predictor of distant recurrence in er-positive, her2-negative breast cancer adds independent information to conventional clinical risk factors. *Clinical Cancer Research*, 17(18):6012–6020, 2011.

[25] The R Project for Statistical Computing. *R: A Language and Environment for Statistical Computing.* R Foundation for Statistical Computing, Vienna, Austria, 2014.

[26] B. Freidlin and E. L. Korn. Biomarker enrichment strategies: matching trial design to biomarker credentials. *Nature Reviews Clinical Oncology*, 11(2):81–90, 2014.

[27] B. Freidlin, L. M. McShane, and E. L. Korn. Randomized clinical trials with biomarkers: design issues. *Journal of the National Cancer Institute*, 102(3):152–160, 2010.

[28] M. Gail and R. Simon. Testing for qualitative interactions between treatment effects and patient subsets. *Biometrics*, 41(2):361–372, 1985.

[29] A. Gelman and H. Stern. The difference between significant and not significant is not itself statistically significant. *American Statistician*, 60(4):328–331, 2006.

[30] A. W. Griffioen, A. Weiss, R. H. Berndsen, U. K. Abdul, M. T. Te Winkel, and P. Nowak-Sliwinska. The emerging quest for the optimal angiostatic combination therapy. *Biochemical Society Transactions*, 42(6):1608–1615, 2014.

[31] M. Hammond and S. E. Taube. Issues and barriers to development of clinically useful tumor markers: a development pathway proposal. In *Seminars in Oncology*, volume 29(3), pages 213–221. Elsevier, 2002.

[32] J. E. Hannay, C. MacLeod, J. Singer, H. P. Langtangen, D. Pfahl, and G. Wilson. How do scientists develop and use scientific software? In *Proceedings of the 2009 ICSE workshop on Software Engineering for Computational Science and Engineering*, pages 1–8. IEEE Computer Society, 2009.

[33] T. J. Hastie, R. J. Tibshirani, and J. H. Friedman. *The Elements of Statistical Learning: Data Mining, Inference, and Prediction.* Springer, New York, NY, USA, 2013.

[34] A. E. Hoerl and R. W. Kennard. Ridge regression: biased estimation for nonorthogonal problems. *Technometrics*, 12(1):55–67, 1970.

[35] J. A. Hoeting, D. Madigan, A. E. Raftery, and C. T. Volinsky. Bayesian model averaging: a tutorial. *Statistical Science*, 14(4):382–401, 1999.

[36] D. Hull, K. Wolstencroft, R. Stevens, C. Goble, M. R. Pocock, P. Li, and T. Oinn. Taverna: a tool for building and running workflows of services. *Nucleic Acids Research*, 34(suppl 2):W729–W732, 2006.

[37] Docker Inc. Build, ship and run any app, anywhere, 2014. http://www.docker.com.

[38] Rstudio Inc. Reproducible Package Management for R, 2014. http://rstudio.github.io/packrat.

[39] K. S. Iwamoto, T. Mizuno, T. Ito, M. Akiyama, N. Takeichi, K. Mabuchi, and T. Seyama. Feasibility of using decades-old archival tissues in molecular oncology/epidemiology. *American Journal of Pathology*, 149(2):399–406, 1996.

[40] H. Janes, M. D. Brown, Y. Huang, and M. S. Pepe. An approach to evaluating and comparing biomarkers for patient treatment selection. *International Journal of Biostatistics*, 10(1):99–121, 2014.

[41] H. Janes, M. D. Brown, and M. S. Pepe. Designing a study to evaluate the benefit of a biomarker for selecting patient treatment. *Statistics in Medicine*, 34(27):3503–3515, 2015.

[42] H. Janes, M. S. Pepe, P. M. Bossuyt, and W. E. Barlow. Measuring the performance of markers for guiding treatment decisions. *Annals of Internal Medicine*, 154(4):253–259, 2011.

[43] L. Jennings, L. Jennings, and M. L. Gulley. Recommended principles and practices for validating clinical molecular pathology tests. *Archives of Pathology & Laboratory Medicine*, 133(5):743–755, 2009.

[44] D. D. Lee and H. S. Seung. Learning the parts of objects by non-negative matrix factorization. *Nature*, 401(6755):788–791, 1999.

[45] J. T. Leek, R. B. Scharpf, H. C. Bravo, D. Simcha, B. Langmead, W. E. Johnson, D. Geman, K. Baggerly, and R. A. Irizarry. Tackling the widespread and critical impact of batch effects in high-throughput data. *Nature Reviews Genetics*, 11(10):733–739, 2010.

[46] M. Lim and T. Hastie. Learning interactions through hierarchical group-lasso regularization. *arXiv preprint arXiv:1308.2719*, 2013.

[47] R. J. A. Little and D. B. Rubin. *Statistical Analysis with Missing Data, 2nd Edition.* John Wiley & Sons, Inc., 2002.

[48] J. Luo, X. Guo, X. Tang, X. Sun, Z. Yang, Y. Zhang, L. Dai, and G. L. Warnock. Intravital biobank and personalized cancer therapy: the correlation with omics. *International Journal of Cancer*, 135(7):1511–1516, 2013.

[49] H. M. Mackey and T. Bengtsson. Sample size and threshold estimation for clinical trials with predictive biomarkers. *Contemporary Clinical Trials*, 36(2):664–672, 2013.

[50] A. Maitournam and R. Simon. On the efficiency of targeted clinical trials. *Statistics in Medicine*, 24(3):329–339, 2005.

[51] S. J. Mandrekar and D. J. Sargent. Clinical trial designs for predictive biomarker validation: theoretical considerations and practical challenges. *Journal of Clinical Oncology*, 27(24):4027–4034, 2009.

[52] J. C. Marioni, C. E. Mason, S. M. Mane, M. Stephens, and Y. Gilad. Rna-seq: an assessment of technical reproducibility and comparison with gene expression arrays. *Genome Research*, 18(9):1509–1517, 2008.

[53] M. N. McCall, B. M. Bolstad, and R. A. Irizarry. Frozen robust multiarray analysis (frma). *Biostatistics*, 11(2):242–253, 2010.

[54] L. M. McShane, M. M. Cavenagh, T. G. Lively, D. A. Eberhard, W. L. Bigbee, P. M. Williams, J. P. Mesirov, M. C. Polley, K. Y. Kim, J. V. Tricoli, et al. Criteria for the use of omics-based predictors in clinical trials. *Nature*, 502(7471):317–320, 2013.

[55] L. M. McShane, M. M. Cavenagh, T. G. Lively, D. A. Eberhard, W. L. Bigbee, P. M. Williams, J. P. Mesirov, M. C. Polley, K. Y. Kim, J. V. Tricoli, et al. Criteria for the use of omics-based predictors in clinical trials: explanation and elaboration. *BMC Medicine*, 11(220):doi:10.1186/1741–7015–11–220, 2013.

[56] L. M. McShane and D. F. Hayes. Publication of tumor marker research results: The necessity for complete and transparent reporting. *Journal of Clinical Oncology*, 30(34):4223–4232, 2012.

[57] C. M. Micheel, S. J. Nass, G. S. Omenn, et al. *Evolution of Translational Omics: Lessons Learned and the Path Forward.* National Academies Press, Washington, D.C., 2012.

[58] K. G. M. Moons, A. P. Kengne, D. E. Grobbee, P. Royston, Y. Vergouwe, D. G. Altman, and M. Woodward. Risk prediction models: II. External validation, model updating, and impact assessment. *Heart*, pages heartjnl–2011, 2012.

[59] K. G. M. Moons, A. P. Kengne, M. Woodward, P. Royston, Y. Vergouwe, D. G. Altman, and D. E. Grobbee. Risk prediction models: I. Development, internal validation, and assessing the incremental value of a new (bio) marker. *Heart*, 98(9):683–690, 2012.

[60] T. Nielsen, B. Wallden, C. Schaper, S. Ferree, S. Liu, D. Gao, G. Barry, N. Dowidar, M. Maysuria, and J. Storhoff. Analytical validation of the pam50-based prosigna breast cancer prognostic gene signature assay and ncounter analysis system using formalin-fixed paraffin-embedded breast tumor specimens. *BMC Cancer*, 14(1):177, 2014.

[61] K. Owzar, W. T. Barry, S. Jung, I. Sohn, and S. L. George. Statistical challenges in preprocessing in microarray experiments in cancer. *Clinical Cancer Research*, 14(19):5959–5966, 2008.

[62] M. Palta. Investigating maximum power losses in survival studies with nonstratified randomization. *Biometrics*, 41(2):497–504, 1985.

[63] H. Pang and S. Jung. Sample size considerations of prediction-validation methods in high-dimensional data for survival outcomes. *Genetic Epidemiology*, 37(3):276–282, 2013.

[64] R. D. Peng. Reproducible research in computational science. *Science*, 334(6060):1226–1227, 2011.

[65] G. A. Pennello. Analytical and clinical evaluation of biomarkers assays: when are biomarkers ready for prime time? *Clinical Trials*, 10(5):653–665, 2013.

[66] M. S. Pepe, R. Etzioni, Z. Feng, J. D. Potter, M. L. Thompson, M. Thornquist, M. Winget, and Y. Yasui. Phases of biomarker development for early detection of cancer. *Journal of the National Cancer Institute*, 93(14):1054–1061, 2001.

[67] M. S. Pepe, H. Janes, G. Longton, W. Leisenring, and P. Newcomb. Limitations of the odds ratio in gauging the performance of a diagnostic, prognostic, or screening marker. *American Journal of Epidemiology*, 159(9):882–890, 2004.

[68] M. C. Polley, B. Freidlin, E. L. Korn, B. A. Conley, J. S. Abrams, and L. M. McShane. Statistical and practical considerations for clinical evaluation of predictive biomarkers. *Journal of the National Cancer Institute*, 105(22):1677–1683, 2013.

[69] H. Rodriguez, Ž. Težak, M. Mesri, S. A. Carr, D. C. Liebler, S. J. Fisher, P. Tempst, T. Hiltke, L. G. Kessler, C. R. Kinsinger, et al. Analytical validation of protein-based multiplex assays: a workshop report by the NCI-FDA interagency oncology task force on molecular diagnostics. *Clinical Chemistry*, 56(2):237–243, 2010.

[70] P. Royston, M. K. Parmar, and D. G. Altman. Visualizing length of survival in time-to-event studies: a complement to Kaplan-Meier plots. *Journal of the National Cancer Institute*, 100(2):92–97, 2008.

[71] P. Royston and W. Sauerbrei. Interactions between treatment and continuous covariates: a step toward individualizing therapy. *Journal of Clinical Oncology*, 26(9):1397–1399, 2008.

[72] D. J. Sargent, B. A. Conley, C. Allegra, and L. Collette. Clinical trial designs for predictive marker validation in cancer treatment trials. *Journal of Clinical Oncology*, 23(9):2020–2027, 2005.

[73] L. Shi, L. H. Reid, W. D. Jones, R. Shippy, J. A. Warrington, S. C.

Baker, P. J. Collins, F. de Longueville, E. S. Kawasaki, et al. The microarray quality control (maqc) project shows inter-and intraplatform reproducibility of gene expression measurements. *Nature Biotechnology*, 24(9):1151–1161, 2006.

[74] R. Simon and D. G. Altman. Statistical aspects of prognostic factor studies in oncology. *British Journal of Cancer*, 69(6):979, 1994.

[75] R. Simon, M. D. Radmacher, K. Dobbin, and L. M. McShane. Pitfalls in the use of DNA microarray data for diagnostic and prognostic classification. *Journal of the National Cancer Institute*, 95(1):14–18, 2003.

[76] R. M. Simon, S. Paik, and D. F. Hayes. Use of archived specimens in evaluation of prognostic and predictive biomarkers. *Journal of the National Cancer Institute*, 101(21):1446–1452, 2009.

[77] J. A. Sparano, R. J. Gray, D. F. Makower, K. I. Pritchard, K. S. Albain, D. F. Hayes, C. E. Geyer, Jr., E. C. Dees, E. A. Perez, J. A. Olson, et al. Prospective validation of a 21-gene expression assay in breast cancer. *New England Journal of Medicine*, 373(21):2005–2014, 2015.

[78] J. A. Sparano and S. Paik. Development of the 21-gene assay and its application in clinical practice and clinical trials. *Journal of Clinical Oncology*, 26(5):721–728, 2008.

[79] K. Specht, T. Richter, U. Müller, A. Walch, M. Werner, and H. Höfler. Quantitative gene expression analysis in microdissected archival formalin-fixed and paraffin-embedded tumor tissue. *American Journal of Pathology*, 158(2):419–429, 2001.

[80] M. Srinivasan, D. Sedmak, and S. Jewell. Effect of fixatives and tissue processing on the content and integrity of nucleic acids. *American Journal of Pathology*, 161(6):1961–1971, 2002.

[81] G. Sun, T. L. Shook, and G. L. Kay. Inappropriate use of bivariable analysis to screen risk factors for use in multivariable analysis. *Journal of Clinical Epidemiology*, 49(8):907–916, 1996.

[82] J. J. Tentler, A. C. Tan, C. D. Weekes, A. Jimeno, S. Leong, T. M. Pitts, J. J. Arcaroli, W. A. Messersmith, and S. G. Eckhardt. Patient-derived tumour xenografts as models for oncology drug development. *Nature Reviews Clinical Oncology*, 9(6):338–350, 2012.

[83] S. M. Teutsch, L. A. Bradley, G. E. Palomaki, J. E. Haddow, M. Piper, N. Calonge, W. D. Dotson, M. P. Douglas, and A. O. Berg. The Evaluation of Genomic Applications in Practice and Prevention (EGAPP) initiative: methods of the EGAPP working group. *Genetics in Medicine*, 11(1):3–14, 2009.

[84] R. Tibshirani. Regression shrinkage and selection via the lasso. *Journal of the Royal Statistical Society: Series B*, 58(1):267–288, 1996.

[85] R. Tibshirani, T. Hastie, B. Narasimhan, and G. Chu. Class prediction by nearest shrunken centroids, with applications to DNA microarrays. *Statistical Science*, 18(1):104–117, 2003.

[86] H. T. Tran, Y. Liu, A. J. Zurita, Y. Lin, K. L. Baker-Neblett, A. Martin, R. A. Figlin, T. E. Hutson, C. N. Sternberg, R. G. Amado, et al. Prognostic or predictive plasma cytokines and angiogenic factors for patients treated with pazopanib for metastatic renal-cell cancer: a retrospective analysis of phase 2 and phase 3 trials. *Lancet Oncology*, 13(8):827–837, 2012.

[87] F. van Maldegem, M. de Wit, F. Morsink, A. Musler, J. Weegenaar, and C. J. M. van Noesel. Effects of processing delay, formalin fixation, and immunohistochemistry on RNA recovery from formalin-fixed paraffin-embedded tissue sections. *Diagnostic Molecular Pathology*, 17(1):51–58, 2008.

[88] T. Voskoglou-Nomikos, J. L. Pater, and L. Seymour. Clinical predictive value of the in vitro cell line, human xenograft, and mouse allograft preclinical cancer models. *Clinical Cancer Research*, 9(11):4227–4239, 2003.

[89] G. Wilson, D. A. Aruliah, C. T. Brown, M. Davis, R. T. Guy, S. H. D. Haddock, K. D. Huff, I. M. Mitchell, M. D. Plumbley, et al. Best practices for scientific computing. *PLoS Biology*, 12(1):e1001745, 2014.

[90] D. M. Witten and R. Tibshirani. Testing significance of features by lassoed principal components. *Annals of Applied Statistics*, 2(3):986–1012, 2008.

[91] J. Wittes. Times to event: why are they hard to visualize? *Journal of the National Cancer Institute*, 100(2):80–81, 2008.

[92] N. R. Wray, J. Yang, B. J. Hayes, A. L. Price, M. E. Goddard, and P. M. Visscher. Pitfalls of predicting complex traits from SNPs. *Nature Reviews Genetics*, 14(7):507–515, 2013.

[93] K. Y. Yeung, R. E. Bumgarner, and A. E. Raftery. Bayesian model averaging: development of an improved multi-class, gene selection and classification tool for microarray data. *Bioinformatics*, 21(10):2394–2402, 2005.

[94] M. Zelen. The randomization and stratification of patients to clinical trials. *Journal of Chronic Diseases*, 27(7):365–375, 1974.

[95] H. Zou and T. Hastie. Regularization and variable selection via the elastic net. *Journal of the Royal Statistical Society: Series B*, 67(2):301–320, 2005.

6

Phase I Trials and Dose-finding

Mark R. Conaway

Nolan A. Wages

CONTENTS

6.1 Background

The primary goal of phase I trials involving cytotoxic agents in oncology is to find the "maximum tolerated dose" (MTD). The MTD is defined as the greatest dose that can be administered to patients with an 'acceptable' level of toxicity. The amount of toxicity at a given dose levels is considered 'acceptable' if the proportion of patients treated at that dose who experience a 'dose-limiting toxicity' (DLT) is less than or equal to a target level of toxicity, usually in the range of 20% to 33%. The definition of a DLT is study specific, and depends on the type of agent being studied.

The majority of statistical designs for these trials focus on choosing an MTD from among a discrete set of pre-chosen dose levels. Each patient is given a single dose level and is observed on a binary outcome specifying whether or not the patient experienced a DLT. Most of the methods for phase I trials were developed with cytotoxic agents in mind, where it is assumed that the probability of toxicity increases with dose. To avoid exposing patients to excessive risks of toxicity, dose levels are allocated to patients sequentially, with a dose level administered to a patient only if there is evidence that dose levels less than the current dose have acceptable levels of toxicity.

The statistical design revolves around two questions: 1) how should doses be allocated to patients as the trial proceeds? and 2) at the end of the trial, what dose should be nominated as the MTD? There are, of course, many other clinical and statistical issues to be made in carrying out a phase I trial, including the choice of dose levels and the definition of a DLT [83]. This chapter focuses primarily on the statistical issues of dose allocation and estimation of the MTD at the end of the study.

This chapter will begin with a discussion of methods for the classical problem of choosing the MTD from a prespecified set of doses, with a binary measure of toxicity, and with the assumption of increasing probability of toxicity with increasing dose. The chapter will then discuss methods that relax one or more of these assumptions, and present methods for dose-finding studies with time-to-event outcomes or ordinal, rather than binary, measures of toxicity. The chapter will also present methods for trials in which more than one endpoint, such as toxicity and efficacy, is of interest, and for studies in which the strict monotonicity assumptions of the classical phase I trial may not hold. Relaxing the monotonicity assumption is required in studies of combinations of agents, in studies with heterogeneous groups of patients, and studies of non-cytotoxic agents.

6.2 Methods for a Single Cytotoxic Agent

In the standard statistical set-up, the MTD is to be chosen from a prespecified set of doses, $d_1 < d_2 < \cdots < d_K$, with the probability that a patient given dose level d_k experiences a DLT denoted by π_k. The majority of design methods are based on the assumption that the probability of a DLT increases with dose, $\pi_1 < \pi_2 < \ldots < \pi_K$. At any point in the trial, we will have observed a number of patients, n_k treated at dose level d_k, and of the patients treated, Y_k have experienced a DLT, $Y_k = 0, 1, \ldots, n_k$, and $k = 1, 2, \ldots, K$. The target level of toxicity is denoted by θ.

Methods in this situation are often broadly categorized as 'rule-based,' in which the dose chosen for the current patient is based on the observed number of toxicities in the cohort of patients treated at the next lower dose, or 'model-based,' in which an assumed parametric model is fit to all the accumulated data and used to guide dose allocation and the estimation of the MTD [48]. In practice, the distinction between rule-based and model-based is not completely clear, as there are methods that use rule-based allocation [43, 87, 88, 114] but use a parametric model or isotonic regression at the end of the trial to estimate the MTD. Other methods [84, 101] are model-based, but start with an initial rule-based stage before using the parametric model to guide the allocation of doses to patients and to estimate the MTD. In this chapter, we will generally categorize methods as rule-based or model-based depending on how patients are allocated to doses.

6.2.1 Rule-based Designs

6.2.1.1 The Standard or 3+3 Design

The most commonly used design in applications is the '3+3' design. Rogatko et al. [82] reviewed phase I clinical trials reported over a 15-year period, from 1991 – 2006 and found that 98% of these trials used some version of the 3+3 design. The version of this design described in [41] bases dose escalation on cohorts of 3 patients enrolled at the current dose. If 0 of the 3 patients experience a DLT, a cohort of 3 patients is enrolled at the next higher dose level. If 1 of the 3 patients experiences a DLT, an additional 3 patients are enrolled at the current dose level; if none of the additional 3 patients experiences a DLT, dose escalation occurs, with the next cohort of 3 patients treated at the next higher dose. If 1 or more of the additional patients has a DLT, dose escalation is stopped and the current dose is labeled the 'maximally administered dose.' If there are only 3 patients observed on the dose immediately below the maximally administered dose, an additional 3 patients are enrolled on the lower dose. When the trial ends, the MTD is usually taken as the highest dose level below the maximally administered dose that has 1 or fewer patients observed to have a DLT. Special consideration needs to be given when the maximally administered dose is the lowest dose level; in this case, the trial may be stopped and all dose levels under consideration declared as 'too toxic,' or more commonly, additional dose levels are added to the trial. Similarly, if the design calls for dose escalation above the greatest prespecified level, the MTD may be taken as the highest level, or additional dose levels may be added.

Despite the prevalence of its use in applications, the 3+3 is generally dismissed in the statistical literature for its poor operating characteristics. Lin and Shih [53] provide an in-depth evaluation of the properties of algorithmic designs in general, including the 3+3 design. The authors present results for 3 scenarios, each with 5 dose levels, and show that if the target toxicity were 25%, the percent of times that the 3+3 correctly selected the true MTD was only 26%, 30%, and 29% in the 3 scenarios. Given that choosing a dose at random, without even doing a trial, would recommend the correct MTD 20% of the time, the results for the 3+3 design are not impressive. Lin and Shih also demonstrate that despite the perception that the 3+3 targets the dose with a 1/3 probability of a DLT, the 3+3 design does not have a fixed target toxicity level.

6.2.1.2 Storer's 2-s tage Designs

Storer [87] provided the first comprehensive study of the statistical properties of the 3+3 design and suggested several alternative rule-based methods for allocating patients to doses. Several of these suggestions are used in other rule-based or model-based methods for phase I trials, such as the use of two-stage designs. The first stage is based on single patient cohorts and is designed for rapid escalation through low toxicity dose levels. Storer also suggested separating the allocation rules from the method for estimating the MTD at the end of the trial. The MTD is estimated from a two-parameter logistic regression model fit to the toxicity data at the end of the trial,

$$\widehat{MTD} = \frac{logit(\theta) - \hat{\alpha}}{\hat{\beta}} \tag{6.1}$$

where $\hat{\alpha}$ and $\hat{\beta}$ are the maximum likelihood estimates of α and β in the logistic regression model $logit(\pi_k) = \alpha + \beta d_k$.

Storer noted that although the 2-parameter logistic model was conceptually reasonable, it could pose computational difficulties for small samples, producing slope estimates that are less than or equal to 0 or infinite. For the 3 assumed dose-toxicity curves he used to evaluate the designs, the slope of the estimated logistic regression curve based on data from the standard 3+3 design 'does not give convergent estimates a usefully large fraction of the time.' Even though this was not a concern with his proposed two-stage designs, Storer's results suggest that combinations of sample size, the true dose-toxicity curve, and the design could create computational difficulties for maximum likelihood estimation in the two-parameter logistic model.

6.2.1.3 Biased Coin Designs

Durham, Flournoy, and Rosenberger [20] describe a method for sequential dose allocation and estimation of the MTD based on random walk methods. If the current patient has been treated at dose level d_k and experiences a DLT, the next patient is treated at dose level d_{k-1}. If the current patient does not experience a DLT, the next patient is treated at the current dose d_k with probability $\frac{\theta}{1-\theta}$ or at dose level d_{k+1} with probability $\frac{1}{1-\theta}$, where θ is the prespecified target level of acceptable toxicity. The trial ends when a prestudy specified total of n patients have been accrued to the study. Durham, Flournoy, and Rosenberger and Stylianou and Flournoy [88] propose several estimators for the MTD at the end of the trial. One of the estimators is based on maximum likelihood logistic regression (6.1) and the authors note, as in [87], that in some cases, existence problems for the MLEs can occur when the conditions in Silvapulle [86] are violated. Other estimators proposed following random walk designs include the mean estimate and the 'empirical mean estimator' (6.2)

$$\widehat{MTD} = \frac{1}{m} \sum_{i=s}^{n+1} X(i) \tag{6.2}$$

where $X(i)$ is the dose administered to the ith patient, $m = n - s + 2$, and $s = \max\{i$: the first i patients having the same response$\}$. The estimator ignores the first set of responses from patients that are all toxicities or non-toxicities. The trimmed estimator has superior properties to the standard mean estimator, especially when the first dose allocated to patients is far from the MTD [88]. Stylianou and Flournoy also suggest two estimators based on isotonic regression [81], a method for estimating the probabilities of toxicities subject to the constraint that the estimated toxicity probabilities are nondecreasing in dose.

There are a number of advantages to the biased coin design [20]. The biased coin design does not rely on an assumed parametric model, the escalation and de-escalation rules are easy to implement, and both the small sample properties and asymptotic distribution theory for the estimators have been derived [21, 22]. Furthermore, the method is coherent in dose escalation and de-escalation. By Cheung's definition [11], a method is coherent for dose escalation if the probability of dose escalation after an observed toxicity is 0; a method is coherent for dose de-escalation if the probability of dose de-escalation is equal to 0 after observing a non-toxicity.

6.2.2 Methods Based on Toxicity Probability Intervals

The 'toxicity probability interval' (TPI) method [113] and its modification, mTPI [114], were developed to combine the simplicity of the 3+3 method, allowing investigators to monitor studies without statistical support, and to allow for the specification of a target toxicity probability. In the mTPI method, the toxicity probabilities $\pi_k, k = 1, 2, \ldots, K$ are assumed to have independent beta distributions with parameters (a_k, b_k). If the current dose is d_k, with n_k patients having been treated at this dose and y_k observed toxicities, the investigators can choose to treat the next patient with a lower dose, d_{k-1}, the same dose as currently used, d_k, or escalate to the next higher dose, d_{k+1}. To make this decision, the mTPI partitions the interval $(0, 1)$ into 3 subintervals, $[0, \theta - \epsilon_1), [\theta - \epsilon_1, \theta + \epsilon_2), [\theta + \epsilon_2, 1)$, where θ is the prespecified target toxicity probability and ϵ_1 and ϵ_2 are prespecified constants. The 'unit probability mass (UPM)' is computed for each subinterval, (l, u), defined as the posterior probability that π_k is in the subinterval, divided by the width of the subinterval,

$$UPM(l, u) = \frac{1}{u - l}[F_{a_k, b_k}(u) - F_{a_k, b_k}(l)] \tag{6.3}$$

where F_{a_k, b_k} is the beta cumulative distribution function with parameters $a_k = a + y_k$ and $b_k = b + n_k - y_k$. The dose is either escalated, remains the same, or is de-escalated depending on whether the interval $[0, \theta - \epsilon_1)$, $[\theta - \epsilon_1, \theta + \epsilon_2)$, or $[\theta + \epsilon_2, 1)$ has the highest UPM, respectively. Additional safety rules are implemented to ensure that the method does not escalate to a dose already deemed overly toxic or if de-escalation is called for from the lowest dose level. As in Storer's designs and the biased coin designs, the rule-based allocation is supplemented by model-based estimation of the toxicity probabilities at the end of the study. For the mTPI, the MTD is taken to be the dose with estimated toxicity probability closest to the target probability, where the estimate of the toxicity probabilities are based on isotonic regression [81]. Recently, Liu and Yuan [54] proposed the Bayesian optimal interval (BOIN) design, which is accompanied by **R** package **BOIN**.

6.3 Model-based Methods

6.3.1 The Continual Reassessment Method

The most widely recognized model-based method for dose-finding trials is the continual reassessment method (CRM) [72]. The original CRM paper proposed a single stage design; a later version [84] is a two-stage design using a rule-based algorithm in the first stage and maximum likelihood estimation in the second stage. An excellent overview of the theoretical properties and guidelines for the practical application of the method are given in [12] and [69]. The CRM assumes a parametric model for the dose-toxicity curve, $F(x, b)$, but it does not require that the model be correct across all the doses under consideration. The model only needs to be sufficiently flexible so that, if x^* denotes the true MTD corresponding to a target value θ, there exists a parameter value b^*

such that $F(x^*, b^*) = \theta$. The original CRM paper discussed one- and two-parameter models, but focused primarily on one-parameter models because the simpler models tended to have better properties in terms of identifying the correct MTD.

The most common implementation of the CRM uses the 'empiric' model,

$$\pi_k = \psi_k^{\exp(a)} \tag{6.4}$$

where $0 < \psi_1 < \psi_2 < \ldots < \psi_K < 1$ are prespecified constants, often referred to as the 'skeleton' values and a is a scalar parameter. The parametrization $exp(a)$ ensures that the probability of toxicity is increasing in dose for all $-\infty < a < \infty$. The original CRM paper [72] provided guidance on eliciting a gamma prior for $exp(a)$ but noted that in many cases, the special case of an exponential prior with mean 1 gave satisfactory performance. The skeleton values can be based on the prior, as suggested in the original CRM paper, or by using the method of Lee and Cheung [50] where the skeleton values are calibrated in a way to give good performance for the CRM across a variety of true dose-response curves.

Once the prior and skeleton values are chosen, the first patient is assigned to the dose level with prior probability closest to the target θ. After that, the CRM allocates patients sequentially, with each patient assigned to the dose level with the model-based estimated probability of toxicity closest to the target. To be specific, suppose that $j-1$ patients have been observed on the trial, with $n_1, n_2, \ldots, n_K$ patients assigned to dose levels $1, 2, \ldots, K$, $\sum_{k=1}^{K} n_k = j - 1$ and with Y_k patients on dose level k, $k = 1, 2, \ldots, K$ having experienced a DLT. With the empiric model (6.4) the likelihood, $L(a; n_k, y_k)$ is

$$L(a; n_k, y_k) = \prod_{k=1}^{K} \psi_k^{y_k \exp(a)} \; (1 - \psi_k^{\exp(a)})^{n_k - y_k} \tag{6.5}$$

If we denote the prior distribution on a by $g(a)$, the posterior density of a, $h(a)$, is proportional to

$$h(a) \propto \int L(a; n_k, y_k) g(a) da \tag{6.6}$$

The updated model-based toxicity probabilities are $\hat{\pi}_k = \psi_k^{\exp(\hat{a})}$, where $(\hat{a})$ can be the posterior mean computed via numerical integration, an approximation to the posterior mean [72], the posterior mode or the posterior median [15]. The jth patient is assigned to the dose level k with the smallest value of $\Delta(\hat{\pi}_k, \theta)$, where $\Delta(u, v)$ is a prespecified measure of distance between u and v. The original paper uses a quadratic distance, $\Delta(u, v) = (u - v)^2$, but asymmetric distance functions, which give greater loss to deviations above the target than below, could also be used. The updating of a and the allocation of patients to the dose with updated toxicity probability closest to the target continues until a prespecified number of patients has been observed. At the end of the study, the MTD is taken to be the dose that the next patient would have received had the trial not ended.

A two-stage version of the CRM is presented by [84]. The first stage uses a rule-based design, and continues until there is heterogeneity in the responses from patients. Once heterogeneity is observed, the trial proceeds as in the original CRM, except that the estimate of the parameter a is based on maximizing the likelihood (6.5). The paper uses a rule-based design using single patient cohorts: if a patient does not experience a DLT, the next patient is treated at the next higher dose level, but the authors note that any rule-based design could be used in stage I until heterogeneity is observed.

Cheung [12] shows that the one-stage Bayesian CRM is coherent, and that the two-stage CRM is coherent as long as it does not produce an incoherent transition between the rule-based and model-based stages. The operating characteristics of the CRM have been evaluated in numerous articles, and it has been shown to have excellent performance in terms of identifying the MTD [2, 73, 102]. The method can be extended naturally to cover more complex dose-finding studies [66, 67].

There are a number of misperceptions concerning the CRM. One is that skeleton values are difficult to specify and that the performance of the method will suffer if the skeleton values are far from the true underlying toxicity probabilities. On the contrary, a change in the skeleton values from ψ_k to ψ_k^c , $c > 0$ does not affect the maximum of the likelihood (6.5), meaning, for example, that using very different sets of skeleton values $\{0.1, 0.2, 0.3, 0.4, 0.5, 0.6\}$, or $\{0.1^3, 0.2^3, \ldots, 0.6^3\}$, or $\{0.1^{0.1}, 0.2^{0.1}, \ldots, 0.6^{0.1}\}$ can produce exactly the same results in the likelihood version and in the Bayesian version, as long as the prior is re-calibrated for each change in the power [35].

This is not to say that the skeleton choice is irrelevant, but rather that skeleton spacing is more important than the actual skeleton values. For example, choosing a set of skeleton values that rise steeply, such as $\{0.01, 0.02, 0.05, 0.50, 0.9, 0.95\}$, will tend to result in recommendations in the steep part of the skeleton. This skeleton will yield excellent properties when the true MTD is in the steep part of the skeleton and poor results otherwise. Skeletons like this can be avoided by using the method of Lee and Cheung [50], or simply spacing out skeleton values over the interval (0,1). Another option is to use the multiple skeleton approach of Yin and Yuan [111], who propose a Bayesian model-averaging (BMA) version of the CRM. Rather than specifying a single skeleton, Yin and Yuan specify multiple skeletons, putting a prior on each set of values. Sequential allocations of patients to doses are made using the BMA estimates of the toxicity probabilities.

Another misperception is that the one-parameter power model is not sufficiently rich to allow accurate estimation of the MTD. The original CRM paper [72] compared one- and two-parameter versions of the method and found that the one-parameter version outperformed the two-parameter version, even when the data were generated from a two-parameter model. Chevret [14] found that the two-parameter model could give slight improvements in estimating the probability of toxicity at the chosen MTD, but only for specific scenarios and certain prior distributions. Paoletti and Kramar [73] generated 5000 dose-toxicity curves and found that the one-parameter power model had superior properties to the two-parameter logistic model and other single parameter models such as a logistic model with either a fixed slope or intercept.

6.3.2 Escalation with Overdose Control (EWOC)

Babb, Rogatko, and Zacks [3] proposed a Bayesian method for sequential dose allocation that is intended to identify the MTD while limiting the proportion of patients exposed to doses with probabilities of toxicity above the chosen target. The method assumes that the true MTD is in the interval $[X_{min}, X_{max}]$ and is based on a 2-parameter model for the probability of a DLT at dose $x \in [X_{min}, X_{max}]$,

$$P(DLT|dose = x) = F(\beta_0 + \beta_1 x) \tag{6.7}$$

where F is a distribution function and $\beta_1 > 0$ so that the probability of a DLT is increasing in x. A prior distribution is assumed for the pair of parameters (β_0, β_1). The first patient is assigned dose X_{min}. The study proceeds as in the CRM method, with the dose for the jth patient being derived from the posterior distribution of (β_0, β_1), combining the prior on (β_0, β_1) and the likelihood-based on the binary responses and dose allocations from the previous $j-1$ patients. The posterior distribution on (β_0, β_1) can be written in terms of the posterior distribution on (p_0, γ), where p_0 is the probability of a DLT at dose X_{min} and γ is the MTD. Integrating over p_0 yields the marginal posterior CDF of the MTD:

$$G(\gamma|Dj-1) = Prob(MTD \leq \gamma \mid D_{j-1}) \tag{6.8}$$

where D_{j-1} denotes all the data up to and including patient $j-1$. If all doses between X_{min} and X_{max} could be used, the next patient would go on the dose x such that $G(x|D_{j-1}) = \alpha$, where α is a prespecified tolerance for overdosing. That is, the patient is allocated to the dose x such that the posterior probability that the dose exceeds the MTD is equal to α. In the more practical case where a set of discrete doses $d_1, d_2, \ldots, d_K$ between X_{min} and X_{max} are available for study, the jth patient would be allocated to the discrete dose that is sufficiently close to the continuous dose choice and where the probability of an overdose is sufficiently close to α:

$$\max_{d_1, d_2, \ldots, d_K} : d_k - x \leq T_1 \quad \text{and} \quad G(d_k|D_{j-1}) - \alpha \leq T_2 \tag{6.9}$$

where T_1 and T_2 are prespecified constants. At the end of the trial, the MTD is chosen as the value that minimizes the expected loss with respect to the posterior distribution of the MTD. This loss is taken as an asymmetric loss function, penalizing overdosing more than underdosing. The authors showed that EWOC and the Bayesian CRM with a symmetric loss function had similar properties for identifying the MTD, and were more efficient than any of the rule-based designs they considered. On average, the EWOC method tended to treat more patients on low and possibly sub-therapeutic dose than did the CRM, but treated fewer patients at dose levels above the MTD than did CRM. Over all the simulations, the average proportion of patients with DLTs with CRM was almost exactly equal to the target level (33%); this proportion was between 25% and 30% for EWOC. Subsequent work [97] refined the prior on (β_0, β_1) and applied the principle of overdose control to a toxicity score rather than a binary measure of toxicity [10]. An excellent overview of EWOC and its extensions is given in [96].

6.3.3 EWOC and CRM

The two methods have an important principle in common, namely, each method sequentially allocates patients to doses in a way that tries to optimize treatment for that patient. Chu, Lin, and Shih [15] show a formal connection between the two methods, noting that using the posterior median, rather than the posterior mean in CRM, is equivalent to EWOC with a symmetric loss function. The authors also propose a hybrid design combining features of CRM and EWOC.

6.3.4 Bayesian 2-Parameter Logistic Models

Wu [108] did not specifically address phase I trials, but he did propose the first use of the two-parameter logistic model (6.1) in a sequential experiment designed to estimate a percentile of a distribution. Gatsonis and Greenhouse [26] considered 2-parameter dose-toxicity models of the form

$$\Pr(\text{toxic response at dose level } x_k) = F(\alpha + \beta x_k) \tag{6.10}$$

with either a logit or probit specification for F. The authors reparameterize the model, and recode the doses so that the lowest dose is 0. Rather than putting priors directly on α and β, Gatsonis and Greenhouse [26] put a prior on $\pi(0) = F(\alpha)$, the probability of a toxicity at the lowest dose, and the MTD, noting that

$$MTD = \frac{F^{-1}(\theta) - \alpha}{\beta} \tag{6.11}$$

where θ is the target toxicity probability. They note that, in order to have a proper posterior distribution, until the first toxicity is observed, the prior for the MTD needs to be informative.

Piantiadosi, Fisher, and Grossman [77] discuss the use of the 2-parameter logistic model parametrized in terms of the steepness of the curve and the dose at which the probability of toxicity is 0.5. They introduce the use of 'pseudo-data priors' [5] in the context of phase I trials, that is, prior information elicited in the form of hypothetical data. For example, the clinicians can be asked to provide the dose that would produce DLTs in 10% of patients. Greater or lesser confidence in their belief could be quantified by stating this as 0.1 of 1 patient, 1 of 10 patients, or 5 of 50 patients. These hypothetical data would then be used in the estimation process. Whitehead and Williamson [107] also propose the use of pseudo-data priors within the context of a 2-parameter logistic model.

Some cautions are in order with the use of the 2-parameter model. Cheung [12] shows that the 2-parameter logistic model can be 'rigid'; the additional flexibility of the 2-parameter model confines the estimation to sub-optimal doses. He presents an example with 0 toxicities out of n_1 patients on dose level 1 and 1 toxicity out of 3 patients on dose level 2. With a target of $\theta = 0.1$, the likelihood-based 2-parameter logistic model will always recommend dose level 1 for all remaining patients, regardless of what happens at dose level 1. Some of the rigidity can be corrected by an appropriate choice of the prior, highlighting, as Gatsonis and Greenhouse [26] pointed out, the importance of the prior in the 2-parameter model.

The use of the 2-parameter model has been recommended in recent papers, despite the problems inherent in the model. Neuenschwander, Brandon and Gsponder [63] reported on a phase I trial in which it appeared that the one-parameter CRM called for escalation after two patients in a cohort of size 2 both experienced DLTs. The authors conjectured that this behavior was due to the use of the one-parameter power model, although it has been pointed out that the behavior is more likely due to a poor choice of skeleton [37], an overly informative prior that puts too much prior probability on high dose levels being the MTD [35], or deviations from the original design that allowed investigators to skip 2 dose levels.

6.3.5 Which Method to Use?

Comparisons of the performance of the methods are complicated by the lack of consensus in the criteria on which the methods should be judged and the necessity of focusing on selected true dose-toxicity scenarios. The primary criterion for evaluation is the 'percent correct selection' (PCS), the proportion of times that the method correctly selects the true MTD, or how often the method selects a dose within a certain range, such as 5 or 10 percentage points of the target toxicity. Comparisons may be also made on the percent of patients treated at the MTD or at doses close to the MTD, or on the basis of the proportion of patients treated at doses above the MTD.

The accuracy index [12] is a useful measure that takes into account the entire distribution of dose recommendations,

$$AI = 1 - K \times \frac{\sum_{k=1}^{K} \rho_k \ \Pr(\text{selecting dose}\, k)}{\sum_{k=1}^{K} \rho_k} \tag{6.12}$$

where ρ_k is a measure of the deviation of the true toxicity probability at dose k from the target θ. Cheung (2011) gives several choices for ρ_k, including an absolute deviation, $\rho_k = |\pi_k - \theta|$ or an asymmetric deviation, $\rho_k = \alpha(\theta - \pi_k)^+ + (1-\alpha)(\pi_k - \theta)^+$. The Accuracy Index has a maximum value of 1, occurring when the design always recommends the correct MTD.

With few exceptions, comparisons among the methods are made based on simulations, using a limited number of true dose-toxicity curves. Even when exact small sample results are available [21, 22, 53], these results depend on the true underlying dose-toxicity curve. This can make comparisons difficult, since every method has some scenarios under which it will perform well. For example, a design that uses no data at all and always delares the MTD to be dose level 2 will do well on all the standard criteria for scenarios that have the true MTD at level 2 and poorly on all other scenarios. It is important, when evaluating a design, to consider the performance across a broad range of scenarios, varying the location of the MTD and the steepness of the dose-toxicity curve.

A tool for evaluating the properties of designs is given in [71, 74]. The benchmark cannot be used in practice because it requires knowledge of the true underlying dose-toxicity curve but it has been shown to be useful in investigating the efficiency of proposed designs [102] in the context of studies with monotone dose-toxicity curves.

Rule-based methods have the practical advantage of being simpler to carry out, but the model-based methods also have some practical advantages over rule-based methods. Model-based methods, either through the time-to-event version or using the proposals in the orignal CRM paper, can enroll patients even if the follow-up period for previously enrolled patients is not yet complete. Model-based methods can accommodate revisions to data errors; on subsequent review, patients thought not to have had DLTs could be found to have had DLTs, or, vice versa, patients thought not to have DLTs could be classified upon further review as having had a DLT. Subsequent allocations can proceed based on models fit to the corrected data. Model-based methods have also been shown to extend naturally to handle more complex dose-finding cases, such as methods for combinations, heterogeneity of patients, or trade-offs between toxicity and efficacy, topics addressed in later sections of this chapter.

6.4 Time-to-event Toxicity Outcomes

The original CRM paper [72] noted that the observation of a toxicity does not occur immediately and there may be patients to be enrolled in the study before all the observations have completed on the prior patients. This paper suggested treating the new patients in the last allocated dose, or given the uncertainty in the dose allocations, treating patients one level above or one level below the most recent model-recommended dose.

Cheung and Chappell [13] proposed an extension known as the 'time-to-event CRM' (TITE-CRM) that allowed for a weighted toxicity model, with weights proportional to the time that the patient has been observed. They consider a number of weight functions, but simulation results suggested that a simple linear weight function of the form $w(u) = u/T$, where T is a fixed length of follow-up observation time for each patient, is adequate. If a patient is observed to have a toxicity at time $u < T$, the follow-up time u is set to equal T.

In choosing the dose allocation for patient j, and using the empiric model (6.4) for the CRM, the TITE-CRM likelihood is given by

$$L(a; y_1, \ldots y_{j-1}, x_1, \ldots x_{j-1}) = \prod_{l=1}^{j-1} \left[\frac{t_l}{T} \psi_{x_l}^{\exp(a)} \right]^{y_l} \left[1 - \frac{t_l}{T} \psi_{x_l}^{\exp(a)} \right]^{1-y_l} \tag{6.13}$$

where $y_1, \ldots y_{j-1}$ are toxicity indicators and $x_1, \ldots x_{j-1}$ are the indices of the dose allocations for the first $j-1$ patients. Note that the likelihood (6.13) is written in terms of the individual patient observations, whereas (6.5) groups patients according to the dose received. If all the subjects were fully observed, $t_l = T$ for all $l = 1, \ldots, j-1$, the likelihood (6.13) reduces to (6.5). Cheung and Chappell investigate this generalization of both the one-stage Bayesian CRM [72] and the two-stage likelihood CRM [84].

Normolle and Lawrence [64] discuss the use of the TITE-CRM in radiation oncology studies, where the toxicities tend to occur late in the follow-up period. Polley [78] observes that in studies with rapid patient accrual and late toxicities, the TITE-CRM can allocate too many patients to overly toxic doses. The paper has a comparison of a modification of the TITE-CRM that was suggested in the original TITE-CRM paper, as well as a modification that incorporates wait times between patient accruals. A version of EWOC with time-to-event endpoints is described in [61, 95].

6.5 Ordinal Outcomes

6.5.1 Rule-based Methods

All of the methods in the previous sections are developed for a binary measure of toxicity indicating whether or not a patient experienced a study-specific "dose-limiting toxicity." In cancer clinical trials, adverse events categories are often based on the National Cancer Institute's Common Terminology Criteria for Adverse Events v4.0 (CTCAE) [62], which assigns grades to adverse events as Mild (grade 1), Moderate (grade 2), Severe (grade 3), Life-threatening (grade 4), or Death related to the adverse event (grade 5). Gordon and Willson [28] proposed a 3-stage rule-based design in which dose escalation or de-escalation across cohorts was guided by the number and severity of the toxicities. Cohort sizes of 1,3, or 6 patients are used in the 3 stages, respectively. At the end of the study, a 2-parameter logistic model is used to model the probability of a grade 3 or greater adverse event as a function of dose. In many cases, the model did not converge, or produced negative estimates of slope. As an alternative, they propose fitting a mean response model [1].

A generalization of the random walk rules of [20] for ordinal toxicity outcomes was proposed by Paul, Rosenberger, and Flournoy (2004) [76]. Instead of a single target toxicity probability, and a single MTD, there are target probabilities $\theta_1 > \theta_2 > \cdots > \theta_C$, one for each of the C categories of the toxicity outcome, and different dose levels, μ_c, that achieve these levels.

$$P(Y \geq c|\mu_c) = \theta_c, \ c = 1, 2, \cdots, C \tag{6.14}$$

where Y is an ordinal toxicity outcome.

Dose allocation of a fixed number of patients n occurs in C stages. At each stage c, $c = 1, 2, \ldots, C$, a single patient at a time is treated and, for $\theta_c \leq 0.5$, dose escalation proceeds as in the binary random walk designs: if a patient experiences a toxicity of grade c or greater, the next patient is treated at the next lower dose level. If the patient experiences no toxicity, or a toxicity of grade less than or equal to $c - 1$, the next patient is treated at the same dose, with probability $1/(1 - \theta_c)$ or with the next higher dose, with probability $\theta_c/(1-\theta_c)$. At the end of the study, the probability of a 'category c or greater' toxicity can be estimated with a proportional odds model, although convergence problems can occur in fitting this model. The authors recommend estimators based on two-dimensional isotonic regression [81], using that the cumulative probabilities in (6.14) are nonincreasing in c and non-decreasing in dose.

6.5.2 Model-based Methods

There are several model-based extensions to the continual reassessment method. Iasonos, Zohar, and O'Quigley [38] developed a method for toxicity measured on a 3-category ordinal scale: none, mild/moderate and severe, and where interest is in limiting the proportion of patients with a severe adverse event. They propose a 2-stage design where escalation in the first stage occurs as long as the sum of observed toxicities is less than 2, where mild/moderate toxicities receive a score of '1', and severe toxicities a score of '2'. Once there is heterogeneity in the toxicity outcomes among patients and the total toxicity score is at least 2, allocation in the second stage is based on the following model,

$$P(Y = 0|\ dose\ k) = 1 - (\psi_k)^{\exp(a)+\exp(b)}$$
$$P(Y = 1|\ dose\ k) = \psi_k^{\exp(a)+\exp(b)} - \psi_k^{\exp(a)}$$
$$P(Y = 2|\ dose\ k) = \psi_k^{\exp(a)}$$

where $0 < \psi_1 < \psi_2 < \ldots < \psi_K < 1$ are pre-chosen 'skeleton' values. As in the CRM for binary outcomes, the $\exp(a)$ and $\exp(b)$ parametrizations are used to ensure monotonicity across dose levels. This model is a direct generalization of the CRM for binary toxicities; the model for severe toxicities $Y = 2$ is the same as (6.4). The authors consider two cases, where both a and b are parameters to be estimated or where b is assumed known. Van Meter and colleagues [99] generalize the CRM method using a continuation ratio model,

$$P(Y = c|Y \geq c; X) = \frac{e^{\alpha+\tau_j+\gamma x}}{1 + e^{\alpha+\tau_j+\gamma x}}, c = 1, \cdots, C-1 \qquad (6.15)$$

where x is the dose, and α, γ, and $\tau_1, \ldots, \tau_{C-1}$ are parameters to be estimated from the data. A similar method is found in Van Meter et al. [98] using a proportional odds model,

$$P(Y \geq c|X) = \frac{e^{\alpha_j+\beta x}}{1 + e^{\alpha_j+\beta x}}, c = 1, \cdots, C-1 \qquad (6.16)$$

To avoid problems of convergence in both the continuation ratio and proportional odds models, Van Meter, Garrett-Mayer, and Bandyopadhyay [98, 99] use a generalization of the pseudo-data approach of Piantadosi, Fisher, and Grossman [77] for ordinal outcomes. Doussau, Thiebault, and Paoletti [18] use a mixed effects proportional odds model for ordinal toxicity grades collected over multiple cycles from each patient. The proportional odds model is also the basis of a version of EWOC for ordinal outcomes [94].

In most cases, the papers that describe methods for ordinal responses report only modest gains in identifying the MTD with the use of ordinal toxicities.

6.5.3 Toxicity Scores

Rather than classifying patients on the basis of a single binary or ordinal toxicity score, several papers have explored the use of a "toxicity score", combining ordinal toxicity grades across multiple types of adverse events. Bekele and Thall [6] note that not all toxicities are equally important and replace the toxicity grade with a "severity weight", elicited from the investigators prior to the study. The severity weights for a patient are summed into a "total toxicity burden" (TTB). Dose allocations and the final estimate of the MTD are based on the posterior distribution of the TTB.

Yuan, Chappell, and Bailey [117] propose the use of an "equivalent toxicity (ET)" score. As in [6] the required information is elicited from the clinicians prior to the study by enumerating all possible outcomes in a cohort of 3 patients in terms of the number of each grade of toxicities and what the clinicians would do in terms of an escalation decision. A score of 1 is assigned to the cutoff grade for defining a DLT; for example, score 1 is assigned to ordinal grade 3. For example, from the response to the hypothetical outcomes from the cohort of 3, it can be determined that in the opinion of the clinicians, two grade 2 toxicities are equivalent to a grade 3 toxicity and a score of 0.5 is assigned to grade 2 toxicities. It was also suggested that a grade 4 and a grade 2 toxicity are equivalent to two grade 3 toxicities, yielding a score of 1.5 for a grade 4 toxicity. Yuan, Chappell, and Bailey normalize the ET scores to be in the range of 0 to 1, and use a one-parameter model similar to that used for the CRM for changes in the distribution of the normalized ET score across doses.

Lee et al. [51] developed a toxicity burden score (TBS) using a regression approach to estimate severity weights. This enables the method to distinguish between toxicity grades and types of toxicities.

6.6 Dose Expansion Cohorts

It is becoming common in phase I studies to enroll an additional set of patients at the dose estimated to be the MTD at the end of the dose-finding stage. The additional set of patients is often termed a 'dose expansion cohort' (DEC) and there are several reasons for the use of a DEC, including obtaining additional data on toxicity or preliminary estimates of efficacy. Additional patients may be needed to assess pharmacokinetics of the agent, or to investigate characteristics such as biomarkers that might enhance the effect of the new therapy. A recent paper [17] reports on trends in 522 adult phase I trials conducted in a single institution over the past 25 years. The authors note a growing trend in the use of DEC typically of size ranging from 6 to 15 patients, and note that few studies justify the number or the aims of the DEC.

Gonen [27] addresses the use of DECs to refine the toxicity estimate at the MTD. He proposes a Bayesian solution for how the toxicity information from patients in the DEC might be used for this objective. Gonen assumes a Beta(α_1, β_1) prior distribution for π, the probability of toxicity at the estimated MTD dose. If N_i patients have been enrolled in cohort i and Y_i

toxicities have been observed among these patients, with $i = 1$ denoting the dose finding cohort and $i = 2$ being the dose expansion cohort, the posterior distribution of π is a Beta(a, b) distribution with parameters $a = \alpha_1 + x_1 + x_2$ and $b = \beta_1 + n_1 - Y_1 + N_2 - Y_2$. From this, one can calculate credible intervals for the probability of toxicity at the estimated MTD and, in particular, compute the posterior probability, $P(\pi > \theta)$, where θ is the target toxicity probability, to decide if the dose needs to be modified for a subsequent phase II trial.

Iasonos and O'Quigley [36] provide one of the first comprehensive assessments of the statistical issues in DECs. They note that patient eligibility often changes with the dose expansion cohort, raising questions as to whether it is appropriate to combine toxicity data from the dose-finding cohort and the DEC, and how efficacy information can be used to derive a recommended phase II dose. Iasonos and O'Quigley discuss five methods for using the DEC to refine the toxicity data and to obtain preliminary estimates of efficacy. The first combines all the data, as in [27], into a single analysis of toxicity. After all the data are collected on the DEC, the data are combined to give a final estimate of the probability of toxicity at the estimated MTD. The MTD can be revised if this estimated probability is too high relative to the target toxicity. The second method allows for revising the MTD prospectively in the dose expansion phase using a dose-finding algorithm applied to the dose-finding cohort and the accumulating data at the estimated MTD. The third option is to use a dose-finding method that takes into account both toxicity and efficacy [68], allocating the first patient in the DEC to the estimated MTD, then allowing patients to be allocated to other doses as safety and efficacy data accumulate. The fourth option is to use more than one dose in the DEC; in a single agent trial, this could mean assigning patients in the DEC to the estimated MTD or to one level above or below the estimated MTD. The assignment to these dose levels could occur at random, or by using a sequential procedure that limits patients being assigned to overly toxic doses. The fifth option explicitly accounts for the different eligibility criteria for patients in the DEC and suggests the use of a "bridging method" [70] that would use the toxicity data from the dose-finding cohort but allow for the MTD in the DEC to be the same, or shifted by one or two levels from the MTD in the dose-finding cohort.

6.7 Dose-finding Based on Safety and Efficacy

In the context of dose-finding trials in oncology, "multiple outcomes" can refer to the assessment of multiple toxicities per patient; these are often combined into a single summary of toxicity burden [6, 51]. More commonly, multiple outcomes refer to a trial with dose-finding based on both safety and efficacy, and in this section, we will present methods for dose-finding with toxicity and response outcomes. The toxicity outcome is denoted by Y_k^T, with $Y_k^T = 1$ if a DLT is observed for a patient at dose level k, and 0 otherwise, and the response outcome is denoted by Y_k^R, with response measured either as a binary or ordinal variable. A general theme of methods in this area is that they try to induce an ordering on the pairs of response and toxicity outcome categories, either by combining categories, specifying trade-off contours, or constructing utility functions.

O'Quigley, Hughes, and Fenton [68] proposed the estimation of the 'most successful dose' (MSD), defined as the dose that maximizes the probability of a clinical response with no toxicity. Both toxicity and response are measured as binary outcomes. In terms of the response and toxicity probabilities, the success probability at dose level k, denoted by π_k^S is

$$\pi_k^S = P(Y_k^R = 1, Y_k^T = 0) = P(Y_k^R = 1 | Y_k^T = 0) P(Y_k^T = 0) \tag{6.17}$$

The authors propose several models for estimating the MSD, including one based on the 'empiric model' (6.4) for the CRM [72]:

$$\pi_k^T = \psi_k^{\exp(a)} \tag{6.18}$$

where $0 < \psi_1 < \psi_2 < \ldots < \psi_K < 1$ is the skeleton for the probability of a DLT at dose level k and a is a parameter to be estimated from the data. A similar model is used for the conditional probabilities of a response, given no toxicity,

$$P(Y_k^R = 1 | Y_k^T = 0) = \phi_k^{\exp(b)} \tag{6.19}$$

where $0 < \phi_1 < \phi_2 < \ldots < \phi_K < 1$ is a set of skeleton values and b is a parameter to be estimated from the data. The assumption is that the toxicity probabilities and the conditional probabilities of a response given no toxicity are monotonic in dose.

Estimates of a and b are updated sequentially as response and toxicity outcomes are observed from patients in the trial. The allocation of the jth patient, based on data from the first $j-1$ patients, is to the dose with the largest estimated value of $\hat{\pi}_k^S$,

$$\hat{\pi}_k^S = \phi_k^{\exp(\hat{b})} [1 - \psi_k^{\exp(\hat{a})}] \tag{6.20}$$

Thall and Russell [93] present a design motivated by a study of autologous bone marrow transplant for patients with advanced hematologic malignancies. Toxicity is measured on a binary scale, efficacy is defined by the severity of graft-versus-host disease (GVHD), measured as 'none' (0), 'moderate' (1), or 'severe' (2) GVHD. Thall and Russell combine the response and toxicity outcomes for a patient treated at dose level k into a 3-level categorical variable Y_k, with $Y_k = 0$ if there is no toxicity and no GVHD; $Y_k = 1$ if there is no toxicity and moderate GVHD; and $Y_k = 2$ if there is a toxicity, or no toxicity and severe GVHD. With this classification, the 6 possible outcomes in the cross classification of response and toxicity are reduced to 3-level ordinal outcome, with the probability that a patient given dose level k has outcome category j denoted by $\theta_j(k)$. A Bayesian proportional odds model is used for the ordinal outcome, with priors elicited for the parameters in the model. As the data accumulate in the trial, Thall and Russell compute the posterior probabilities that current dose levels have an unacceptably low efficacy rate,

$$P(\theta_1(k) < \theta_1^*|data) > \gamma_1 \tag{6.21}$$

or an unacceptably high toxicity rate,

$$P(\theta_2(k) > \theta_2^*|data) > \gamma_2 \tag{6.22}$$

where θ_j^* and $\gamma_j, j = 1, 2$ are prespecified thresholds. Escalation or de-escalation for the next patient depends on whether the posterior probabilities indicate acceptable toxicity or sufficient efficacy.

Thall and Cook [89] consider both the trinary outcome case of Thall and Russell [93] and a full cross classification of the response outcome Y_k^R and the toxicity outcome Y_k^T, each measured as a binary variable, for a patient treated at dose level k. Prior to the study, Thall and Cook give specific guidelines on how to elicit from the clinicians, prior to the study, a contour of 'equally desirable' pairs in terms of the probability of a toxicity π_k^T and the probability of a response π_k^R. The contour is used to induce an ordering on the doses, as determined from a trade-off of toxicity and efficacy, and this ordering guides the allocation of doses to patients. Thall, Nguyen, and Estey [92] generalize this method to include patient-specific covariates.

Several papers use utility functions to express the trade-off between response and toxicity [55, 91]. Loke et al. assign utility weights to the four possible cross-classifications of a binary response and a binary toxicity outcome. Thall et al. (2013) construct a utility function for response and toxicity, each measured as a 'time-to-event' outcome. In each case, accumulating data is used to allocate patients to doses to maximize the expected utility.

6.8 Combinations of Agents

There has been an increasing interest in investigating the potential of drug combinations for patient treatment. The motivation to treat with drug combinations stems from the desire to improve the response of the patient, especially those who have been resistant to traditional treatment. Multi-agent trials present the significant challenge of finding the MTD combination (MTDC), or combinations, of the agents being tested with the typically small sample sizes involved in phase I clinical trials. Many authors have developed dose-

TABLE 6.1: Treatment labels for dose combinations

Combos	d_1	d_2	d_3	d_4	d_5	d_6
BMS-214662	80	80	120	160	160	225
Paclitaxel	135	175	175	175	225	175

finding methods, a thorough review of which is given in Harrington et al. [29].

As previously noted, a key assumption to phase I methods for single-agent trials is the monotonicity of the dose-toxicity curve. In this case, the curve is said to follow a "simple order" because the ordering of DLT probabilities for any pair of doses is known and administration of greater doses of the agent can be expected to produce DLTs in increasing proportions of patients. In studies testing combinations of agents, the probabilities of DLT associated with the dose combinations often follow a "partial order" in that there are pairs of dose combinations for which the ordering of the probabilities is not known. As an example of a partial order, consider a phase I trial of BMS-214662 in combination with Paclitaxel and Carboplatin in patients with advanced cancer [23]. The trial investigated escalating doses of BMS-214662 in combination with escalating doses of Paclitaxel, along with a fixed dose of Carboplatin. The six combinations are labeled, $d_1, \ldots, d_6$ as in Table 6.1. For d_1 to d_5, the dose of one agent remains fixed, while the dose of the other agent is escalated. Therefore, with regards to the probability of DLT at each combination, it is reasonable to assume that $\pi_1 < \pi_2 < \pi_3 < \pi_4 < \pi_5$. For d_5 and d_6, the dose of BMS-214662 is escalated, while the dose of Paclitaxel is de-escalated. It may not be reasonable to assume that d_5 is less toxic than d_6. It could be that $\pi_5 < \pi_6$ or $\pi_5 > \pi_6$, creating a partial order.

6.8.1 Assumption of a Single Ordering

A traditional approach is to prespecify an escalation path in the drug combination matrix and apply the 3+3 algorithm along this path. However, such an approach is essentially using only one path, and it can miss more promising dose combinations located outside of the path. Two-dimensional search strategies, based on A+B and A+B+C designs, are described in Fan et al. [24], Braun and Alonzo [7], and Lee and Fan [49]. Another one-dimensional approach taken in early work in model-based dose-finding for drug combinations was to reduce the problem to a complete order by laying out an a priori ordering of the combinations, where the initial ordering is based on single agent toxicity profiles. Korn and Simon [46] present a graphical method, called the "tolerable dose diagram," based on single agent toxicity profiles, for guiding the escalation strategy in combination. Kramar, Lebecq, and Candahl [47] also lay out an a priori ordering for the combinations, and estimate the

MTDC using a parametric model for the probability of a DLT as a function of the doses of the two agents in combination. The disadvantage of this approach is that it limits the number of combinations that can be considered and could produce highly misleading results if the assumed ordering is incorrect.

6.8.2 Specifying Multiple Possible Orderings

Rather than work with a single ordering, another approach to dealing with added complexity is to specify multiple possible orderings and appeal to established model selection techniques. Taking into account these known and unknown relationships between combinations in the Dy et al. [23] example, we can formulate two possible orderings of the toxicity profile

$$\pi_1 < \pi_2 < \pi_3 < \pi_4 < \pi_5 < \pi_6$$

$$\pi_1 < \pi_2 < \pi_3 < \pi_4 < \pi_6 < \pi_5.$$

Two methods making use of this approach are Conaway, Dunbar, and Peddada [16] and Wages, Conaway and O'Quigley [100].

The method proposed by Conaway et al. [16] is a two-stage design based on the estimation procedure of Hwang and Peddada [34]. The initial stage is designed to quickly escalate through treatment combinations that are non-toxic (in single patient cohorts until first DLT is observed) and then the second stage implements the Hwang and Peddada [34] estimates. Throughout the second stage, the toxic response data for treatment combination d_k is of the form $Y = \{Y_k; k = 1, \ldots, K\}$ with Y_k equal to the number of observed toxicities from patients treated with combination d_k. Let $\mathcal{A}$ denote the set of treatments that have been administered thus far in the trial such that $\mathcal{A} = \{(k : n_k > 0\}$, where n_k denotes the number of patients treated on each combination. Using a Beta(α_k, β_k) prior for the π_k, the DLT probabilities are updated only for $k \in \mathcal{A}$ so that

$$\hat{\pi}_k = \frac{Y_k + \alpha_k}{n_k + \alpha_k + \beta_k}.$$

The estimation procedure of Dunbar, Conaway, and Peddada [19] is applied to the updated posterior means $\hat{\pi}_k$ for $k \in \mathcal{A}$.

The CRM for partial orders (POCRM) is based on utilizing a class of working models that correspond to possible orderings of the toxicity probabilities for the combinations. In general, suppose there are M possible orderings being considered which are indexed by m. For a particular ordering, we model the true probability of toxicity, π_k, corresponding to combination d_k, via a power model

$$\pi_k = \psi_{km}^{\exp(a_m)}; \qquad m = 1, \ldots, M,$$

where the ψ_{km} represent the skeleton of the model under ordering m. Wages et al. [100, 101] propose an escalation method that, after each inclusion, estimates a single ordering, m^*, that is most consistent with the observed data, according to some model selection criteria. The authors then use the estimate $\hat{a}_{m^*}$ to estimate DLT probabilities for each combination under ordering m^* so that $\hat{\pi}_k \approx \psi_{km^*}^{\exp(\hat{a}_{m^*})}$.

After each inclusion, the estimated toxicity probabilities $\hat{\pi}_k$ are obtained for each method using the estimation procedures above. In principle, the next entered patient is then allocated to the dose combination with estimated toxicity probability closest to the target toxicity rate so that $|\hat{\pi}_k - \theta|$ is minimized. The trial stops once enough information accumulates about the MTD. The Conaway et al. [16] method was implemented in a phase I trial investigating induction therapy with VELCADE and Vorinostat in patients with surgically resectable non-small cell lung cancer (NSCLC) [44]. The POCRM builds off of the well-known CRM and is likely to be more easily understood by clinicians and review boards. It also has the ability to be carried out using widely available software (**R** package **pocrm** [105]). Wages, Conaway, and O'Quigley [103] extended the TITE-CRM to the partially ordered case.

6.8.3 Use of More Flexible Models

The methods of Conaway et al. [16] and Wages et al. [100] take an "underparameterized" approach, and, in the case of POCRM, rely upon several single parameter models from a CRM class of models. Additional parameters can be utilized to further increase flexibility and account for possible interactive effects the two agents may have on the DLT probabilities. Thall et al. [90] proposed a 2-parameter model for the toxicity probabilities of the dose combinations and a toxicity equivalence contour for two-agent combinations. Wang and Ivanova [106] proposed a logistic-type regression for dose combinations that used the doses of the two agents as the covariates. Yin and Yuan [109, 110] developed a Bayesian adaptive design based on latent 2×2 tables [109] and a copula-type model [110] for two agents. Braun and Wang [9] proposed a hierarchical Bayesian model for the probability of toxicity at each combination. Hirakawa *et al.* [30] proposed a dose-finding method based on the shrunken predictive probability of toxicity for the two agents. Baily et al. [4] outlined a two-dimensional Bayesian dose-finding procedure employing a logistic regression model. Shi and Yin [85] proposed an extension of EWOC to the drug combination setting.

Like the POCRM, a recent article by Braun and Jia [8] aimed to more directly utilize the CRM framework in developing a method for combinations, a method the authors termed generalized CRM (gCRM). Generally speaking, separate CRM models are employed to individually investigate each dose of one agent (Agent A) with the doses of the other agent (Agent B). The individual CRM models each contain the same slope parameter that measures how the doses of Agent A affects the DLT probabilities. Each model also contains an additional intercept parameter that can be different between the models in order to describe the effect of Agent B on DLT probabilities. The intercepts of the various models are connected through the use of Bayesian methods, from which the DLT probabilities and MTDC are estimated [8]. The added mathematical complexity in using more flexible models may hinder the implementation of these methods in practice.

6.8.4 Finding Multiple MTDCs

Papers by Thall *et al.* [90] and Wang and Ivanova [106] differ from many others in their view of what constitutes an "MTD" for a combination. Many of the methods referenced above produce a *single* MTDC that is estimated to have acceptable toxicity. Thall *et al.* [90] and Wang and Ivanova [106] note that, unlike the simply ordered (monotone) case, there is no unique MTDC. The set of dose combinations with acceptable toxicity forms an equivalence contour in two dimensions. Another method designed to select multiple MTDCs is that of Yin and Yuan [115]. They propose a method that has elements of parallel phase I designs and partial orders. For agent, A, with dose levels $A_1 < \cdots < A_J$ and agent B, with dose levels $B_1 < \cdots < B_K$, Yuan and Yin [115] divide up the trial into a series of subtrials. A single subtrial is denoted by $A_i B_{(s \to t)}$ meaning that in the subtrial, agent A is held fixed at dose A_i and agent B ranges in dose from B_s to B_t, with $s \leq t$. They start with a subtrial $A_1 B_{(1 \to s)}$ with A at its lowest dose. Agent B starts at the lowest dose B_1 and escalates, depending on the observed toxicities, to level B_s. Yuan and Yin [115] use the results of this subtrial to plan the next subtrial, $A_2 B_{(s \to t)}$, where the dose levels of B are, in part, determined from the previous subtrial. Their approach relies heavily on ordering assumptions, noting that if dose $A_1 B_k$ is found to be too toxic, the next subtrial $A_2 B_{(s \to t)}$ should only treat patients at dose levels of B less than B_k. Finally, a recent editorial in *Journal of Clinical Oncology* by Mandrekar [60] described the identification of multiple MTDCs using the method of Ivanova and Wang [39] in a phase I study of neratinib in combination with temsirolimus in patients with human epidermal growth factor receptor 2-dependent and other solid tumors [25]. Recently, Mander and Sweeting [57] proposed a curve-free (nonparametric) method, based on a product of independent beta probabilities, for identifying a maximum tolerated contour. Their method has available software for implementation that includes **R** package **pipe.design**.

6.9 Patient Heterogeneity

In some dose-finding trials, there are several groups of patients, and the goal is to estimate an MTD within each group. For example, Ramanathan et al. [80] stratifies patients into 'none', 'mild', 'moderate,' or 'severe' liver dysfunction at baseline. A similar classification is used by LoRusso et al. [56]. In each of these cases, the group structure was not used in the design, in that parallel phase I studies were conducted within each group and the design did not account for the expectation that the MTD would be lower in the more severely impaired patients at baseline.

Ignoring the group structure can lead to at least 2 problems: reversals and inefficiency. By "reversals", we mean that the MTDs in the groups can contradict what is known clinically. For example, the parallel designs might recommend a greater dose level as the MTD in the most severely impaired group compared to a less severely impaired group. By inefficiency, we mean that a design that takes into account the known clinical relationship might recommend the correct MTDs in the groups a greater proportion of times.

O'Quigley, Shen, and Gamst [42] proposed a generalization of the CRM [72] for two groups. Although they consider a number of models, we can illustrate their method with the empiric model (6.4), with skeleton values $0 < \psi_1 < \ldots < \psi_K < 1$. In group 1, the probability of a DLT at dose level k is $\psi_k^{\exp(a)}$; in group 2, the probability is $\psi_k^{\exp(a+b)}$. A value of $b = 0$ means no group effect. It is possible to induce an ordering in the groups by the appropriate use of prior information for the parameter b. Legedza and Ibrahim [52] propose a related method, augmenting the dose-toxicity model for a vector of patient characteristics and putting a prior on the coefficient in the dose-toxicity model.

The 'shift model' [65, 70] is a way of generalizing the CRM to two ordered groups. To illustrate this method, we assume that DLT probabilities are at least as great in group B as in group A. One way to interpret the notion of "at least as much toxicity in group B than in group A" is to say that we anticipate that the MTD in group B will be L dose levels less than in group A, with $L = 0, 1, 2, \cdots, K$. Using the simple power model, the DLT probability at dose level k in group A are equal to $\psi_k^{\exp(a)}$. A shift of $L = 0$ means that the DLT probabilities are the same in the two groups. If $L = 1$, the probability of a DLT in group B at dose level k is equal to $\psi_{k+1}^{\exp(a)}$. The method uses the data from all group-dose combinations to estimate the parameter a and the magnitude of the shift L, $L = 0, 1, 2, \ldots, K$.

Yuan and Chappell [116] propose a generalization of the CRM that is a hybrid of the single agent-single group CRM and isotonic regression methods described by Robertson, Wright, and Dykstra [81]. As in the single agent CRM, the working model and the data within each group are used to estimate the DLT probabilities at each dose for that group. Using standard algorithms for estimation under order restrictions [81], the resulting DLT probability estimates within each dose level are modified so that there are no reversals, meaning no dose levels where a lower risk group has greater DLT probability estimates than a higher risk group. It is possible that this process across groups will create reversals within groups across dose levels, producing modified estimates that are not increasing with dose. Yuan and Chappell would then iterate back and forth between modifying estimates across groups within dose levels and across dose levels within groups. Ivanova and Wang [40] also use isotonic estimates in their designs for bivariate outcomes in two ordered groups.

6.10 Non-cytotoxic Agents

In dose-finding trials of cytotoxic agents, the goal of identifying the MTD is usually determined by considering information on toxicity only, with the assumption that the highest safe dose also provides the most promising outlook for efficacy. Therefore, the design is generally driven by the assumption of monotone increasing dose-toxicity and dose-efficacy relationships. By contrast, many molecularly targeted agents (MTAs) are essentially considered safe and higher doses do not necessarily produce greater efficacious response. Trials of MTAs therefore challenge accepted dose-finding methods because minimal toxicity may be observed over the doses under consideration and higher doses may not result in greater efficacious response [45, 75]. Dose-efficacy relationships may exhibit non-monotone patterns, such as increasing at low doses and either decreasing or plateauing at higher levels. Therefore, the goal of the trial shifts to identifying the optimal biological dose (OBD), which is defined as the dose with acceptable toxicity that maximizes efficacious response.

6.10.1 Locating the OBD

The assumption of monotonicity with regards to dose-toxicity relationships is usually appropriate for MTAs, yet this assumption for dose-efficacy curves may fail. For these types of therapies, dose-efficacy curves could follow a non-monotone pattern, such as a unimodal or plateau relationship. In general, suppose a trial is investigating a set $d_1, \ldots, d_K$, of K doses and that the probability of efficacious response at dose d_k is denoted π_k^R. In the presence of unimodal (including monotone increasing and monotone decreasing) or plateau dose-efficacy relationships, the primary objective of the trial is to find the optimal dose, $d_\nu \in \{d_1, \ldots, d_K\}$, defined such that

$$\pi_1^R \leq \cdots \leq \pi_\nu^R \geq \cdots \geq \pi_K^R. \tag{6.23}$$

In other words, π_ν^R corresponds to the dose d_ν where the peak of the unimodal relationship occurs, or where the dose-efficacy curve begins to plateau. Using the terminology of Hwang and Peddada [34], π_ν^R is said to be a *nodal* parameter (or a node) in that it is known that $\pi_\nu^R \geq \pi_k^R$ for all $k \neq \nu$. Order restriction (6.23) is referred to as an *umbrella* ordering with the node of the umbrella occurring at d_ν. For instance, if the node occurs at the highest dose, we have a monotone increasing dose-efficacy relationship. In actuality, we do not know where in the dose range this node occurs and we must account for this uncertainty. The node could occur at any of the K available dose levels, with non-decreasing efficacy probabilities for doses before the node and non-increasing efficacy probabilities for doses after the node.

In locating the OBD, accepted early-phase designs are challenged by the use of non-traditional endpoints that accompany cytostatic agents. The potential growth of targeted therapies will be driven by the need to define suitable measures of biologic effect and finding ways to incorporate them into early-phase designs. Although the relationship between clinical outcome and biologic activity may not be clear, it is generally assumed that the absence of targeted effect will accompany a lack of clinical efficacy. Before a targeted agent can be taken into large-scale trials to test for clinical efficacy, early-phase trials are needed to establish that the therapy can produce a biologic activity with the *potential* to translate to clinical benefit. Protocol-specific endpoints give the investigator a measure of targeted effect that serves as a driving factor in early-phase trial design.

A discussion of the challenges presented by non-toxicity endpoints in phase I trial design of targeted agents is presented in [45, 75]. Unlike cytotoxic agents, the effects of these agents will likely be cytostatic, which will require measures of anti-tumor activity other than those used as traditional endpoints, such as tumor shrinkage. Surrogate markers of efficacy, such as measurement of target inhibition or pharmacokentic endpoints, will be necessary. Incorporation of these endpoints can be challenging due to the fact that (1) it may be difficult to define the desired biological effect, and (2) once defined, these endpoints may lack reliable, validated assays, making them practically difficult to measure.

Despite the emergence of molecularly targeted agents in oncology drug development, there are relatively few statistical methods for designing phase I trials of these agents [59]. Assuming minimal toxicity over the therapeutic dose range, Hunsberger et al. [33] described two practical phase I designs for identifying the OBD for molecularly targeted agents. Zhang, Sargent, and Mandrekar [119] introduced a trinomial continual reassessment method (Tri-CRM) that utilizes a continuation ratio to model toxicity and efficacy simultaneously. Mandrekar, Cui, and Sargent [58] extended this method to account for combinations for two agents. Polley and Cheung [79] outlined a two-stage design for finding the OBD that implements a futility interim analysis. Recently, Hoering, LeBlanc, and Crowley and Hoering et al. [31, 32] proposed methods for early phase trials of targeted agents that uses a traditional dose-finding method to find the MTD in phase I, and then subsequently allocates patients in phase II to the MTD [31] or a small set of doses at and around the MTD [32] based on a randomization scheme. Yin, Zheng, and Xu [112] described a two-stage dose-finding design for cytostatic agents. Zang et al. [118] described several methods for locating the OBD of MTAs, which consisted of designs based on isotonic regression and local logistic models. Wages and Tait [104] recently proposed a method for identifying the OBD that combines features of CRM and order-restricted inference.

6.11 Summary

This chapter presented both rule-based and model-based methods for the classical dose-finding problem of choosing the MTD from a prespecified set of doses, with a binary measure of toxicity, and with the assumption of increasing probability of toxicity with increasing dose. Our recommendation in this context is to use model-based methods with a simple parametric model; these methods have excellent performance across a broad range of dose-toxicity scenarios. In addition, the use of these methods can allow for revisions of previously collected DLT information because of late toxicities or for errors in the classification of adverse events as DLTs.

Much of the discussion in this chapter centered on methods developed to address more complex dose-finding trials, such as those that involve time-to-event outcomes, combinations of agents, heterogeneous groups of patients, or non-cytotoxic agents. The evaluation of the various proposed methods suggests that even in more complex trials, methods based on simple parametric models, alone or in combination with order restrictions, tend to have the best properties across a range of dose-toxicity scenarios. The development of methods for dose-finding trials remains an active area of research, as methods are being developed to meet the practical demands of recent advances in cancer treatment.

Bibliography

[1] A. Agesti. *Analysis of Ordinal Categorical Data, 2nd Edition.* John Wiley & Sons, Inc., New York, NY, USA, 2010.

[2] C. Ahn. An evaluation of phase I cancer clinical trial designs. *Statistics in Medicine*, 17:1537–1549, 1998.

[3] J. Babb, A. Rogatko, and S. Zacks. Cancer phase I clinical trials: efficient dose escalation with overdose controli. *Statistics in Medicine*, 17:1103–1120, 1998.

[4] S. Bailey, B. Neuenschwander, G. Laird, and M. Branson. A Bayesian case study in oncology phase I combination dosefinding using logistic regression with covariates. *Journal of Biopharmaceutical Statistics*, 19:469–484, 2009.

[5] E. Bedrick, R. Christensen, and W. Johnson. A new perspective on priors for generalized linear models. *Journal of the American Statistical Association*, 91:1450–1460, 1996.

[6] B. Bekele and P. Thall. Dose-finding based on multiple toxicities in a soft tissue sarcoma trial. *Journal of the American Statistical Association*, 99:26–35, 2004.

[7] T. Braun and T. Alonzo. Beyond the 3+3 method: expanded algorithms for dose-escalation in phase I oncology trials of two agents. *Clinical Trials*, 8:247–259, 2011.

[8] T. Braun and N. Jia. A generalized continual reassessment method for two-agent phase I trials. *Statistics in Biopharmaceutical Research*, 5:105–115, 2013.

[9] T. Braun and S. Wang. A hierarchical Bayesian design for phase I trials of novel combinations of cancer therapeutic agents. *Biometrics*, 66:805–812, 2010.

[10] Z. Chen, M. Tighiouart, and J. Kowalski. Dose escalation with overdose control using a quasi-continuous toxicity score in cancer phase I clinical trials. *Contemporary Clinical Trials*, 33:949–958, 2012.

[11] Y. K. Cheung. Coherence principles in dose-finding studies. *Biometrika*, 92:203–215, 2005.

[12] Y. K. Cheung. *Dose Finding by the Continual Reassessment Method.* Chapman and Hall/CRC Biostatistics Series, 2011.

[13] Y. K. Cheung and R. Chappell. Sequential designs for phase I clinical trials with late-onset toxicities. *Biometrics*, 56:1177–1182, 2010.

[14] S. Chevret. The continual reassessment method in cancer phase I clinical trials: a simulation study. *Statistics in Medicine*, 12:1093–1108, 1993.

[15] P.-L. Chu, Y. Lin, and W.J. Shih. Unifying CRM and EWOC designs for phase I cancer clinical trials. *Journal of Statistical Planning and Inference*, 139:1146–1163, 2009.

[16] M. Conaway, S. Dunbar, and S. Peddada. Designs for single- or multiple-agent phase I trials. *Biometrics*, 60:661–669, 2004.

[17] S. E. Dahlberg, G. I. Shapiro, J. W. Clark, and B. E. Johnson. Evaluation of statistical designs in phase I expansion cohorts: The Dana-Farber/Harvard Cancer Center experience. *Journal of the National Cancer Institute*, 106(7):dju163, 2014.

[18] A. Doussau, R. Thiebault, and X. Paoletti. Dose-finding design using mixed-effect proportional odds model for longitudinal graded toxicity data in phase I oncology clinical trials. *Statistics in Medicine*, 32:5430–5447, 2013.

[19] S. Dunbar, M. Conaway, and S. Peddada. On improved estimation of parameters subject to order restrictions. *Statistics and Applications*, 3:121–128, 2001.

[20] S. Durham, N. Flournoy, and W. Rosenberger. A random walk rule for phase 1 clinical trials. *Biometrics*, 53(2):745–760, 1997.

[21] S. D. Durham and N. Flournoy. Random walks for quantile. In S. S. Gupta and J. O. Berger, editors, *Statistical Decision Theory and Related Topics V*, pages 467–476. Springer-Verlag, New York, 1994.

[22] S. D. Durham and N. Flournoy. Up-and-down designs I: Stationary treatment distributions. In N. Flournoy and W. F. Rosenberger, editors, *Adaptive Designs*, pages 139–157. Institute of Mathematical Statistics Hayward, California, 1995.

[23] G. K. Dy, L. M. Bruzek, G. A. Croghan, S. Mandrekar, C. Erlichman, P. Peethambaram, H. C. Pitot, L. J. Hanson, J. M. Reid, A. Furth, et al. A phase I trial of the novel farnesyl protein transferase inhibitor, BMS-214662, in combination with paclitaxel and carboplatin in patients with advanced cancer. *Clinical Cancer Research*, 11:1877–1883, 2005.

[24] S. Fan, A. Venook, and Y. Lu. Design issues in dose-finding phase I trials for combination of two agents. *Journal of Biopharmaceutical Statistics*, 19:509–523, 2009.

[25] L. Gandhi, R. Bahleda, S. M. Tolaney, E. L. Kwak, J. M. Cleary, S. S. Pandya, A. Hollebecque, R. Abbas, R. Ananthakrishnan, A. Berkenblit, et al. Phase I study of neratinib in combination with temsirolimus in patients with human epidermal growth factor receptor 2-dependent and other solid tumors. *Journal of Clinical Oncology*, 32:65–67, 2014.

[26] C. Gatsonis and J. Greenhouse. Bayesian methods for phase I clinical trials. *Statistics in Medicine*, 11:1377–1389, 1992.

[27] M. Gonen. A Bayesian evaluation of enrolling additional patients at the maximum tolerated dose in phase I trials. *Contemporary Clinical Trials*, 26:131–140, 2005.

[28] N. Gordon and J. Willson. Using toxicity grades in the design and analysis of cancer phase I clinical trials. *Statistics in Medicine*, 11:2063–2075, 1992.

[29] J. Harrington, G. Wheeler, M. Sweeting, A. Mander, and D. Jodrell. Adaptive designs for dual-agent phase I dose-escalation studies. *Nature Reviews Clinical Oncology*, 10:277–288, 2013.

[30] A. Hirakawa, C. Hamada, and S. Matsui. A dose-finding approach based on shrunken predictive probability for combinations of two agents in phase I trials. *Statistics in Medicine*, 32:4515–4525, 2013.

[31] A. Hoering, M. LeBlanc, and J. Crowley. Seamless phase I/II trial design for assessing toxicity and efficacy for targeted agents. *Clinical Cancer Research*, 17:640–646, 2011.

[32] A. Hoering, A. Mitchell, M. LeBlanc, and J. Crowley. Early phase trial design for assessing several dose levels for toxicity and efficacy for targeted agents. *Clinical Trials*, 10:422–429, 2013.

[33] S. Hunsberger, L. Rubinstein, J. Dancey, and E. Korn. Dose escalation trial designs based on a molecularly targeted endpoint. *Statistics in Medicine*, 24:2171–2181, 2005.

[34] J. Hwang and S. Peddada. Confidence interval estimation subject to order restrictions. *The Annals of Statistics*, 22:67–93, 1994.

[35] A. Iasonos and J. O'Quigley. Interplay of priors and skeletons in two-stage continual reassessment method. *Statistics in Medicine*, 31(30):4321–4336, 2012.

[36] A. Iasonos and J. O'Quigley. Design considerations for dose-expansion cohorts in phase I trials. *Journal of Clinical Oncology*, 31(31):4014–4021, 2013.

[37] A. Iasonos and J. O'Quigley. Adaptive dose-finding studies: a review of model-guided phase I clinical trials. *Journal of Clinical Oncology*, 32:2505–2511, 2014.

[38] A. Iasonos, S. Zohar, and J. O'Quigley. Incorporating lower grade toxicity information into dose finding designs. *Clinical Trials*, 8:370–379, 2011.

[39] A. Ivanova and K. Wang. Non-parametric approach to the design and analysis of two-dimensional dose-finding trials. *Statistics in Medicine*, 23:1861–1870, 2004.

[40] A. Ivanova and K. Wang. Bivariate isotonic design for dose-finding with ordered groups. *Statistics in Medicine*, 25:2018–2026, 2006.

[41] S. Ivy, L. Siu, E. Garrett-Mayer, and L. Rubinstein. Approaches to phase 1 clinical trial design focused on safety, efficiency, and selected patient populations: a report from the Clinical Trial Design Task Force of the National Cancer Institute Investigational Drug Steering Committee. *Clinical Cancer Research*, 16(6):1726–1736, 2010.

[42] O'Quigley J., L. Shen, and A. Gamst. Two sample continual reassessment method. *Journal of Biopharmaceutical Statistics*, 9:17–44, 1999.

[43] Y. Ji, Y. Li, and B. Bekele. Dose-finding in phase I clinical trials based on toxicity probability intervals. *Clinical Trials*, 4:235–244, 2007.

[44] D. R. Jones, C. A. Moskaluk, H. H. Gillenwater, G. R. Petroni, S. G. Burks, J. Philips, P. K. Rehm, J. Olazagasti, B. D. Kozower, and Y. Bao. Phase I trial of induction histone deacetylase and proteasome inhibition followed by surgery in non-small cell lung cancer. *Journal of Thoracic Oncology*, 7:1683–1690, 2012.

[45] E. Korn. Nontoxicity endpoints in phase I trial designs for targeted, non-cytotoxic agents. *Journal of the National Cancer Institute*, 96:977–978, 2004.

[46] E. Korn and R. Simon. Using tolerable-dose diagrams in the design of phase I combination chemotherapy trials. *Journal of Clinical Oncology*, 11:794–801, 1993.

[47] A. Kramar, A. Lebecq, and E. Candalh. Continual reassessment methods in phase I trials of the combination of two agents in oncology. *Statistics in Medicine*, 18:1849–864, 1999.

[48] C. Le Tourneau, J. Lee, and L. Siu. Dose escalation methods in phase I clinical trials. *Journal of the National Cancer Institute*, 101:708–720, 2009.

[49] B. Lee and S. Fan. A two-dimensional search algorithm for dose-finding trials of two agents. *Journal of Biopharmaceutical Statistics*, 22:1802–818, 2012.

[50] S. Lee and Y.K. Cheung. Model calibration in the continual reassessment method. *Clinical Trials*, 6:227–238, 2009.

[51] S. Lee, D. Hershman, P. Martin, J. Leonard, and Y.K. Cheung. Toxicity burden score: a novel approach to summarize multiple toxic effects. *Annals of Oncology*, 23:537–541, 2012.

[52] A. Legezda and J. Ibrahim. Heterogeneity in phase I clinical trials: prior elicitation and computation using the continual reassessment method. *Statistics in Medicine*, 20:867–882, 2001.

[53] Y. Lin and W. Shih. Statistical properties of traditional algorithm-based designs for phase I cancer clinical trials. *Biostatistics*, 2(2):203–215, 2001.

[54] S. Liu and Y. Yuan. Bayesian optimal interval designs for phase I clinical trials. *Journal of the Royal Statistical Society: Series C*, 64:507–523, 2015.

[55] Y.-C. Loke, S.-B. Tan, Y. Cai, and D. Machin. A Bayesian dose finding design for dual endpoint phase I trials. *Statistics in Medicine*, 25:3–22, 2006.

[56] P. LoRusso, K. Venkatakrishnan, R. Ramanathan, J. Sarantopoulos, D. Mulkerin, S. Shibata, A. Hamilton, A. Dowlati, S. Mani, M. Rudek, C. Takimoto, R. Neuwirth, D. Esseltine, and P. Ivy. Pharmacokinetics and safety of bortezomib in patients with advanced malignancies and varying degrees of liver dysfunction: Phase I NCI Organ Dysfunction Working Group Study NCI-6432. *Clinical Cancer Research*, 18(10):1–10, 2012.

[57] A. Mander and M. Sweeting. A product of independent beta probabilities dose escalation design for dual-agent phase I trials. *Statistics in Medicine*, 34:1261–1276, 2015.

[58] S. Mandrekar, Y. Cui, and D. Sargent. An adaptive phase I design for identifying a biologically optimal dose for dual agent drug combinations. *Statistics in Medicine*, 26:2317–2330, 2007.

[59] S. Mandrekar, R. Qin, and D. Sargent. Model-based phase I designs incorporating toxicity and efficacy for single and dual agent drug combinations: methods and challenges. *Statistics in Medicine*, 29:1077–1083, 2010.

[60] S. J. Mandrekar. Dose-finding trial designs for combination therapies in oncology. *Journal of Clinical Oncology*, 32:68–75, 2014.

[61] A. Mauguen, M. Le Deleya, and S. Zohar. Dose-finding approach for dose escalation with overdose control considering incomplete observations. *Statistics in Medicine*, 30:1584–1594, 2011.

[62] National Cancer Institute. NCI Common Terminology Criteria for Adverse Events (CTCAE) v.4. http://evs.nci.nih.gov/ftp1/CTCAE/About.html.

[63] B. Neuenschwander, M. Branson, and T. Gsponder. Critical aspects of the Bayesian approach to phase I cancer trials. *Statistics in Medicine*, 27:2420–2439, 2008.

[64] D. Normolle and T. Lawrence. Designing dose-escalation trials with late-onset toxicities using the time-to-event continual reassessment method. *Journal of Clinical Oncology*, 24:4426–4433, 2006.

[65] J. O'Quigley. Phase I and phase I/II dose finding algorithms using continual reassessment method. In J. Crowley and D. Ankherst, editors, *Handbook of Statistics in Clinical Oncology, 2nd Edition*. Chapman and Hall/CRC Biostatistics Series, 2006.

[66] J. O'Quigley and M. Conaway. Continual reassessment and related dose-finding designs. *Statistical Science*, 25(2):202–216, 2010.

[67] J. O'Quigley and M. Conaway. Extended model-based designs for more complex dose-finding studies. *Statistics in Medicine*, 30:2062–2069, 2011.

[68] J. O'Quigley, M. Hughes, and Fenton T. Dose-finding design for HIV studies. *Biometrics*, 57:1018–1029, 2001.

[69] J. O'Quigley and A. Iasonos. Dose-finding designs based on the continual reassessment method. In J. Crowley and A. Hoering, editors, *Handbook of Statistics in Clinical Oncology, 3rd Edition*, pages 21–52. Chapman and Hall/CRC Biostatistics Series, 2012.

[70] J. O'Quigley and A. Iasonos. Bridging solutions in dose-finding problems. *Journal of Biopharmaceutical Statistics*, 6(2):185–197, 2014.

[71] J. O'Quigley, X. Paoletti, and J. Maccario. Nonparametric optimal design in dose finding studies. *Biostatistics*, 3(1):51–56, 2002.

[72] J. O'Quigley, M. Pepe, and L. Fisher. Continual reassessment method: a practical design for phase I clinical trials in cancer. *Biometrics*, 46(1):33–48, 1990.

[73] X. Paoletti and A. Kramar. A comparison of model choices for the continual reassessment method in phase I cancer trials. *Statistics in Medicine*, 28:3012–3028, 2009.

[74] X. Paoletti, J. O'Quigley, and J. Maccario. Design efficiency in dose finding studies. *Computational Statistics and Data Analysis*, 45:197–214, 2004.

[75] W. Parulekar and E. Eisenhauer. Phase I trial design for solid tumors studies of targeted, non-cytotoxic agents: theory and practice. *Journal of the National Cancer Institute*, 96:970–978, 2004.

[76] R. Paul, W. Rosenberger, and N. Flournoy. Quantile estimation following non-parametric phase I clinical trials with ordinal response. *Statistics in Medicine*, 23:2483–2495, 2004.

[77] S. Piantadosi, S. Fisher, and S. Grossman. Practical implementation of a modified continual reassessment method for dose-finding trials. *Cancer Chemotherapy and Pharmacology*, 41:429–436, 1998.

[78] M. Polley. Practical modifications to the time-to-event continual reassessment method for phase I cancer trials with fast patient accrual and late-onset toxicities. *Statistics in Medicine*, 30:2130–2143, 2011.

[79] M. Polley and Y.K. Cheung. Two-stage designs for dose-finding trials with a biologic endpoint using stepwise tests. *Biometrics*, 64:232–241, 2008.

[80] R. Ramanathan, M. Egorin, C. Takimoto, S. Remick, J. Doroshow, P. LoRusso, D. Mulkerin, J. Grem, A. Hamilton, A. Murgo, D. Potter, C. Belani, M. Hayes, B. Peng, and P. Ivy. Phase I and pharmacokinetic study of imatinib mesylate in patients with advanced malignancies and varying degrees of liver dysfunction: a study by the National Cancer Institute Organ Dysfunction Working Group. *Journal of Clinical Oncology*, 26:563–569, 2008.

[81] T. Robertson, F.T. Wright, and R. Dykstra. *Order Restricted Statistical Inference.* J. Wiley New York, 1988.

[82] A. Rogatko, D. Schoeneck, W. Jonas, M. Tighiouaet, F. Khuri, and A. Porter. Translation of innovative designs into phase I trials. *Journal of Clinical Onocology*, 25(31):4982–4986, 2007.

[83] A. Senderowicz. Information needed to conduct first-in-human oncology trials in the United States: A view from a former FDA medical reviewer. *Clinical Cancer Research*, 16(6):1719–1725, 2010.

[84] L. Shen and J. O'Quigley. Continual reassessment method: A likelihood approach. *Biometrics*, 52(2):673–684, 1996.

[85] Y. Shi and G. Yin. Escalation with overdose control for phase I drug combination trials. *Statistics in Medicine*, 32:4400–4412, 2013.

[86] M. Silvapulle. On the existence of maximum likelihood estimators for the binomial response model. *Journal of the Royal Statistical Society: Series B*, 43:310–313, 1981.

[87] B. Storer. Design and analysis of phase I clinical trials. *Biometrics*, 45(3):925–937, 1989.

[88] M. Stylianou and N. Flournoy. Dose finding using the biased coin up-and-down design and isotonic regression. *Biometrics*, 58:171–177, 2002.

[89] P. Thall and J. Cook. Dose-finding based on efficacy-toxicity trade-offs. *Biometrics*, 60:684–693, 2004.

[90] P. Thall, R. Millikan, P. Mueller, and S. Lee. Dose-finding with two agents in phase I oncology trials. *Biometrics*, 59:487–496, 2003.

[91] P. Thall, H. Nguyen, T. Braun, and M. Qazilbash. Using joint utilities of the times to response and toxicity to adaptively optimize schedule-dose regimes. *Biometrics*, 69:673–682, 2013.

[92] P. Thall, H. Nguyen, and E. Estey. Patient-specific dose finding based on bivariate outcomes and covariates. *Biometrics*, 64:1126–1136, 2008.

[93] P. Thall and K. Russell. A strategy for dose-finding and safety monitoring based on efficacy and adverse outcomes in phase I/II clinical trials. *Biometrics*, 54(1):251–264, 1998.

[94] M. Tighiouart, G. Cook-Wiens, and A. Rogatko. Escalation with overdose control using ordinal toxicity grades for cancer phase I clinical trials. *Journal of Probability and Statistics*, 2012:ID317634, 2012.

[95] M. Tighiouart, Y. Liu, and A. Rogatko. Escalation with overdose control using time to toxicity for cancer phase I clinical trials. *PLOS ONE*, 9(3):e93070, 2014.

[96] M. Tighiouart and A. Rogatko. Dose finding with escalation with overdose control (EWOC) in cancer clinical trials. *Statistical Science*, 25(2):217–226, 2014.

[97] M. Tighiouart, A. Rogatko, and J. Babb. Flexible Bayesian methods for cancer phase I clinical trials.dose escalation with overdose control. *Statistics in Medicine*, 24:2183–2196, 2005.

[98] M. Van Meter, E. Garrett-Mayer, and D. Bandyopadhyay. Proportional odds model for dose-finding clinical trial designs with ordinal toxicity grading. *Statistics in Medicine*, 30:2070–2080, 2011.

[99] M. Van Meter, E. Garrett-Mayer, and D. Bandyopadhyay. Dose-finding clinical trial design for ordinal toxicity grades using the continuation ratio model: an extension of the continual reassessment method. *Clinical Trials*, 9:303–313, 2012.

[100] N. Wages, M. Conaway, and J. O'Quigley. Continual reassessment method for partial ordering. *Biometrics*, 67:1555–1563, 2011.

[101] N. Wages, M. Conaway, and J. O'Quigley. Dose-finding design for multi-drug combinations. *Clinical Trials*, 8:380–389, 2011.

[102] N. Wages, M. Conaway, and J. O'Quigley. Performance of two-stage continual reassessment method relative to an optimal benchmark. *Clinical Trials*, 10:862–875, 2013.

[103] N. Wages, M. Conaway, and J. O'Quigley. Using the time-to-event continual reassessment method in the presence of partial orders. *Statistics in Medicine*, 32:131–141, 2013.

[104] N. Wages and C. Tait. Seamless phase I/II adaptive design for oncology trials of molecularly targeted agents. *Journal of Biopharmaceutical Statistics*, 25(5):903–920, 2015.

[105] N. Wages and N. Varhegyi. POCRM: an R-package for phase I trials of combinations of agents. *Computer Methods and Programs in Biomedicine*, 112:211–218, 2013.

[106] K. Wang and A. Ivanova. Two-dimensional dose finding in discrete dose space. *Biometrics*, 61:217–222, 2005.

[107] J. Whitehead and D. Williamson. Bayesian decision procedures based on logistic regression models for dose-finding studies. *Journal of Biopharmaceutical Statistics*, 8:445–467, 1998.

[108] C. Wu. Efficient sequential designs with binary data. *Journal of the American Statistical Association*, 80:974–984, 1985.

[109] G. Yin and Y. Yuan. A latent contingency table approach to dose finding for combination of two agents. *Biometrics*, 65:866–875, 2005.

[110] G. Yin and Y. Yuan. Bayesian dose finding in oncology for drug combinations by copula regression. *Journal of the Royal Staistical Society: Series C*, 58:211–224, 2009.

[111] G. Yin and Y. Yuan. Bayesian model averaging continual reassessment method in phase I clinical trials. *Journal of the American Statistical Association*, 104:954–968, 2009.

[112] G. Yin, S. Zheng, and J. Xu. Two-stage dose finding for cytostatic agents in phase I oncology trials. *Statistics in Medicine*, 32:644–660, 2013.

[113] J. Yuan, Y. Li, and B. Bekele. Dose-finding in phase I clinical trials based on toxicity probability intervals. *Clinical Trials*, 4:235–244, 2007.

[114] J. Yuan, P. Liu, Y. Li, and B. Bekele. A modified toxicity probability interval method for dose-finding trials. *Clinical Trials*, 7:653–663, 2010.

[115] Y. Yuan and G. Yin. Sequential continual reassessment method for two-dimensional dose finding. *Statistics in Medicine*, 27:5664–5678, 2008.

[116] Z. Yuan and R. Chapell. Isotonic designs for phase I cancer clinical trials with multiple risk groups. *Clinical Trials*, 1(6):499–508, 2004.

[117] Yuan Z., R. Chappell, and H. Bailey. The continual reassessment method for multiple toxicity grades: a Bayesian quasi-likelihood approach. *Biometrics*, 63:173–179, 2007.

[118] Y. Zang, J. Lee, and Y. Yuan. Adaptive designs for identifying optimal biological dose for molecularly targeted agents. *Clinical Trials*, 11:319–327, 2014.

[119] W. Zhang, D. Sargent, and S. Mandrekar. An adaptive dose-finding design incorporating both toxicity and efficacy. *Statistics in Medicine*, 25:2365–2383, 2006.

7

Design and Analysis of Phase II Cancer Clinical Trials

Sin-Ho Jung

CONTENTS

7.1 Introduction

Cancer clinical trials investigate the efficacy and toxicity of experimental cancer therapies. If an appropriate dose level of an experimental drug is determined from a phase I trial, the drug's anticancer activity is assessed through phase II clinical trials. Phase II clinical trials screen out inefficacious experimental therapies before they proceed to further investigation through large scale phase III trials. In order to expedite this process, phase II trials traditionally use a single-arm design to treat patients with experimental therapies only. The efficacy of an experimental therapy is compared with that of a standard therapy using historical controls. The most popular primary endpoint of phase II cancer clinical trials is tumor response which is measured by the change in tumor size before and during treatment. If the size of a target tumor, defined as the largest diameter of the tumor, decreases by at least 30%

compared to that at the baseline, a partial response is declared. A complete response is defined as complete disappearance of the tumor. Overall response is defined as partial or complete response.

Phase II trials generally require shorter study periods than phase III trials. Consequently, phase II trials have small sample sizes, so that exact statistical methods are preferable to asymptotic methods for their design and analysis. Various exact methods have been published for phase II trials with binary outcomes such as tumor response. For ethical reasons, two-stage designs are commonly used for phase II cancer clinical trials. A typical single-arm two-stage trial with a futility (a_1) and a superiority (b_1) stopping value and a stage 2 rejection value (a) are conducted as follows.

- Stage 1: Treat n_1 patients and count the number of responders X_1.
  - If $X_1 \leq a_1$, then reject the experimental therapy and stop the trial.
  - If $X_1 \geq b_1$, then accept the experimental therapy and stop the trial.
  - If $a_1 < X_1 < b_1$, then proceed to the second stage.
- Stage 2: Treat an additional n_2 patients and count the number of responders X_2.
  - If $X_1 + X_2 \leq a$, then reject the experimental therapy.
  - Otherwise, accept the experimental therapy for further investigation.

We usually do not stop the trial early for superiority since there is no ethical issue to continue treating patients with an efficacious therapy and we want to collect as much data as possible to use when designing a subsequent phase III trial. In this case, we choose $b_1 = n_1 + 1$.

The design and analysis of phase II trials require exact statistical methods accounting for the two-stage design and small sample sizes. The most popular design for phase II cancer clinical trials has been a two-stage design with futility stopping only based on Simon's [22] minimax or optimality criterion. But most publications reporting the results of phase II trials fail to appropriately address these issues. When the above two-stage phase II trial is completed, we should be able to accept or reject the experimental therapy based on the critical values and sample sizes, (a_1, b_1, a, n_1, n_2). In a usual clinical trial, we would recruit slightly more patients than required to make up for possible attrition due to ineligibility and dropout. As a result, the observed sample size tends to be different from that specified by the design. In a typical two-stage phase II trial, the sample size at the stopping stage is different from (usually larger, but rarely smaller, than) the planned one. In this case, the critical values at the stopping stage become meaningless. This is one reason why investigators are not able to draw clear conclusions from their phase II trials. To address this issue, we propose to extend the two-stage testing rule by calculating a p-value or a confidence interval of the true response rate (RR). These methods exactly coincide with the two-stage testing rule if the observed sample sizes are identical to the prespecified (n_1, n_2). In this chapter, we discuss further design and analysis methods for single-arm phase II trials with tumor response as the primary endpoint.

In spite of these adjustments, single-arm phase II trials have intrinsic shortcomings. Single-arm phase II trials are appropriate only when reliable and valid data for an existing standard therapy are available for the same patient population. Furthermore, the response assessment method in the historical control data should be identical to the one that will be used for a new study. If no historical control data satisfying these conditions exist or the existing data are too small to represent the whole patient population, we have to consider a randomized phase II clinical trial with a prospective control to be compared with the experimental therapy under investigation. Cannistra [2] recommends a randomized phase II trial if a single-arm design is subject to any of the above issues. Readers may refer to Gan et al. [10] about more issues associated with which design to choose between a single-arm phase II trial and a randomized phase II trial. In this chapter, we discuss randomized phase II trials based on Fisher's exact test [9].

7.2 Single-arm Phase II Trials

7.2.1 Optimal Two-stage Designs

In this section, we focus on the popular two-stage single-arm phase II trial designs with a futility interim test only, i.e., $b_1 = n_1+1$. These designs are defined by the number of patients to be treated during stages 1 and 2, n_1 and n_2, and rejection values a_1 and a $(a_1 < a)$, so that we specify them by $(a_1/n_1, a/n)$, where $n = n_1 + n_2$ is the maximal sample size. The values of $(a_1/n_1, a/n)$ are determined based on prespecified design parameters as described below. Let p_0 denote the maximum unacceptable probability of response which is usually chosen by the RR of a historical control, and p_1 the minimum acceptable probability of response with $p_0 < p_1$. For the true RR p of the experimental therapy, we want to test $H_0 : p \leq p_0$ against $H_1 : p > p_0$. Given (p_0, p_1), we can calculate the type I error probability α and power $1 - \beta$ of a two-stage design $(a_1/n_1, a/n)$ based on the fact that the number of responders from the two stages, X_1 and X_2, are independent binomial random variables.

Suppose that we want to find a two-stage design with a type I error probability no larger than α^* and a power no smaller than $1 - \beta^*$ for given (p_0, p_1) values. The quantities $(p_0, p_1, \alpha^*, \beta^*)$ are the design parameters. Given (p_0, p_1), there are infinitely many 2-stage designs satisfying the $(\alpha^*, 1 - \beta^*)$-constraint. Noting that the sample size of a two-stage trial is a random variable taking n_1 or n, we can calculate the expected sample size of the trial given a true RR of the experimental therapy. Simon [22] proposes two criteria to select a good two-stage design among these candidate designs. The minimax design minimizes the maximal sample size, n, among the designs satisfying the $(\alpha^*, 1-\beta^*)$-constraint. On the other hand, the so-called "optimal" design minimizes the expected sample size under $H_0 : p = p_0$, denoted as EN.

While the minimax and the optimal designs have both been widely used, other two-stage designs have been largely ignored. Oftentimes, the two criteria result in very different two-stage designs, i.e., the minimax design may have an excessively large EN as compared to the optimal design and the optimal design may have an excessively large maximal sample size n as compared to the minimax design. This results from the discrete nature of the exact binomial method.

Example 1: For the design parameters $(p_0, p_1, \alpha^*, 1-\beta^*) = (0.1, 0.3, 0.05, 0.85)$, the minimax design is given by $(a_1/n_1, a/n) = (2/18, 5/27)$ and the optimal design by $(1/11, 6/35)$. The maximal sample size n for the minimax design is less than that for the optimal design by 8. However, the expected sample size EN under H_0 for the optimal design is 18.3 which is only slightly smaller than EN = 20.4 for the minimax design. Thus, we may consider choosing the minimax design since, compared to the optimal design, it largely saves the maximal sample size while sacrificing the expected sample size by only about 2. In this case, there exists a practical compromise without changing the statistical operating characteristics appreciably. For the same design parameters $(p_0, p_1, \alpha^*, 1-\beta^*) = (0.1, 0.3, 0.05, 0.85)$, the design given by $(a_1/n_1, a/n) = (1/13, 5/28)$ requires only one more patient in the maximal sample size n than the minimax design but its expected sample size EN under H_0 is very comparable to that of the optimal design (18.7 vs 18.3).

This design is a good compromise between the minimax design and the optimal design [15]. There are other designs that satisfy the given design specifications. Such designs are called admissible designs and an algorithm to identify them has been proposed [16]. Simon's minimax and optimal designs belong to the family of admissible designs. An interactive computer program to find admissible designs is available at www.dukecancerinstitute.org/research/shared-resources/biostatistics/clinical-trial-design-systems/.

Figure 7.1 is a snapshot of this program for Example 1. It displays the plot of EN against n for various designs with $n \leq 37$. Simon's minimax design given by $(a_1/n_1, a/n) = (2/18, 5/27)$ is the leftmost point in the figure and the optimal design by $(1/11, 6/35)$ is at the very bottom. The program provides specification of a design $(a_1/n_1, a/n)$ along with $(\alpha, 1-\beta)$, EN, and the probabilities of early termination for $p = p_0$ and p_1 when the circle representing a candidate design, actually (n, EN), is clicked with a pointer.

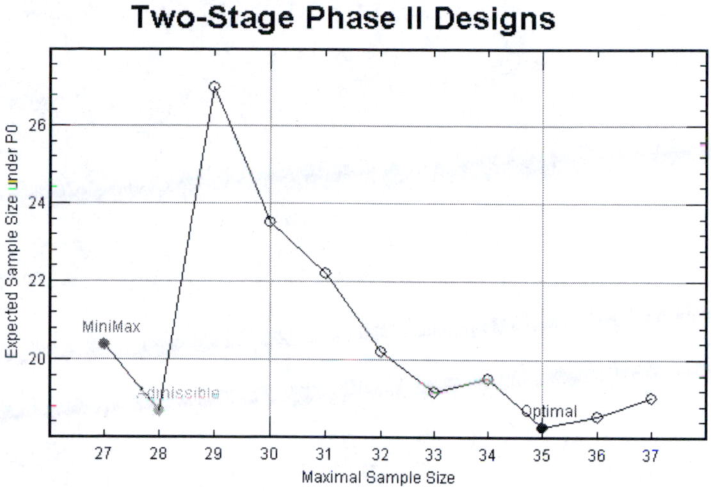

FIGURE 7.1: Two-stage designs for$(p_0, p_1, \alpha, \beta) = (.1, .3, .05, .15)$ with $N = 37$.

In this section, we have considered two-stage designs with a futility stopping value only. Also available are optimal multistage designs with both futility and superiority stopping boundaries by minimizing the average of expected sample sizes under H_0 and H_1 [4]. The computer program mentioned above also provides minimax, optimal and admissible designs with both futility and superiority stopping boundaries.

7.2.2 Estimation of Response Rate

In a two-stage phase II trial, let M (=1 or 2) denote the stopping stage, and S the cumulative number of responders by the stopping stage, i.e., $S = X_1$ if $M = 1$ and $S = X_1 + X_2$ if $M = 2$. The most popular estimator of RR p for $(M, S) = (m, s)$ is the sample proportion, i.e.,

$$\hat{p} = \begin{cases} s/n_1 & \text{if } m = 1 \\ s/(n_1 + n_2) & \text{if } m = 2 \end{cases}$$

By not reflecting the two-stage design aspect of the trial, this estimator, called the maximum likelihood estimator (MLE), is always negatively biased for standard two-stage trials with futility stopping only [16]. As a result, if p_0 of a future trial is chosen by the sample proportion of a historical control taken from a previous two-stage phase II trial, then it will underestimate the true RR of the historical control and result in a higher chance of false positivity for the future trial.

For $(M, S) = (m, s)$, the uniformly minimum variance unbiased estimator

(UMVUE) of p for two-stage phase II trials is given by

$$\tilde{p} = \begin{cases} s/n_1 & \text{if } m = 1 \\ \dfrac{\sum_{x_1=(a_1+1)\vee(s-n_2)}^{s\wedge(b_1-1)} \binom{n_1-1}{x_1-1}\binom{n_2}{s-x_1}}{\sum_{x_1=(a_1+1)\vee(s-n_2)}^{s\wedge(b_1-1)} \binom{n_1}{x_1}\binom{n_2}{s-x_1}} & \text{if } m = 2 \end{cases} \quad (7.1)$$

where $a \wedge b = \min(a, b)$ and $a \vee b = \max(a, b)$ [16]. Note that the UMVUE and the MLE are identical if the trial stops after stage 1, i.e., $m = 1$.

For a true RR of p, the probability mass function (PMF) of (M, S), $f(m, s|p) = Pr(M = m, S = s)$, is given as

$$\begin{aligned} f(m, s|p) &= p^s(1-p)^{n_1-s}\binom{n_1}{s} \\ &\quad \text{if } m = 1, 0 \leq s \leq a_1 \text{ or } b_1 \leq s \leq n_1 \text{ and} \\ f(m, s|p) &= p^s(1-p)^{n_1+n_2-s}\sum_{x_1=a_1+1}^{(b_1-1)\wedge s}\binom{n_1}{x_1}\binom{n_2}{s-x_1} \\ &\quad \text{if } m = 2, a_1 + 1 \leq s \leq b_1 - 1 + n_2 \end{aligned} \quad (7.2)$$

Since the UMVUE of p is a function of (M, S), its PMF is derived from $f(m, s|p)$.

Example 2: Under $(p_0, p_1, \alpha^*, 1-\beta^*) = (0.2, 0.4, 0.05, 0.8)$, Simon's optimal two-stage design with a futility stopping value only is given as $(a_1/n_1, a/n) = (3/13, 12/43)$. Table 7.1 gives the UMVUE and the MLE for observations (m, s) for the two-stage design and their PMF for various RR values. When $m = 1$, two estimates are exactly the same as noted earlier. When $m = 2$, the MLE is much smaller than UMVUE for small s values. Jung and Kim [16] show that the UMVUE has a comparable variance as compared to the MLE overall.

In order to account for ineligible or unevaluable patients, we often accrue slightly more (or possibly less) patients than the planned sample size at the stopping stage, especially in multicenter trials (e.g., [11][12]). But, this does not become any issue in the calculation of the UMVUE, since it does not require specification of the critical values (a_m, b_m) at the stopping stage m, where $a_2 = a$ and $b_2 = a+1$. If the study is terminated after stage 1 (i.e., $m = 1$), then the UMVUE is calculated by regarding the observed number of stage 1 patients as n_1. If the study is proceeded to the second stage (i.e., $m = 2$), then the UMVUE in (1) depends only on the rejection values for stage 1 (a_1, b_1) and the number of patients for the two stages (n_1, n_2). When $m = 2$, the interim test is always conducted using (a_1, b_1) when exactly n_1 patients have response data as planned. However, the number of stage 2 patients may be slightly different from n_2. In this case, we calculate the UMVUE by regarding the observed number of patients for stage 2 as n_2 with (n_1, a_1, b_1) fixed by the design.

TABLE 7.1: UMVUE, MLE, and probability mass function for true p for each observation in a two-stage design with $(a_1/n_1, a/n) = (3/13, 12/43)$

				$f(m, s \mid p)$ for p				
m	s	UMVUE	MLE	0.1	0.2	0.3	0.4	0.5
1	0	0.000	0.000	0.254	0.055	0.010	0.001	0.000
1	1	0.077	0.077	0.367	0.179	0.054	0.011	0.002
1	2	0.154	0.154	0.245	0.268	0.139	0.045	0.010
1	3	0.231	0.231	0.100	0.246	0.218	0.111	0.035
2	4	0.308	0.093	0.001	0.000	0.000	0.000	0.000
2	5	0.312	0.116	0.004	0.002	0.000	0.000	0.000
2	6	0.317	0.140	0.007	0.006	0.001	0.000	0.000
2	7	0.322	0.163	0.008	0.015	0.002	0.000	0.000
2	8	0.328	0.186	0.006	0.027	0.006	0.000	0.000
2	9	0.335	0.209	0.004	0.038	0.015	0.001	0.000
2	10	0.343	0.233	0.002	0.043	0.030	0.003	0.000
2	11	0.351	0.256	0.001	0.041	0.049	0.008	0.000
2	12	0.360	0.279	0.000	0.033	0.068	0.018	0.001
2	13	0.371	0.302	0.000	0.023	0.081	0.033	0.003
2	14	0.382	0.326	0.000	0.014	0.084	0.054	0.006
2	15	0.395	0.349	0.000	0.007	0.076	0.076	0.013
2	16	0.409	0.372	0.000	0.003	0.062	0.096	0.025
2	17	0.424	0.395	0.000	0.001	0.044	0.107	0.042
2	18	0.440	0.419	0.000	0.001	0.029	0.108	0.063
2	19	0.458	0.442	0.000	0.000	0.017	0.098	0.085
2	20	0.477	0.465	0.000	0.000	0.009	0.080	0.105
2	21	0.496	0.488	0.000	0.000	0.004	0.059	0.116
2	22	0.517	0.512	0.000	0.000	0.002	0.040	0.118
2	23	0.538	0.535	0.000	0.000	0.001	0.025	0.108
2	24	0.560	0.558	0.000	0.000	0.000	0.014	0.091
2	25	0.582	0.581	0.000	0.000	0.000	0.007	0.069
2	26	0.605	0.605	0.000	0.000	0.000	0.003	0.048
2	27	0.628	0.628	0.000	0.000	0.000	0.001	0.030
2	28	0.651	0.651	0.000	0.000	0.000	0.001	0.017
2	29	0.674	0.674	0.000	0.000	0.000	0.000	0.009
2	30	0.698	0.698	0.000	0.000	0.000	0.000	0.004
2	31	0.721	0.721	0.000	0.000	0.000	0.000	0.002
2	32	0.744	0.744	0.000	0.000	0.000	0.000	0.001
2	33	0.767	0.767	0.000	0.000	0.000	0.000	0.000
2	34	0.791	0.791	0.000	0.000	0.000	0.000	0.000
2	35	0.814	0.814	0.000	0.000	0.000	0.000	0.000
2	36	0.837	0.837	0.000	0.000	0.000	0.000	0.000
2	37	0.861	0.861	0.000	0.000	0.000	0.000	0.000
2	38	0.884	0.884	0.000	0.000	0.000	0.000	0.000
2	39	0.907	0.907	0.000	0.000	0.000	0.000	0.000
2	40	0.930	0.930	0.000	0.000	0.000	0.000	0.000
2	41	0.954	0.954	0.000	0.000	0.000	0.000	0.000
2	42	0.977	0.977	0.000	0.000	0.000	0.000	0.000
2	43	1.000	1.000	0.000	0.000	0.000	0.000	0.000

Example 2 (revisited): Suppose that a phase II trial was designed for Simon's optimal two-stage design with a futility stopping value only as $(a_1/n_1, a/n) = (3/13, 12/43)$ under $(p_0, p_1, \alpha^*, 1-\beta^*) = (0.2, 0.4, 0.05, 0.8)$, but it was completed with $s = 7$ responders from a total of 45 patients after stage 2. Then, by using $(a_1, n_1) = (3, 13)$ and conditioning n_2 at $32 (= 45 - 13)$, we have $(a_1 + 1) \vee (s - n_2) = (3 + 1) \vee (7 - 32) = 4$ and $s \wedge (b_1 - 1) = 7 \wedge (14 - 1) = 13$. Hence, from (7.1), the UMVUE is calculated by

$$\tilde{p} = \frac{\sum_{x_1=4}^{7} \binom{12}{x_1-1}\binom{32}{7-x_1}}{\sum_{x_1=4}^{7} \binom{13}{x_1}\binom{32}{7-x_1}} = \frac{1,362,988}{4,241,380} = 0.321$$

while the MLE is only $\hat{p} = 7/45 = 0.156$.

Jennison and Turnbull [13] proposed a confidence interval method for RR for multistage clinical trials. Jung and Kim [16] prove that the ordering of the sample space Jennison and Turnbull [13] used to calculate their confidence intervals is identical to that of (M, S) in terms of the magnitude of the UMVUE.

7.2.3 Confidence Interval

Jung and Kim [16] prove that the ordering of the sample space for (M, S) in terms of the magnitude of the UMVUE is identical to that by Jennison and Turnbull [13]; see also [1] and [24]. In other words, we have

$$\begin{aligned} &\tilde{p}(1,0) < \tilde{p}(1,1) < \cdots < \tilde{p}(1,a_1) \\ &< \tilde{p}(2, a_1+1) < \cdots < \tilde{p}(2, b_1 - 1 + n_2) \\ &< \tilde{p}(1, b_1) < \cdots < \tilde{p}(1, n_1) \end{aligned} \tag{7.3}$$

where $\tilde{p}(m, s)$ denotes the UMVUE for $(M, S) = (m, s)$. Hence, the confidence intervals calculated according to [6] and the stochastic ordering based on the magnitude of the UMVUE are identical to those by [13].

With the UMVUE $\tilde{p}(m, s)$, an exact $100(1-\alpha)\%$ equal tail confidence interval (p_L, p_U) for p is given by

$$\Pr(\tilde{p}(M,S) \geq \tilde{p}(m,s) | p = p_L) = \alpha/2$$

and

$$\Pr(\tilde{p}(M,S) \leq \tilde{p}(m,s) | p = p_U) = \alpha/2,$$

where the probabilities are calculated using the PMF of (M, S) as defined in (7.2). Confidence limits p_L and p_U can be obtained by the bisection method to solve the equations.

Example 3: Suppose that we observed $(m, s) = (2, 7)$ from a two-stage study with lower boundaries only, $(n_1, n_2, a_1, a) = (13, 30, 3, 12)$. In this case, we have $b_1 = n_1 + 1 = 14$, $(a_1 + 1) \vee (s - n_2) = (3 + 1) \vee (7 - 30) = 4$, and $s \wedge (b_1 - 1) = 7 \wedge (14 - 1) = 7$. From (1), the UMVUE is

$$\tilde{p}(2,7) = \frac{\sum_{x_1=4}^{7} \binom{13-1}{x_1-1}\binom{30}{7-x_1}}{\sum_{x_1=4}^{7} \binom{13}{x_1}\binom{30}{7-x_1}} = .322.$$

Using (7.2), we have

$$\Pr(\tilde{p}(M,S) \geq .322 | p = .103) = .025,$$

$$\Pr(\tilde{p}(M,S) \leq .322 | p = .538) = .025$$

so that a 95% confidence interval on p is given as (.103, .538), which is the same as the one according to [13]. In contrast, a naive exact 95% confidence interval by [6] ignoring the two-stage aspect of the study design is given as (.068, .307). Note that the latter is narrower than the former by ignoring the group sequential feature of the study. Furthermore, the former is slightly shifted to the right from the latter to reflect the fact that the study has been continued to stage 2 after observing more responders than $a_1 = 3$ in stage 1. The popularly used asymptotic confidence interval $\hat{p} \pm 1.96\sqrt{\hat{p}(1 - \hat{p})/n} = (.052, .273)$ with 95% significance level is even narrower and further shifted to the left than the naive exact confidence interval.

The Jennison-Turnbull confidence interval based on the stochastic ordering (7.3) has a desirable property: given (p_0, α^*), the testing result based on the two-stage design $(a_1/n_1, a/n)$ exactly coincides with that based on the one-sided confidence interval with significance level $100(1 - \alpha^*)$%, i.e., we reject $H_0 : p = p_0$ by the two-stage design if and only if the lower confidence limit is larger than p_0. This property is very valuable especially when the observed sample size for the stopping stage is different from the sample size specified by the study design. In this case, the two-stage design does not provide us a proper testing rule any more since the rejection values, (a_1, b_1) or a, are meaningful only when the number of patients are identical to the prespecified sample size. But we can calculate a Jennison-Turnbull confidence interval of RR by treating the observed sample size at the stopping stage like the planned sample size. This is possible since (7.2) and (7.3) do not require specification of the rejection values at the stopping stage. Various confidence interval methods have been proposed for multistage designs (e.g., [8][23]), but no other confidence intervals have this property.

Example 4: Kim et al. [20] published a phase II trial of concurrent chemoradiotherapy for newly diagnosed patients with limited-stage extranodal natural killer/T-cell lymphoma, nasal type. The primary endpoint is complete response (CR) rate. The study had Simon's [22] optimal two-stage design $(a_1/n_1, a/n) = (4/6, 22/27)$ under $(p_0, p_1, \alpha^*, 1 - \beta^*) = (0.7, 0.9, 0.05, 0.8)$. The trial proceeded to the second stage to treat a total of 30 eligible and evaluable patients of which 27 achieved CR. Since the observed maximal sample size is different from the planned one, the rejection value $a = 22$ was of no use to determine the positivity of the study. The authors concluded the study to be positive without statistical ground. Noting this, Shimada and Suzuki [21] claimed that this trial was a negative study by calculating an asymptotic confidence interval with 2-sided 95% significance level and showing that it covers $p_0 = 0.7$. This claim is misleading since their interval (i) has a two-sided $100(1-\alpha) = 95\%$ confidence level while the two-stage design has 1-sided $\alpha = 5\%$, (ii) ignores the two-stage feature of the trial, and (iii) is using a large-sample approximation. Kim et al. [19] defended their conclusion by showing that the 1-sided 95% Jennison-Turnbull confidence interval $(0.762, 1]$ is above $p_0 = 0.7$.

7.2.4 p-Value Calculation

In a phase II trial, we conduct a statistical test to reject or accept the experimental therapy. If we reject or fail to reject the null hypothesis, we should be able to provide a p-value as a measure of how strong evidence the decision is against the null hypothesis. However, publications from phase II trials rarely report p-values to support their conclusions. In most of the publications, it is not even clear if the investigators decide to accept their therapies or not.

Using the stochastic ordering of UMVUE (7.3), Jung et al. [15] propose a p-value method for 2-stage phase II clinical trials. Noting that a p-value is defined as the probability of observing an extreme test statistic value toward the direction of H_1 when H_0 is true, they propose to calculate the probability of observing a UMVUE value larger than that obtained from the study under H_0. Let $\tilde{p}$ denote the UMVUE of the RR observed from a two-stage phase II trial specified by (a_1, b_1, a, n_1, n_2). Given $(M, S) = (m, s)$, the p-value $= Pr\{\tilde{p}(M, S) \geq \tilde{p}(m, s)|p_0\}$ based on UMVUE can be calculated as

$$\text{p-value} = \begin{cases} \sum_{j=s}^{n_1} f(1, j|p_0) & \text{if } m = 1, s \geq b_1 \\ 1 - \sum_{j=0}^{s-1} f(1, j|p_0) & \text{if } m = 1, s \leq a_1 \\ \sum_{j=b_1}^{n_1} f(1, j|p_0) + \sum_{j=s}^{b_1-1+n_2} f(2, j|p_0) & \text{if } m = 2 \end{cases} \tag{7.4}$$

Jung et al. [17] show that, if the observed sample size at each stage is identical to that specified by the design, the decision by the two-stage design exactly matches with that by the p-value compared with the α value. As discussed in the previous section, the confidence interval by [13] also has this property.

Example 5: For $H_0 : p_0 = .4$ vs. $H_1 : p_1 = .6$, the two-stage design $(n_1, n_2, a_1, b_1, a) = (34, 5, 17, 35, 20)$ is the Simon's minimax design among those with $(\alpha^*, 1 - \beta^*) = (0.05, 0.8)$ and a futility stopping boundary only. Table 7.2 displays the p-values and the PMF at $p_0 = 0.4$ for each sample point in the descending order for UMVUE. For example, for $(m, s) = (2, 19)$, we calculate the UMVUE by

$$\tilde{p} = \frac{\sum_{x_1=(17+1)\vee(19-5)}^{19\wedge(35-1)} \binom{34-1}{x_1-1}\binom{5}{19-x_1}}{\sum_{x_1=(17+1)\vee(19-5)}^{19\wedge(35-1)} \binom{34}{x_1}\binom{5}{19-x_1}} = \frac{\binom{33}{17}\binom{5}{1}+\binom{33}{18}\binom{5}{0}}{\binom{34}{18}\binom{5}{1}+\binom{34}{19}\binom{5}{0}} = 0.5337$$

Hence, when $(m, s) = (2, 19)$ is observed, we calculate the p-value based on UMVUE as

$$\Pr(\tilde{p}(M,S) \geq .5337|p_0) = \sum_{j=19}^{39} f(2, j|p_0)$$

$$= .0129 + .0219 + .0217 + .0145 + .0075 + .0033 + .0013 + .0005 + .0002 + .0000 + \cdots + .0000$$

$$= .0838$$

Since p-value $> \alpha^*(= 0.05)$, we fail to reject H_0. Since $s = 19$ after stage $2(= m)$ is smaller than $a = 20$, we fail to reject H_0 by the two-stage testing rule also. Table 7.2 also reports the p-values based on the ordering by MLE values and the p-values calculated by ignoring the fact that the two-stage design aspect, denoted as 'naive'. Note that the p-values based on the UMVUE and MLE orderings are different for large s values with $m = 1$ and for small s values with $m = 2$. This occurs because of the difference between the UMVUE-ordering and the MLE-ordering for the small s values with $m = 2$. The naive p-values are quite different from the p-values based on the UMVUE-ordering too.

The strength of the above p-value method is that it can be extended to the cases where the observed sample size at the stopping stage is different from that specified by the design. This becomes possible because the PMF $f(m, s|p)$ and the UMVUE depend on the stopping boundaries only up to stage $m - 1$, i.e., $\{(a_k, b_k), 1 \leq k \leq m-1\}$, where $a_2 = b_2 - 1$ denotes a, the rejection value at the second stage. Suppose that a study is stopped after stage $m = 1$ with $S = s$ responders from n_1 patients that may be different from the stage 1 sample size specified by the design. Then, (7.4) can be modified to calculate a p-value

$$\text{p-value} = \begin{cases} \sum_{j=s}^{n_1} p^s(1-p)^{n_1-s}\binom{n_1}{s} & m = 1, \text{ stopped for superiority} \\ 1 - \sum_{j=0}^{s-1} p^s(1-p)^{n_1-s}\binom{n_1}{s} & m = 1, \text{ stopped for futility} \end{cases}$$

Note that the p-value with $m = 1$ is calculated as if the study had a single-stage design with sample size n_1, so that it does not require specification of stopping values (a_1, b_1).

On the other hand, suppose that the study proceeded to the second stage,

TABLE 7.2: UMVUE and MLE, and p-value using these estimators for a two-stage design of $(n_1, n_2, a_1, b_1, a) = (34, 5, 17, 35, 20)$ with $p_0 = 0.4$

			Estimate		p-value		
m	s	$f(m, s \mid p_0)$	UMVUE	MLE	UMVUE	MLE	Naive
1	0	0.0000	0.0000	0.0000	1.0000	1.0000	1.0000
1	1	0.0000	0.0294	0.0294	1.0000	1.0000	1.0000
1	2	0.0000	0.0588	0.0588	1.0000	1.0000	1.0000
1	3	0.0001	0.0882	0.0882	1.0000	1.0000	1.0000
1	4	0.0003	0.1176	0.1176	0.9999	0.9999	0.9999
1	5	0.0010	0.1471	0.1471	0.9997	0.9997	0.9997
1	6	0.0034	0.1765	0.1765	0.9986	0.9986	0.9986
1	7	0.0090	0.2059	0.2059	0.9952	0.9952	0.9952
1	8	0.0203	0.2353	0.2353	0.9862	0.9862	0.9862
1	9	0.0391	0.2647	0.2647	0.9659	0.9659	0.9659
1	10	0.0652	0.2941	0.2941	0.9268	0.9268	0.9268
1	11	0.0948	0.3235	0.3235	0.8617	0.8617	0.8617
1	12	0.1211	0.3529	0.3529	0.7669	0.7669	0.7669
1	13	0.1366	0.3824	0.3824	0.6458	0.6458	0.6458
1	14	0.1366	0.4118	0.4118	0.5092	0.5092	0.5092
1	15	0.1214	0.4412	0.4412	0.3726	0.3726	0.3726
1	16	0.0961	0.4706	0.4706	0.2512	0.2478	0.2512
1	17	0.0679	0.5000	0.5000	0.1550	0.1388	0.1550
2	18	0.0033	0.5294	0.4615	0.0872	0.2512	0.2653
2	19	0.0129	0.5337	0.4872	0.0838	0.1517	0.1713
2	20	0.0219	0.5403	0.5128	0.0709	0.0709	0.1021
2	21	0.0217	0.5508	0.5385	0.0490	0.0490	0.0559
2	22	0.0145	0.5672	0.5641	0.0273	0.0273	0.0280
2	23	0.0075	0.5897	0.5897	0.0128	0.0128	0.0128
2	24	0.0033	0.6154	0.6154	0.0053	0.0053	0.0053
2	25	0.0013	0.6410	0.6410	0.0020	0.0020	0.0020
2	26	0.0005	0.6667	0.6667	0.0007	0.0007	0.0007
2	27	0.0002	0.6923	0.6923	0.0002	0.0002	0.0002
2	28	0.0000	0.7179	0.7179	0.0001	0.0001	0.0001
2	29	0.0000	0.7436	0.7436	0.0000	0.0000	0.0000
2	30	0.0000	0.7692	0.7692	0.0000	0.0000	0.0000
2	31	0.0000	0.7949	0.7949	0.0000	0.0000	0.0000
2	32	0.0000	0.8205	0.8205	0.0000	0.0000	0.0000
2	33	0.0000	0.8462	0.8462	0.0000	0.0000	0.0000
2	34	0.0000	0.8718	0.8718	0.0000	0.0000	0.0000
2	35	0.0000	0.8974	0.8974	0.0000	0.0000	0.0000
2	36	0.0000	0.9231	0.9231	0.0000	0.0000	0.0000
2	37	0.0000	0.9487	0.9487	0.0000	0.0000	0.0000
2	38	0.0000	0.9744	0.9744	0.0000	0.0000	0.0000
2	39	0.0000	1.0000	1.0000	0.0000	0.0000	0.0000

i.e., $m = 2$. In this case, the stage 1 decision will be made based on (a_1, b_1, n_1) as specified by the design, but the sample size for the second stage may be slightly different from n_2 that is specified by the design. In this case, based on observed values of (n_2, s), we calculate

$$\text{p-value} = \sum_{j=b_1}^{n_1} p^s(1-p)^{n_1-s}\binom{n_1}{s} + \sum_{j=s}^{b_1-1+n_2} p^s(1-p)^{n_1+n_2-s} \sum_{x_1=a_1+1}^{(b_1-1)\wedge s} \binom{n_1}{x_1}\binom{n_2}{s-x_1}$$

when $m = 2$. This p-value does not require specification of a either. We can reject H_0 and accept the study therapy when p-value $< \alpha^*$ regardless of the observed sample size at the stopping stage.

It is easy to show that the ordering of MLE depends on the critical values at the stopping stage. Hence, we can not calculate an MLE-based p-value if the sample size at the stopping stage is different from that specified by the design. Furthermore, the decision rule based on the MLE-based p-value may not match with that based on the two-stage testing rule whether the observed sample is identical to the planned one or not.

Example 4 (revisited): In Example 4, with 27 CRs out of $n = 30$ patients after the second stage, the p-value is 0.0093 by [17] for $p_0 = 0.7$ and $(a_1, n_1) = (4, 6)$. Since p-value $< \alpha^*$, this is another justification that [20] is a positive study.

In summary, it is obvious from (7.3) that UMVUE gives p-value satisfying the properties: (a) the p-values in the acceptance region of H_0 are larger than those in the rejection region, and (b) the p-value for the critical value matches with the type I error probability α of the two-stage testing. As mentioned above, the critical values of a two-stage design can not be used for testing if the realized sample size at the stopping stage is different from that specified at the design. In this case, we can conduct a statistical test by calculating the p-value with the sample size at the stopping stage conditioned on the observed value and checking if it is smaller than the prespecified α level or not. In the previous section, we show that the Jennison-Turnbull confidence interval also can be used for this purpose. This property makes the p-value, together with the Jennison-Turnbull confidence interval, very useful for the analysis of two-stage phase II trials. Other p-value methods for multistage design do not have these desirable properties [3, 7].

Green and Dahlberg [11] and Herndon [12] have also considered under- or over-accrual of patients in each stage and proposed some ad hoc approaches to the selection of rejection values depending on the realized sample sizes. Chen and Ng [5] considered a set of combinations for possible sample sizes for stages 1 and 2 (n_1, n_2) and provided the rejection values (a_1, a) to minimize the maximal sample size or the average expected sample assuming that each combination in the set has the same probability to be observed. The latter approach has some undesirable properties: (i) If the combination of realized sample sizes does not belong to the prespecified set, it does not provide valid rejection values; (ii) For each combination of (n_1, n_2), rejection values (a_1, a) are given. For each n_1 value, there are multiple n_2 values with their own a_1 values. So, it is not clear which rejection value a_1 should be used for a realized n_1 after stage 1. Furthermore, suppose that we observed a combination (n_1, n_2) through two stages. Then, we will use a that is assigned to this combination, but a_1 that have been used after stage 1 may be different from the stage 1 rejection value assigned to this combination of sample sizes.

7.3 Randomized Phase II Trials

Let p_X and p_Y denote the RRs of an experimental and a control arms, respectively. In a randomized phase II trial, we want to test $H_0 : p_X \leq p_Y$ against $H_1 : p_X > p_Y$. The null distribution of the binomial test statistic depends on the common RR $p_X = p_Y$; see [14]. Consequently, if the true RRs are different from the specified ones, the testing based on binomial distributions may not maintain the type I error close to the specified design value. In order to avoid this issue, Jung [14] proposes to control the type I error rate at $p_X = p_Y = 1/2$, called MaxTest. This results in a strong conservativeness when the true RR is different from 50%. Asymptotic tests avoid specification of $p_X = p_Y$ by replacing them with their consistent estimators, but the sample sizes of phase II trials usually are not large enough for a good large sample approximation.

Fisher's [9] exact test has been a popular testing method for comparing two sample binomial proportions with small sample sizes. In a randomized phase II trial setting, Fisher's exact test is based on the distribution of the number of responders on one arm conditioning on the total number of responders which is a sufficient statistic of $p_X = p_Y$ under H_0. Hence, the rejection value of Fisher's exact test does not require specification of the common RRs $p_X = p_Y$ under H_0. In this section, we propose two-stage randomized phase II trial designs based on Fisher's exact test.

7.3.1 Single-stage Design

If patient accrual is fast or it takes a lengthy time (say, longer than 6 months) for response assessment, we may consider using a single-stage design. Suppose that n patients are randomized to each arm, and let X and Y denote the number of responders in arms x (experimental) and y (control), respectively. Let $q_k = 1 - p_k$ for arm $k(= \mathrm{x}, \mathrm{y})$. Then the frequencies (and RRs in the parentheses) can be summarized as in Table 7.3.

At the design stage, n is prespecified. Fisher's exact test is based on the conditional distribution of X given the total number of responders $Z = X+Y$

TABLE 7.3: Frequencies (and RRs in the parentheses) of a single-stage randomized phase II trial

		Arm 1	Arm 2	Total
Response	Yes	x (p_X)	y (p_Y)	z
	No	$n-x$ (q_X)	$n-y$ (q_Y)	$2n-z$
Total		n	n	

with a probability mass function

$$f(x|z,\theta) = \frac{\binom{n}{x}\binom{n}{z-x}\theta^x}{\sum_{i=m_-}^{m_+}\binom{n}{i}\binom{n}{z-i}\theta^i}$$

for $m_- \leq x \leq m_+$, where $m_- = \max(0, z-n)$, $m_+ = \min(z,n)$, and $\theta = p_X q_Y/(p_Y q_X)$ denotes the odds ratio.

Suppose that we want to limit the type I error rate to be no larger than α^*. Given $X+Y=z$, we reject $H_0 : p_X = p_Y$ (i.e., $\theta = 1$) in favor of $H_1 : p_X > p_Y$ (i.e., $\theta > 1$) if $X - Y \geq a$, where a is the smallest integer satisfying

$$\alpha(z) \equiv \text{P}(X - Y \geq a|z, H_0) = \sum_{x=\langle(z+a)/2\rangle}^{m_+} f(x|z, \theta = 1) \leq \alpha^*,$$

where $\langle c\rangle$ is the round-up integer of c. Hence, the critical value a depends on the total number of responders z. Under $H_1 : \theta = \theta_1(> 1)$, the power conditional on $X+Y=z$ is given by

$$1 - \beta(z) \equiv \text{P}(X - Y \geq a|z, H_1) = \sum_{x=\langle(z+a)/2\rangle}^{m_+} f(x|z, \theta_1)$$

We propose to choose n so that the marginal power is no smaller than a specified power level $1-\beta^*$, i.e.,

$$\text{E}\{1-\beta(Z)\} = \sum_{z=0}^{2n}\{1-\beta(z)\}g(z) \geq 1-\beta^*$$

where $g(z)$ is the probability mass function of $Z = X+Y$ under $H_1 : p_X > p_Y$ that is given as

$$g(z) = \sum_{x=m_-}^{m_+}\binom{n}{x}p_X^x q_X^{n-x}\binom{n}{z-x}p_Y^{z-x}q_Y^{n-z+x}$$

for $z = 0, 1, \cdots, 2n$. Note that the marginal type I error rate is controlled below α^* since the conditional type I error rate is controlled below α^* for any z value.

Given a type I error rate and a power $(\alpha^*, 1-\beta^*)$ and a specific alternative hypothesis $H_1 : (p_X, p_Y)$, we find a sample size n as follows.

Algorithm for Single-stage Design:

1. For $n = 1, 2, \cdots$,

   (a) For $z = 0, 1, \cdots, 2n$, find the smallest $a = a(z)$ such that

   $$\alpha(z) = \text{P}(X - Y \geq a|z, \theta = 1) \leq \alpha^*$$

   and calculate the power conditional on $X + Y = z$ for the chosen $a = a(z)$

   $$1 - \beta(z) = \text{P}(X - Y \geq a|z, \theta_1)$$

   (b) Calculate the marginal power $1 - \beta = \text{E}\{1 - \beta(Z)\}$.

2. Find the smallest n such that $1 - \beta \geq 1 - \beta^*$.

Given a fixed n, Fisher's test, which is based on the conditional distribution, is valid under $\theta = 1$ (i.e., controls the type I error rate exactly), and its power conditional on the total number of responders depends only on the odds ratio θ_1 under H_1. However, the marginal power, and hence the sample size n, depends on (p_X, p_Y), so that we need to specify (p_X, p_Y) at the design stage. If (p_X, p_Y) are misspecified, the trial may be over- or under-powered but the type I error in data analysis will always be appropriately controlled.

7.3.2 Two-stage Design

For ethical and economical reasons, clinical trials are often conducted using multiple stages. Phase II trials usually enter small number of patients, so that the practical number of stages is two at the most. We consider designs with the same features as popular two-stage phase II trial designs, with an early stopping rule when the experimental therapy has a low probability achieving additional benefits to the patients.

Suppose that n_l $(l = 1, 2)$ patients are randomized to each arm during stage $l(= 1, 2)$. Let $n_1 + n_2 = n$ denote the maximal sample size for each arm, and X_l and Y_l denote the number of responders during stage l in arms x and y, respectively, $X = X_1 + X_2$ and $Y = Y_1 + Y_2$.

At the design stage, n_l are appropriately prespecified. Note that X_1 and X_2 are independent, and, given $X_l + Y_l = z_l$, X_l has the conditional probability mass function,

$$f_l(x_l|z_l, \theta) = \frac{\binom{n_l}{x_l}\binom{n_l}{z_l - x_l}\theta^{x_l}}{\sum_{i=m_{l-}}^{m_{l+}} \binom{n_l}{i}\binom{n_l}{z_l - i}\theta^i}$$

for $m_{l-} \leq x_l \leq m_{l+}$, where $m_{l-} = \max(0, z_l - n_l)$ and $m_{l+} = \min(z_l, n_l)$.

We consider a two-stage randomized phase II trial whose rejection values are chosen conditional on z_1 and z_2 as follows.

Stage 1: Randomize n_1 patients to each arm; observe x_1 and y_1.

a. Given $z_1(= x_1 + y_1)$, find a stopping value $a_1 = a_1(z_1)$.
b. If $x_1 - y_1 \geq a_1$, proceed to stage 2.
c. Otherwise, stop the trial.

Stage 2: Randomize n_2 patients to each arm; observe x_2 and y_2 ($z_2 = x_2 + y_2$).

a. Given (z_1, z_2), find a rejection value $a = a(z_1, z_2)$.
b. Accept the experimental arm if $x - y \geq a$.

Now, the question is how to choose rejection values (a_1, a) conditioning on (z_1, z_2).

7.3.2.1 Choice of a_1 and a

In this section, we assume that n_1 and n_2 are given. As the first stage stopping value, we propose to use $a_1 = 0$. Most standard optimal two-stage phase II trials also stop early when the observed RR from stage 1 is no larger than the specified RR under H_0; refer to [22] and [16] for single-arm trial cases and [14] for randomized trial cases.

With a_1 fixed at 0, we choose the second stage rejection value a conditioning on (z_1, z_2). Given type I error rate α^*, a is chosen as the smallest integer satisfying

$$\alpha(z_1, z_2) \equiv \mathrm{P}(X_1 - Y_1 \geq a_1, X - Y \geq a | z_1, z_2, \theta = 1) \leq \alpha^*$$

We calculate $\alpha(z_1, z_2)$ by

$$\mathrm{P}(X_1 \geq (a_1 + z_1)/2, X_1 + X_2 \geq (a + z_1 + z_2)/2 | z_1, z_2, \theta = 1) =$$

$$\sum_{x_1=m_{1-}}^{m_{1+}} \sum_{x_2=m_{2-}}^{m_{2+}} I\{x_1 \geq (a_1 + z_1)/2, x_1 + x_2 \geq (a + z_1 + z_2)/2\} f_1(x_1|z_1, 1) f_2(x_2|z_2, 1),$$

where $I(\cdot)$ is the indicator function.

Under $H_1 : \theta = \theta_1$, the power conditional on (z_1, z_2) is obtained by

$$1 - \beta(z_1, z_2) = \mathrm{P}(X_1 - Y_1 \geq a_1, X - Y \geq a | z_1, z_2, \theta_1) =$$

$$\sum_{x_1=m_{1-}}^{m_{1+}} \sum_{x_2=m_{2-}}^{m_{2+}} I\{x_1 \geq (a_1 + z_1)/2, x_1 + x_2 \geq (a + z_1 + z_2)/2\} f_1(x_1|z_1, \theta_1) f_2(x_2|z_2, \theta_1)$$

Note that, as in the single-stage case, the calculation of type I error rate $\alpha(z_1, z_2)$ and rejection values (a_1, a) does not require specification of the common RR $p_X = p_Y$ under H_0, and that the conditional power $1 - \beta(z_1, z_2)$ requires specification of the odds ratio θ_1 under H_1, but not the RRs for the two arms, p_X and p_Y.

7.3.2.2 Choice of n_1 and n_2

We now investigate how to choose sample sizes n_1 and n_2 at the design stage based on some optimality criteria.

Given (α^*, β^*), we propose to choose n_1 and n_2 so that the marginal power is maintained above $1 - \beta^*$ while controlling the conditional type I error rate for any (z_1, z_2) below α^* as described in Section 3.2.1. For stage $l(= 1, 2)$, the marginal distribution of $Z_l = X_l + Y_l$ has a probability mass function

$$g_l(z_l) = \sum_{x_l=m_{l-}}^{m_{l+}} \binom{n_l}{x_l} p_{\mathrm{X}}^{x_l} q_{\mathrm{X}}^{n_l - x_l} \binom{n_l}{z_l - x_l} p_{\mathrm{Y}}^{z_l - x_l} q_{\mathrm{Y}}^{n_l - z_l + x_l}$$

for $z_l = 0, \cdots, 2n_l$. Under $H_0 : p_{\mathrm{X}} = p_{\mathrm{Y}} = p_0$, this is expressed as

$$g_{0l}(z_l) = p_0^{z_l} q_0^{2n_l - z_l} \sum_{x_l=m_{l-}}^{m_{l+}} \binom{n_l}{x_l} \binom{n_l}{z_l - x_l}$$

Noting that Z_1 and Z_2 are independent, we can choose n_1 and n_2 so that the marginal power is no smaller than a specified level $1 - \beta^*$, i.e.,

$$1 - \beta \equiv \sum_{z_1=0}^{2n_1} \sum_{z_2=0}^{2n_2} \{1 - \beta(z_1, z_2)\} g_1(z_1) g_2(z_2) \geq 1 - \beta^*$$

The marginal type I error is calculated by

$$\alpha \equiv \sum_{z_1=0}^{2n_1} \sum_{z_2=0}^{2n_2} \alpha(z_1, z_2) g_{01}(z_1) g_{02}(z_2)$$

Since the conditional type I error rate is controlled below α^* for any (z_1, z_2), the marginal type I error rate is no larger than α^*.

Although we do not have to specify the RRs for testing, we need to do so when choosing (n_1, n_2) at the design stage. If the specified RRs are different from the true ones, then the marginal power may be different from that expected. But in this case, our proposed test is still valid in the sense that it always controls both the conditional and marginal type I error rates below the specified level. Given (n_1, n_2) and $a_1 = 0$ and under H_0, the conditional probability of early termination given z_1 and the marginal probability of early termination

$$\mathrm{PET}_0(z_1) = \mathrm{P}(X_1 - Y_1 < a_1 | z_1, H_0) = \sum_{x_1=m_{1-}}^{[(a_1+z_1)/2]-1} f_1(x_1 | z_1, \theta = 1)$$

and

$$\mathrm{PET}_0 = \mathrm{E}\{\mathrm{PET}_0(Z_1) | H_0\} = \sum_{z_1=0}^{2n_1} \mathrm{PET}_0(z_1) g_{01}(z_1)$$

respectively. Then, among those (n_1, n_2) satisfying the $(\alpha^*, 1 - \beta^*)$-condition, the Simon-type [22] minimax and the optimal designs can be chosen as follows.

- *Minimax design* chooses (n_1, n_2) with the smallest maximal sample size $n(= n_1 + n_2)$.

- *Optimal design* chooses (n_1, n_2) with the smallest marginal expected sample size EN under H_0, where

$$\text{EN} = n_1 \times \text{PET}_0 + n \times (1 - \text{PET}_0)$$

Tables 7.4–7.7 report the sample sizes (n, n_1) of the minimax and optimal two-stage designs for $\alpha^* = 0.15$ or 0.2, $1 - \beta^* = 0.8$ or 0.85, and various combinations of (p_X, p_Y) under H_1. For comparison, we also list the sample size n of the single-stage design under each setting. Note that the maximal sample size of the minimax is slightly smaller than or equal to the sample size of the single-stage design. If the experimental therapy is inefficacious, however, the expected sample sizes of minimax and optimal designs are much smaller than the sample size of the single-stage design. We also observe from Tables 7.4 and 7.7 that the sample sizes under $(\alpha^*, 1 - \beta^*) = (0.15, 0.8)$ are similar to those under $(\alpha^*, 1 - \beta^*) = (0.2, 0.85)$.

Jung [14] proposed a randomized phase II design method based on the binomial test, called MaxTest in this chapter, by controlling the type I error rate at $p_X = p_Y = 50\%$. Since the type I error rate of the two-sample binomial test is maximized at $p_X = p_Y = 50\%$, this test will be conservative if the true RR under H_0 is different from 50%.

7.3.3 Numerical Studies

Jung and Sargent [18] compare the performance of our Fisher's exact test with that of MaxTest. All the calculations in this section are based on exact distributions, not on simulations. Figure 7.2 displays the type I error rate and power in the range of $0 < p_Y < 1 - \Delta$ for single-stage designs with $n = 60$ per arm, $\Delta = p_X - p_Y = 0.15$ or 0.2 under H_1, and $\alpha = 0.1$, 0.15 or 0.2 under $H_0 : p_X = p_Y$. The solid lines are for Fisher's test and the dotted lines are for MaxTest; the lower two lines represent type I error rate and the upper two lines represent power. As is well known, Fisher's test controls the type I error conservatively over the range of p_Y. The conservativeness gets slightly stronger with small p_Y values close to 0. MaxTest controls the type I error accurately around $p_Y = 0.5$, but becomes more conservative for p_Y values far from 0.5, especially with small p_Y values. For $\alpha = 0.1$, Fisher's test and MaxTest have similar power around $0.2 \leq p_Y \leq 0.4$ except that MaxTest is slightly more powerful for $p_Y \approx 0.4$. Otherwise, Fisher's test is more powerful. The difference in power between the two methods becomes larger with $\Delta = 0.15$. We observe similar trends overall, but the difference in power becomes smaller with $\Delta = 0.2$, especially when combined with a large $\alpha(= 0.2)$.

TABLE 7.4: Single-stage designs, and minimax and optimal two-stage Fisher designs for $(\alpha^*, 1-\beta^*) = (.15, .8)$

			Single-stage Design			Minimax Two-stage Design				Optimal Two-stage Design			
p_y	p_x	θ	n	α	$1-\beta$	(n, n_1)	α	$1-\beta$	EN	(n, n_1)	α	$1-\beta$	EN
.05	.15	3.353	79	.0827	.8005	(78, 40)	.0823	.8001	63.00	(81, 26)	.0836	.8008	60.83
	.2	4.750	45	.0631	.8075	(44, 17)	.0620	.8033	35.11	(44, 17)	.0620	.8033	35.11
	.25	6.333	29	.0450	.8109	(29, 11)	.0448	.8014	23.96	(29, 11)	.0448	.8014	23.96
.1	.25	3.000	56	.0884	.8033	(56, 25)	.0896	.8003	43.46	(58, 19)	.0925	.8016	42.80
	.3	3.857	36	.0747	.8016	(36, 16)	.0783	.8009	28.41	(37, 12)	.0800	.8024	28.03
.15	.3	2.429	65	.1036	.8023	(65, 36)	.1036	.8004	52.42	(69.22)	.1060	.8009	49.48
	.35	3.051	41	.0879	.8025	(41, 19)	.0919	.8010	32.01	(42, 14)	.0925	.8016	30.99
.2	.35	2.154	74	.1076	.8054	(74, 42)	.1097	.8001	59.74	(79, 26)	.1133	.8003	56.17
	.4	2.667	46	.0953	.8074	(46, 23)	.1016	.8007	36.19	(49, 14)	.1061	.8019	34.81
.25	.4	2.000	83	.1149	.8022	(81, 37)	.1147	.8005	61.35	(84, 30)	.1155	.8006	60.21
	.45	2.455	47	.0986	.8056	(47, 27)	.1007	.8005	38.25	(50, 17)	.1053	.8003	36.10
.3	.45	1.909	85	.1112	.8005	(85, 65)	.1115	.8000	75.76	(95, 27)	.1210	.8004	65.02
	.5	2.333	53	.1121	.8015	(49, 26)	.1100	.8007	38.88	(52, 19)	.1113	.8014	37.82
.35	.5	1.857	86	.1155	.8006	(86, 66)	.1153	.8000	76.73	(95, 32)	.1186	.8002	66.78
	.55	2.270	54	.1009	.8026	(54, 21)	.1169	.8016	39.62	(55, 19)	.1168	.8012	39.43
.4	.55	1.833	87	.1228	.8032	(87, 59)	.1216	.8004	74.05	(94, 35)	.1205	.8000	67.36
	.6	2.250	54	.1015	.8013	(54, 22)	.1150	.8017	39.95	(56, 18)	.1147	.8006	39.56
.45	.6	1.833	87	.1265	.8032	(87, 59)	.1252	.8004	74.03	(94, 35)	.1234	.8000	67.32
	.65	2.270	54	.1043	.8026	(54, 21)	.1151	.8016	39.53	(55, 19)	.1148	.8012	39.33
.5	.65	1.857	86	.1263	.8006	(86, 66)	.1260	.8000	76.69	(95, 32)	.1235	.8002	66.63
	.7	2.333	53	.1033	.8015	(49, 26)	.1147	.8007	38.77	(52, 19)	.1126	.8014	37.62
.55	.7	1.909	85	.1237	.8005	(85, 65)	.1234	.8000	75.70	(96, 26)	.1203	.8010	64.87
	.75	2.455	47	.1114	.8056	(47, 27)	.1240	.8005	38.09	(50, 17)	.1221	.8003	35.75
.6	.75	2.000	83	.1173	.8022	(81, 37)	.1134	.8005	61.08	(84, 30)	.1193	.8006	59.83
	.8	2.667	46	.1208	.8074	(46, 23)	.1163	.8007	35.87	(50, 12)	.1145	.8011	34.13
.65	.8	2.154	74	.1150	.8054	(74, 42)	.1214	.8001	59.46	(81, 23)	.1213	.8006	55.56
	.85	3.051	41	.1020	.8025	(41, 19)	.1004	.8010	31.48	(43, 12)	.1060	.8024	30.12
.7	.85	2.429	65	.1088	.8023	(65, 36)	.1083	.8004	51.98	(69, 22)	.1139	.8009	48.57
	.9	3.857	36	.1023	.8016	(36, 16)	.1068	.8009	27.53	(38, 9)	.1075	.8004	26.45
.75	.9	3.000	56	.1098	.8033	(56, 25)	.1099	.8003	42.52	(59, 17)	.1110	.8016	41.30
	.95	6.333	29	.0929	.8109	(29, 11)	.0919	.8014	21.76	(30, 7)	.0949	.8022	21.32
.8	.95	4.750	45	.0948	.8075	(44, 17)	.1036	.8033	32.81	(46, 11)	.1041	.8007	32.23
.85	.95	3.353	79	.1065	.8005	(78, 40)	.1071	.8001	61.38	(83, 22)	.1098	.8011	57.67

TABLE 7.5: Single-stage designs, and minimax and optimal two-stage Fisher designs for $(\alpha^*, 1-\beta^*) = (.15, .85)$

			Single-stage Design			Minimax Two-stage Design				Optimal Two-stage Design			
p_y	p_x	θ	n	α	$1-\beta$	(n, n_1)	α	$1-\beta$	EN	(n, n_1)	α	$1-\beta$	EN
.05	.15	3.353	92	.0868	.8502	(92, 48)	.0870	.8500	74.20	(94, 35)	.0881	.8502	71.17
	.2	4.750	51	.0677	.8526	(51, 24)	.0676	.8506	41.27	(52,18)	.0678	.8505	40.61
	.25	6.333	35	.0531	.8581	(34, 11)	.0516	.8506	27.56	(34, 11)	.0516	.8506	27.56
.1	.25	3.000	65	.0952	.8529	(65, 37)	.0950	.8502	53.18	(68, 24)	.0963	.8501	50.29
	.3	3.857	41	.0785	.8515	(41, 21)	.0823	.8500	33.09	(42, 16)	.0847	.8502	32.14
.15	.3	2.429	78	.1058	.8521	(78, 48)	.1067	.8502	64.71	(82, 29)	.1091	.8506	59.40
	.35	3.051	49	.0948	.8541	(49, 23)	.0976	.8506	38.15	(51, 17)	.1004	.8527	37.28
.2	.35	2.154	88	.1113	.8518	(88, 43)	.1120	.8502	67.92	(93, 32)	.1147	.8500	66.49
	.4	2.667	52	.0990	.8506	(52, 29)	.0992	.8506	42.01	(56, 18)	.1062	.8506	40.16
.25	.4	2.000	94	.1132	.8511	(94, 68)	.1133	.8502	82.03	(102, 37)	.1203	.8503	72.98
	.45	2.455	59	.1067	.8535	(59, 30)	.1122	.8503	46.22	(62, 19)	.1129	.8506	43.71
.3	.45	1.909	104	.1210	.8504	(100, 55)	.1200	.8501	79.37	(107, 39)	.1209	.8503	76.34
	.5	2.333	60	.1034	.8524	(60, 39)	.1062	.8501	50.53	(65, 22)	.1138	.8510	46.31
.35	.5	1.857	106	.1148	.8508	(106, 79)	.1148	.8501	93.40	(114, 39)	.1252	.8503	80.04
	.55	2.270	61	.1089	.8551	(61, 37)	.1082	.8507	50.16	(65, 24)	.1112	.8504	46.96
.4	.55	1.833	107	.1178	.8520	(107, 74)	.1170	.8500	91.60	(115, 45)	.1205	.8500	83.00
	.6	2.250	61	.1147	.8538	(61, 38)	.1132	.8500	50.57	(66, 23)	.1138	.8502	47.07
.45	.6	1.833	107	.1214	.8520	(107, 74)	.1203	.8500	91.59	(115, 45)	.1196	.8500	82.95
	.65	2.270	61	.1184	.8551	(61, 37)	.1163	.8507	50.11	(65, 24)	.1156	.8504	46.86
.5	.65	1.857	106	.1215	.8508	(106, 79)	.1210	.8501	93.36	(114, 39)	.1240	.8503	79.88
	.7	2.333	60	.1176	.8524	(60, 39)	.1163	.8501	50.45	(65, 22)	.1151	.8510	45.07
.55	.7	1.909	104	.1180	.8504	(100, 55)	.1159	.8501	79.22	(107, 39)	.1234	.8503	76.08
	.75	2.455	59	.1145	.8535	(59, 30)	.1104	.8503	46.00	(62, 19)	.1114	.8506	43.28
.6	.75	2.000	94	.1205	.8511	(94, 68)	.1256	.8502	81.91	(102, 37)	.1277	.8503	72.57
	.8	2.667	52	.0999	.8506	(52, 29)	.1071	.8506	41.72	(56, 18)	.1147	.8506	39.56
.65	.8	2.154	88	.1180	.8518	(88, 43)	.1146	.8502	67.52	(93, 32)	.1178	.8500	65.68
	.85	3.051	49	.1158	.8541	(49, 23)	.1160	.8506	37.60	(52, 15)	.1155	.8519	36.31
.7	.85	2.429	78	.1141	.8521	(78, 48)	.1190	.8502	64.33	(84, 26)	.1201	.8503	58.49
	.9	3.857	41	.0980	.8515	(41, 21)	.1000	.8500	32.34	(43, 14)	.1050	.8514	30.87
.75	.9	3.000	65	.1082	.8529	(65, 37)	.1102	.8502	52.50	(69, 22)	.1150	.8500	48.76
	.95	6.333	35	.1019	.8581	(34, 11)	.0997	.8506	24.75	(35, 7)	.1016	.8505	24.43
.8	.95	4.750	51	.0983	.8526	(51, 24)	.1021	.8506	39.45	(53, 15)	.1073	.8518	37.47
.85	.95	3.353	92	.1065	.8502	(92, 48)	.1101	.8500	72.52	(98, 27)	.1140	.8503	67.92

TABLE 7.6: Single-stage designs, and minimax and optimal two-stage Fisher designs for $(\alpha^*, 1-\beta^*) = (.2, .8)$

			Single-stage Design			Minimax Two-stage Design				Optimal Two-stage Design			
p_y	p_x	θ	n	α	$1-\beta$	(n, n_1)	α	$1-\beta$	EN	(n, n_1)	α	$1-\beta$	EN
.05	.15	3.353	65	.1078	.8031	(65, 36)	.1121	.8005	53.73	(68, 24)	.1152	.8004	52.14
	.2	4.750	38	.0799	.8040	(38, 15)	.0813	.8007	30.73	(38, 15)	.0813	.8007	30.73
	.25	6.333	26	.0509	.8050	(25, 10)	.0481	.8005	20.98	(25, 10)	.0481	.8005	20.98
.1	.25	3.000	48	.1200	.8043	(47, 19)	.1222	.8002	36.08	(47, 19)	.1222	.8002	36.08
	.3	3.857	30	.0991	.8012	(30, 19)	.1022	.8005	25.71	(31, 13)	.1066	.8024	24.43
.15	.3	2.429	54	.1343	.8005	(54, 40)	.1349	.8003	47.88	(60, 18)	.1445	.8015	42.94
	.35	3.051	35	.1220	.8057	(34, 15)	.1209	.8022	26.46	(35, 13)	.1221	.8020	26.44
.2	.35	2.154	63	.1512	.8003	(62, 29)	.1491	.8011	47.66	(65, 23)	.1507	.8002	47.09
	.4	2.667	39	.1264	.8005	(39, 26)	.1342	.8005	33.40	(40, 14)	.1408	.8001	29.46
.25	.4	2.000	67	.1424	.8028	(67, 47)	.1467	.8001	54.95	(73, 24)	.1582	.8003	51.75
	.45	2.455	41	.1295	.8101	(40, 35)	.1292	.8000	37.78	(45, 12)	.1477	.8001	31.59
.3	.45	1.909	68	.1518	.8006	(68, 55)	.1517	.8001	62.04	(75, 30)	.1570	.8003	55.02
	.5	2.333	41	.1392	.8034	(41, 28)	.1389	.8002	35.25	(45, 16)	.1445	.8003	32.72
.35	.5	1.857	69	.1631	.8012	(69, 54)	.1625	.8001	62.10	(76, 32)	.1602	.8010	56.29
	.55	2.270	42	.1515	.8092	(42, 25)	.1479	.8004	34.50	(46, 16)	.1491	.8003	33.20
.4	.55	1.833	70	.1713	.8043	(70, 50)	.1692	.8005	60.81	(77, 32)	.1656	.8010	56.78
	.6	2.250	42	.1581	.8079	(42, 26)	.1545	.8007	34.90	(45, 18)	.1528	.8007	33.32
.45	.6	1.833	70	.1751	.8043	(70, 50)	.1727	.8005	60.80	(77, 32)	.1685	.8010	56.75
	.65	2.270	42	.1618	.8092	(42, 25)	.1572	.8004	34.46	(46, 16)	.1549	.8003	33.11
.5	.65	1.857	69	.1746	.8012	(69, 54)	.1737	.8001	62.07	(76, 32)	.1686	.8010	56.19
	.7	2.333	41	.1601	.8034	(41, 28)	.1581	.8002	35.19	(45, 16)	.1542	.8003	32.53
.55	.7	1.909	68	.1716	.8006	(68, 55)	.1711	.8001	62.00	(77, 28)	.1651	.8022	55.11
	.75	2.455	41	.1589	.8101	(41, 23)	.1559	.8000	37.74	(45, 12)	.1505	.8001	31.17
.6	.75	2.000	67	.1660	.8028	(67, 47)	.1638	.8001	57.84	(73, 24)	.1601	.8003	51.37
	.8	2.667	39	.1491	.8005	(39, 26)	.1472	.8005	33.23	(40, 14)	.1430	.8001	28.98
.65	.8	2.154	63	.1522	.8003	(62, 29)	.1531	.8011	47.31	(65, 23)	.1599	.8002	46.58
	.85	3.051	35	.1311	.8057	(34, 15)	.1425	.8022	25.94	(36, 11)	.1458	.8003	25.71
.7	.85	2.429	54	.1466	.8005	(54, 40)	.1518	.8003	47.68	(60, 18)	.1590	.8015	42.03
	.9	3.857	30	.1386	.8012	(30, 19)	.1427	.8005	25.27	(33, 7)	.1428	.8008	22.99
.75	.9	3.000	48	.1446	.8043	(47, 19)	.1427	.8002	35.09	(48, 17)	.1458	.8009	35.09
	.95	6.333	26	.1305	.8050	(25, 10)	.1249	.8005	19.04	(26, 6)	.1267	.8007	18.65
.8	.95	4.750	38	.1392	.8040	(38, 15)	.1406	.8007	28.60	(40, 9)	.1419	.8017	28.16
.85	.95	3.353	65	.1411	.8031	(65, 36)	.1410	.8005	52.42	(70, 20)	.1483	.8010	49.45

TABLE 7.7: Single-stage designs, and minimax and optimal two-stage Fisher designs for $(\alpha^*, 1-\beta^*) = (.2, .85)$

			Single-stage Design			Minimax Two-stage Design				Optimal Two-stage Design			
p_y	p_x	θ	n	α	$1-\beta$	(n, n_1)	α	$1-\beta$	EN	(n, n_1)	α	$1-\beta$	EN
.05	.15	3.353	81	.1148	.8535	(78, 37)	.1197	.8503	62.00	(81, 29)	.1214	.8501	61.52
	.2	4.750	44	.0897	.8459	(44, 19)	.0924	.8504	35.50	(44, 19)	.0924	.8504	35.50
	.25	6.333	30	.0618	.8542	(30, 11)	.0621	.8519	24.68	(30, 11)	.0621	.8519	24.68
.1	.25	3.000	56	.1292	.8511	(56, 36)	.1301	.8501	47.58	(59, 21)	.1321	.8503	43.97
	.3	3.857	35	.1046	.8545	(35, 19)	.1097	.8521	28.76	(37, 12)	.1132	.8502	28.03
.15	.3	2.429	65	.1411	.8523	(65, 35)	.1411	.8506	52.01	(69, 26)	.1453	.8508	50.85
	.35	3.051	43	.1294	.8577	(42, 19)	.1344	.8508	32.60	(43, 16)	.1345	.8511	32.19
.2	.35	2.154	74	.1469	.8528	(74, 51)	.1497	.8502	63.64	(80, 30)	.1575	.8507	58.22
	.4	2.667	45	.1298	.8559	(45, 27)	.1349	.8501	37.22	(48, 18)	.1443	.8505	35.50
.25	.4	2.000	80	.1575	.8515	(78, 50)	.1530	.8500	65.29	(84, 36)	.1567	.8515	62.60
	.45	2.455	46	.1402	.8514	(46, 32)	.1398	.8501	39.81	(50, 20)	.1453	.8508	37.18
.3	.45	1.909	87	.1531	.8506	(87, 68)	.1561	.8501	78.21	(92, 36)	.1670	.8503	66.87
	.5	2.333	53	.1468	.8501	(50, 29)	.1568	.8510	40.70	(52, 21)	.1547	.8500	38.57
.35	.5	1.857	89	.1541	.8533	(89, 63)	.1537	.8502	76.97	(93, 40)	.1660	.8501	68.97
	.55	2.270	54	.1392	.8523	(53, 27)	.1589	.8503	41.47	(55, 23)	.1599	.8506	40.96
.4	.55	1.833	89	.1600	.8508	(89, 71)	.1595	.8501	80.61	(96, 39)	.1686	.8516	70.12
	.6	2.250	54	.1405	.8510	(53, 28)	.1569	.8501	41.85	(57, 21)	.1563	.8502	41.25
.45	.6	1.833	89	.1637	.8508	(89, 71)	.1632	.8501	80.60	(96, 39)	.1713	.8516	70.08
	.65	2.270	54	.1437	.8523	(53, 27)	.1564	.8503	41.41	(55, 23)	.1559	.8506	40.88
.5	.65	1.857	89	.1649	.8533	(89, 63)	.1627	.8502	76.92	(92, 50)	.1604	.8502	72.67
	.7	2.333	53	.1426	.8501	(50, 29)	.1548	.8510	40.60	(52, 21)	.1559	.8500	38.40
.55	.7	1.909	87	.1610	.8506	(87, 68)	.1603	.8501	78.15	(92, 36)	.1664	.8503	66.64
	.75	2.455	46	.1437	.8514	(46, 32)	.1616	.8501	39.70	(50, 20)	.1659	.8508	36.89
.6	.75	2.000	80	.1485	.8515	(78, 50)	.1621	.8500	65.14	(85, 34)	.1692	.8502	62.01
	.8	2.667	45	.1664	.8559	(45, 27)	.1615	.8501	36.99	(48, 18)	.1576	.8505	35.02
.65	.8	2.154	74	.1672	.8528	(74, 51)	.1679	.8502	63.45	(82, 27)	.1627	.8501	57.62
	.85	3.051	43	.1544	.8577	(42, 19)	.1439	.8508	32.05	(44, 14)	.1473	.8505	31.35
.7	.85	2.429	65	.1480	.8523	(65, 35)	.1503	.8506	51.56	(69, 26)	.1591	.8508	50.09
	.9	3.857	35	.1286	.8545	(35, 19)	.1362	.8521	28.13	(37, 12)	.1461	.8502	26.71
.75	.9	3.000	56	.1536	.8511	(56, 36)	.1545	.8501	47.08	(59, 21)	.1538	.8503	42.70
	.95	6.333	30	.1408	.8542	(30, 11)	.1373	.8519	22.36	(31, 7)	.1386	.8519	21.94
.8	.95	4.750	44	.1290	.8549	(44, 19)	.1429	.8504	33.53	(46, 14)	.1451	.8520	33.02
.85	.95	3.353	81	.1506	.8535	(78, 37)	.1496	.8503	60.17	(83, 26)	.1516	.8506	58.94

Figure 7.3 displays the type I error rate and power of two-stage designs with $n_1 = n_2 = 30$ per arm. We observe that, compared to MaxTest, Fisher's test controls the type I error more accurately in the most range of p_Y values. If $\alpha = 0.1$, Fisher's test is more powerful than MaxTest over the range of $p_Y < 0.2$ or $p_Y > 0.6$. But with a larger α, such as 0.15 or 0.2, MaxTest is more powerful in the range of p_Y between 0.2 and 0.6. As in the single-stage design case, the difference in power diminishes as Δ and α increase. While Fisher's exact test is more powerful than the binomial test in single-stage designs, their performance is comparable in two-stage designs. With a_1 value fixed at 0, the two-stage designs based on Fisher's exact test are not fully optimal. A fully optimal choice of a_1 value will depend on z_1 and the two-stage design using the optimal a_1 value is believed to outperform the two-stage designs based on binomial test in single-stage design case. We will develop an efficient algorithm to identify fully optimal two-stage designs using Fisher's exact test in our future study.

Readers may refer to [18] for the cases where two arms have an unbalanced allocation.

7.4 Discussion

The most popular design for a phase II cancer clinical trial is a single-arm two-stage design. Most publications reporting the results of these trials do not use appropriate statistical methods for data analysis. These trials are specified by sample sizes and critical values for two stages. Often the number of patients treated at each stage is different from that specified by the design. In this case, the critical values become meaningless. Possibly due to this reason, publications reporting phase II trials often are not clear if they accept or reject the treatments under study, or they accept or reject them without a solid statistical ground.

When analyzing a phase III clinical trial this issue is avoided by conducting statistical analysis conditioning on the observed sample size. Phase III trials usually have large sample sizes and the statistical methods using large sample approximation do not require prespecification of a sample size. In fact, we can use the same approach for the analysis of phase II trials with small sample sizes, but most investigators are not familiar with them. To this end, we propose to use p-value and confidence interval methods for two-stage phase II clinical trials. The theory behind these methods is identical to that of two-stage design of phase II clinical trials, so that any of these methods lead to the same conclusions if the sample size at the stopping stage is the same as that specified by the design. This is possible because all of these methods are based on the UMVUE of RR. If the observed sample size for the stopping stage is different from that specified by the design, then the testing based on

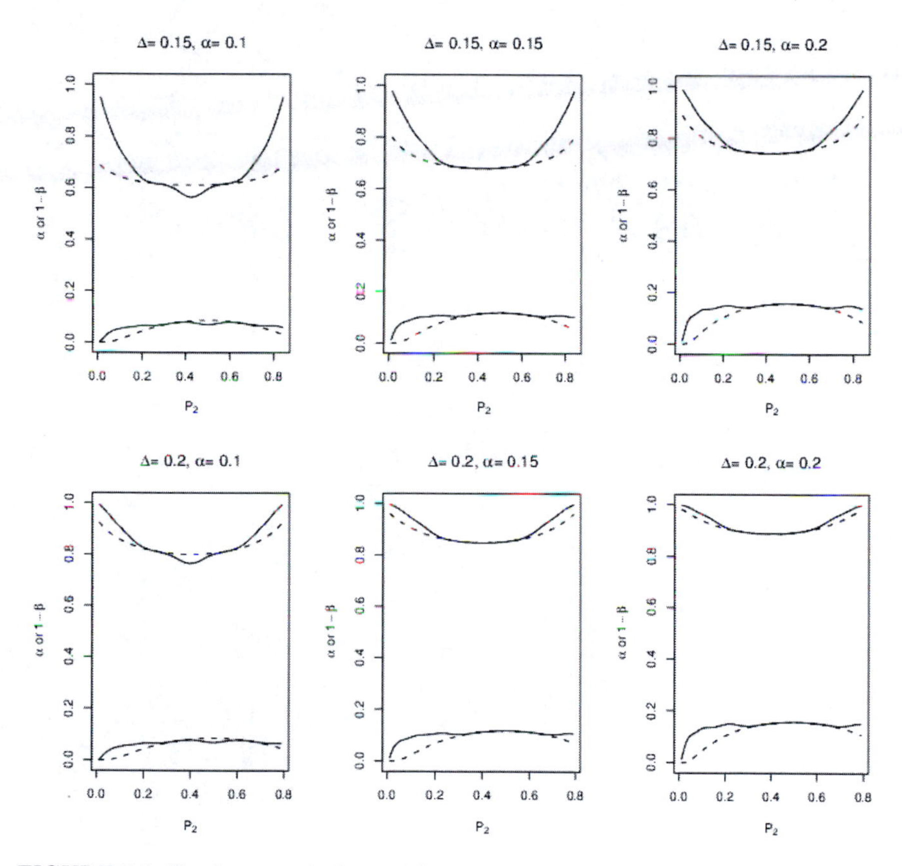

FIGURE 7.2: Single-stage designs with $n = 60$ per arm: Type I error rate and power for Fisher's test (solid lines) and MaxTest (dotted lines).

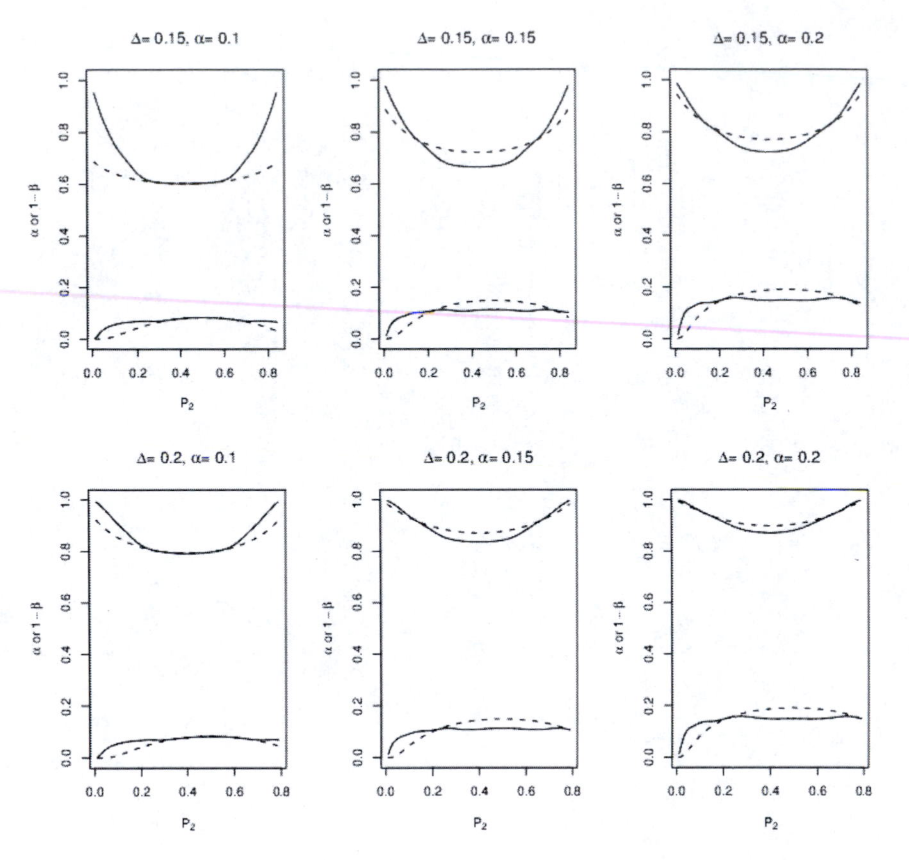

FIGURE 7.3: Two-stage designs with $n_1 = n_2 = 30$ per arm: Type I error rate and power for Fisher's test (solid lines) and MaxTest (dotted lines).

two-stage critical values is of no use while one can calculate unbiased p-value and confidence interval by extending the UMVUE calculation to this case.

We have extended the search algorithm of two-stage phase II trial designs beyond Simon's minimax and optimal designs. The new designs, called admissible designs, closely satisfy both the minimax and optimality criteria of Simon.

We also have investigated randomized phase II trials for evaluating the efficacy of an experimental therapy compared to a prospective control. Although we demonstrate the proposed method using response as the endpoint, the method can be applied to any binomial endpoint, e.g., the proportion of patients progression-free at a fixed time point (say 6 months). We have limited our discussions to single-stage and two-stage designs that are most commonly used for phase II cancer clinical trials, but all of the methods discussed in this chapter can be extended to phase II trials with any number of stages.

Bibliography

[1] P. Armitage. Numerical studies in the sequential estimation of a binomial parameter. *Biometrika*, 45(1-2):1–15, 1958.

[2] S. A. Cannistra. Phase II trials in journal of clinical oncology. *Journal of Clinical Oncology*, 27(19):3073–6, 2009.

[3] M. N. Chang, A. L. Gould, and S. M. Snapinn. p-values for group sequential testing. *Biometrika*, 82:650–654, 1995.

[4] M. N. Chang, T. M. Therneau, H. S. Wieand, and S. S. Cha. Designs for group sequential phase II clinical trials. *Biometrics*, 43(4):865–74, 1987.

[5] T. T. Chen and T. H. Ng. Optimal flexible designs in phase II clinical trials. *Statistics in Medicine*, 17(20):2301–12, 1998.

[6] C. J. Clopper and E. S. Pearson. The use of confidence or fiducial limits illustrated in the case of the binomial. *Biometrika*, 26(4):404–413, 1934.

[7] T. D. Cook. p-value adjustment in sequential clinical trials. *Biometrics*, 58(4):1005–11, 2002.

[8] D. E. Duffy and T. J. Santner. Confidence intervals for a binomial parameter based on multistage tests. *Biometrics*, 43(1):81–93, 1987.

[9] R. A. Fisher. The logic of inductive inference. *Journal of the Royal Statistical Society*, 98(1):39–82, 1935.

[10] H. K. Gan, A. Grothey, G. R. Pond, M. J. Moore, L. L. Siu, and D. Sargent. Randomized phase II trials: inevitable or inadvisable? *Journal of Clinical Oncology*, 28(15):2641–7, 2010.

[11] S. J. Green and S. Dahlberg. Planned versus attained design in phase II clinical trials. *Statistics in Medicine*, 11(7):853–62, 1992.

[12] J. E. Herndon 2nd. A design alternative for two-stage, phase II, multicenter cancer clinical trials. *Controlled Clinical Trials*, 19(5):440–50, 1998.

[13] C. Jennison and B. W. Turnbull. Confidence intervals for a binomial parameter following a multistage test with application to mil-std 105d and medical trials. *Technometrics*, 25(1):49–58, 1983.

[14] S. H. Jung. Randomized phase II trials with a prospective control. *Statistics in Medicine*, 27(4):568–83, 2008.

[15] S. H. Jung, M. Carey, and K. M. Kim. Graphical search for two-stage designs for phase II clinical trials. *Controlled Clinical Trials*, 22(4):367–72, 2001.

[16] S. H. Jung and K. M. Kim. On the estimation of the binomial probability in multistage clinical trials. *Statistics in Medicine*, 23(6):881–96, 2004.

[17] S. H. Jung, K. Owzar, S. L. George, and T. Lee. p-value calculation for multistage phase II cancer clinical trials. *Journal of Biopharmaceutical Statistics*, 16(6):765–75; discussion 777–83, 2006.

[18] S. H. Jung and D. J. Sargent. Randomized phase II cancer clinical trials. *Journal of Biopharmaceutical Statistics*, 24(4):802–16, 2014.

[19] S. Kim, S. Jung, and W. Kim. Reply to K. Shimada et al. *Journal of Clinical Oncology*, 28(14):e230, 2010.

[20] S. J. Kim, K. Kim, B. S. Kim, C. Y. Kim, C. Suh, J. Huh, S. W. Lee, J. S. Kim, J. Cho, G. W. Lee, K. M. Kang, H. S. Eom, H. R. Pyo, Y. C. Ahn, Y. H. Ko, and W. S. Kim. Phase II trial of concurrent radiation and weekly cisplatin followed by VIPD chemotherapy in newly diagnosed, stage IE to IIE, nasal, extranodal NK/T-Cell Lymphoma: Consortium for Improving Survival of Lymphoma study. *Journal of Clinical Oncology*, 27(35):6027–32, 2009.

[21] K. Shimada and R. Suzuki. Concurrent chemoradiotherapy for limited-stage extranodal natural killer/t-cell lymphoma, nasal type. *Journal of Clinical Oncology*, 28(14):e229; author reply e230, 2010.

[22] R. Simon. Optimal two-stage designs for phase II clinical trials. *Controlled Clinical Trials*, 10(1):1–10, 1989.

[23] W. Y. Tsai, Y. Chi, and C. M. Chen. Interval estimation of binomial proportion in clinical trials with a two-stage design. *Statistics in Medicine*, 27(1):15–35, 2008.

[24] A. A. Tsiatis, G. L. Rosner, and C. R. Mehta. Exact confidence intervals following a group sequential test. *Biometrics*, 40(3):797–803, 1984.

Part III

Late Phase Clinical Trials

8

Sample Size for Survival Trials in Cancer

Edward Lakatos

CONTENTS

8.1 Introduction

There are copious formulas for sample size calculation designed for dealing with what is a vast variety of possible experimentation. This chapter will focus on one small corner of that methodology: sample size calculations for oncology survival clinical trials. Such trials present many challenges. These emanate largely from the difficulties in controlling the experiment. Unlike experiments on plots of land or laboratory animals, the treatment of patients is much more complex. In oncology trials, patients may experience adverse reactions severe enough that treatment must be suspended or abandoned on a patient by patient basis. And patients may discontinue trial participation entirely. In preventive oncology trials, patients may be given a bottle of pills, to be taken, say, twice a day. Perhaps they will take those pills as prescribed, or most of them, or perhaps very few. Maybe they will return to the clinic for their next scheduled exams to pick up another bottle of pills. Maybe not. Recruitment of patients into a trial is one of the more difficult aspects of trial management. Recruitment patterns usually involve a slow start up. Often clinical sites must be added to attempt to meet recruitment goals. As will be discussed below, slow recruitment may compromise power.

A large portion of the sample size literature for survival trials is based on methods that assume exponential models. In oncology trials, non-constant and non-proportional hazards are the rule rather than the exception. This chapter focuses on methods for calculating sample size in a realistic way that accounts for the complexities of dealing with patients as well as real life oncology survival trials for which the hazards are rarely constant or proportional.

Issues of oncology trial design, some of which were mentioned above, anticipate what may take place once the trial is underway. Those issues do not vanish when the trial is underway. Yet typical methods for mid-trial corrections, such as sample size re-estimation or futility assessment, make no attempt to deal with those issues. So if real-world considerations lead to a 20% increase in sample size at the design stage, most during-the-trial methods would result in a sample size that ignores those very same real-world considerations, leading to underpowered sample size adjustments. But even if those design stage issues are addressed at the time of an interim, there are many issues that are unique to sample size modification or futility during the trial which have no analogue during the design stage. Some of these issues will also be discussed.

In this chapter, a number of examples are provided which are meant to be thought-provoking. For instance, in Section 3b, an example is presented of a group-sequential clinical trial for which the sample size for the "same" trial, but with a fixed sample design, is larger than that of the group-sequential design. Although one might be tempted to dismiss such examples as unlikely, that would miss the point. Just as a counter example raises questions regarding the validity of what might seem like a reasonable proof, these examples are designed to cast doubt on the validity of conventional ways of thinking. In the example of the trial for which the sample size of the group-sequential version is smaller than that of the fixed design, the immediate implication is that the increase in sample size due to using a group-sequential rather than fixed design is not an intrinsic factor of the group-sequential design. In other words, the degree of sample size inflation of a group-sequential procedure compared to the fixed also depends on the non-proportionality of the hazards. Since non-proportionality is common in oncology trials, the inflation factor concept should be viewed skeptically.

The Markov model for clinical trials [8, 9] provides statistical methodology for dealing with non-proportional hazards and other time-dependent processes such as non-compliance, loss to follow-up, and non-uniform recruitment. That model is used throughout this chapter to compare and contrast the implications of assuming constant rates and isolated processes versus assuming the actual time-dependent interdependent processes.

The structure of this chapter is as follows. The chapter begins with an introduction to some common types of non-proportional hazards and their implications for sample size, power, trial length, recruitment length, etc. The effect of non-proportional hazards on two well-known paradigms is then presented. Up to this point in the chapter, the discussion of sample size has been restricted to the design stage. The next section focuses on mid-trial sample size issues, especially sample size re-estimation in the presence of non-proportional hazards, and futility. All of these issues are presented and discussed prior to explaining how the Markov model for clinical trials works, which is presented in the next to last section. This is followed by a discussion section.

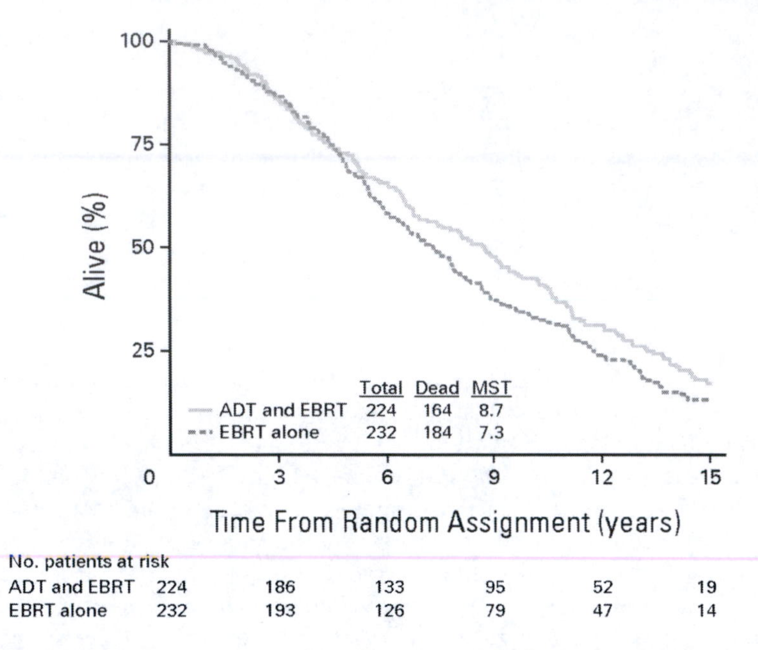

No. patients at risk						
ADT and EBRT	224	186	133	95	52	19
EBRT alone	232	193	126	79	47	14

FIGURE 8.1: Kaplan-Meier curves from Roach et al. [20] which exhibit a threshold lag. Reprinted with permission.

8.2 Departures f rom Proportionality

Survival trials in oncology abound with non-proportionality. While the non-proportionality can manifest itself in many ways, two of the most common are the treatment lag and anti-lag. This section opens with examples of non-proportional hazards from three actual trials. This is followed by constructed examples which isolate the effects of one or two factors at a time to illustrate the effects of those specific factors.

8.2.1 Treatment Lag

With a treatment lag, rather than being fully effective immediately, the treatment effect increases until a maximum level is attained. The threshold lag is a special case: there is essentially no separation of the survival curves for some time period, but immediately after that period, the treatment is fully effective. Basically, there are two zones: a "null" zone immediately after randomization, and an "alternative" zone starting at the time the treatment is fully effective (Figure 8.1).

Table 8.1 lists time periods and corresponding annual failure rates similar

TABLE 8.1: Treatment lag: Failure rates similar to death-specific mortality rates in Roach et al. [20] (Figure 3) of prostate cancer.

	Annual Failure Rates	
Year	Control	Experimental
0-1	.035	.035
1-2	.253	.253
2-4	.406	.406
4-6	.632	.331
6-15	.348	.271

to those of the Kaplan-Meier [6] curves of Figure 3 (Disease-Specific Mortality (DSM)) (here Figure 8.1) of Roach et al. [20] in a trial of Neoadjuvant Androgen Deprivation Therapy and External Radiotherapy. There is no apparent separation of the survival curves before year 4. In these survival curves, for each treatment arm, there are 3 levels of the hazard in the null zone.

Undoubtedly, there are a variety of mechanisms giving rise to delayed treatment effects. In preventive oncology, with treatments such as dietary modification, it has been conjectured that already existing, but subclinical tumors will continue to emerge for perhaps 1–2 years, despite dietary changes. The concept is that dietary changes will reduce the incidence of new tumors, which might take years before becoming visible. For examples of threshold lags in prostate cancer see Lu and Pajak [13] as well as Roach et al. [20].

8.2.2 Treatment Anti-lag

A treatment anti-lag occurs when initially the survival curves separate indicative of a clear early treatment effect, but after some time point, there is no further separation, i.e., the curves are "parallel." If the treatment effect (hazard ratio) presents at "exactly" two levels, one during the initial zone of separation, and a null zone beginning at the end of the initial zone with no further separation, this is called a threshold anti-lag. The curves in Figure 8.2 exhibit this pattern.

8.2.3 Both Lag and Anti-lag

The survival curves in Figure 8.3 exhibit both treatment lag and anti-lag characteristics. While exponential survival curves will always meet when the survival probability approaches 0 in both treatment arms, the survival probability is 40% when the survival curves in Figure 8.3 meet. Examples of this phenomenon appear in [1] (carcinoma of the head and neck), and [16, 19] (ovarian cancer).

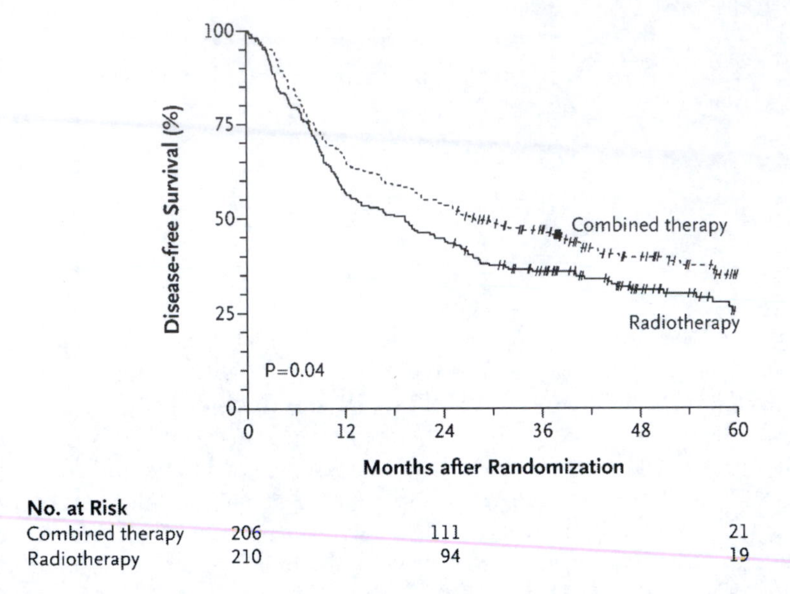

FIGURE 8.2: Kaplan-Meier curves from Cooper et al. [3] which exhibit a threshold anti-lag. Reprinted with permission.

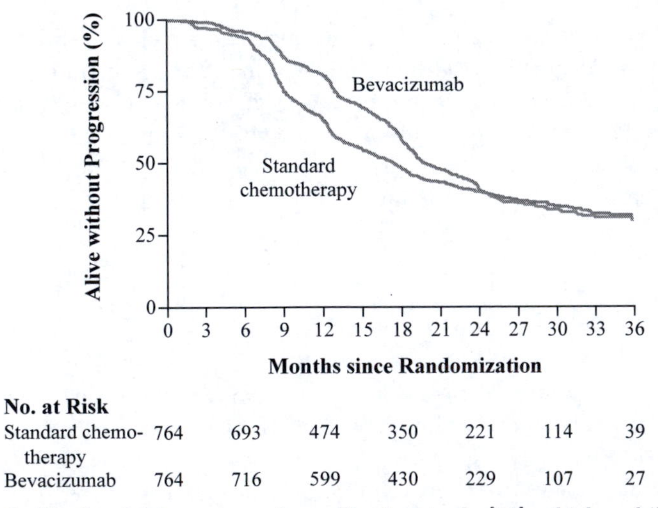

FIGURE 8.3: Kaplan-Meier curves from Perrin et al. [16] which exhibit a both threshold lag and anti-lag characteristics. Reprinted with permission.

8.2.4 Sample Size Implications

During the course of designing a trial, if there are one or more completed previous trials which have enough in common with the current trial, those trial(s) could be used to derive background information for planning the current trial. Published survival curves from such previous trials are extremely valuable for this purpose. The discussion that follows assumes that such published survival curves are available.

8.2.4.1 Implications for Treatment Lag — Real World Example

Figure 8.1 was based on a trial of patients with prostate cancer that lasted 12 years with recruitment complete in about 51 months. Although the Markov model approach is designed to handle complex situations with loss to follow-up and other complicating factors, to examine the effects of the treatment lag, loss to follow-up was not considered in the calculations below.

For all calculations, the significance level was set at 0.05 2-sided, and power at 90%. For time-dependent rates, STOPP® software, developed by the author, was used. For comparisons of proportions, PASS® was used. (Although not used here, PASS® also includes modules for calculating sample sizes for time-dependent rates using the Lakatos [8, 9] Markov model approach.)

Using the time-varying rates from Table 8.1, the sample size needed, based on using the logrank statistic [14, 17], is 993 patients total, 971 events. Sample size can also be calculated assuming constant risk, still assuming the analysis will use the logrank statistic. From Roach et al. [20], the observed DSM event rates at 10 years were 23.3% and 35.6%. Assuming exponential distributions, the corresponding yearly event rates are 2.618% and 4.305%. The total sample size for the logrank statistic, using STOPP® software and assuming constant 4, is 566 patients, 165 events. In this example, for which proportional hazards are clearly not justified, the assumption of constant hazards results in the calculated number of events being only 17% (165/971) of the required number of events based on calculations capable of addressing the time-dependent hazards.

The sample size assuming 10 year DSM event rates as above at 23.3% and 35.6%, but based on using a comparison of proportions rather than the logrank, is 574 patients total (PASS®). This substantial reduction in sample size compared with the logrank (993) when there is a threshold lag is not unexpected. The logrank statistic uses the entire curve and, for this reason, is usually assumed to be more efficient than the proportions test. However, with a threshold lag, the logrank statistic must combine or "average" the early zone of no treatment effect with the post-lag zone when the treatment effect is positive. The resultant "average" is smaller than had the no treatment effect period not been included. The power of the logrank statistic when the possibility of a threshold lag exists can be improved by using an appropriately weighted version of that statistic [24].

TABLE 8.2: Annual failure rates for two constructed trials with threshold lag and threshold anti-lag characteristics.

Time Period	Annual Failure Rates			
	Treatment Lag		Treatment Anti-lag	
(Months)	Control	Experimental	Control	Experimental
0-12	.20	.20	.20	.15
13-30	.20	.15	.20	.20
Failure Rate (0-30)	.428	.373	.428	.392
Average Annual Rate	.20	.170	.20	.181

8.2.4.2 Exploring the Implications of Treatment Lag and Anti-lag in a Controlled Setting

The time-varying failure rates in published Kaplan-Meier [6] curves are often complex. Besides the fact that it may take time for the effects of treatments to measurably impact progression or survival, patients may discontinue therapy. Further, if an experimental treatment has an early impact, this may (or may not) result in an imbalance in the two treatment arms, with the higher risk patients failing disproportionately in the control group, but remaining at risk in the experimental arm. In order to explore and compare some of the implications for sample size and power of treatment lag and anti-lag without the more complex time varying failure rates, much simpler patterns of failure rates are now assumed (see Table 8.2).

The general shape of the survival curves corresponding to probabilities in Table 8.2 is similar to those presented in Figure 8.1 (Treatment Lag) and Figure 8.2 (Treatment Anti-lag).

8.2.4.3 Sample Size and Power Calculations

The sample sizes below were derived using two approaches. First, the Markov model approach [8, 9] fully utilizing the time-dependent information in Table 8.2 was used. The other approach calculated constant hazards for each of the two arms, from the time-dependent information in Table 8.2. The Markov approach was also used to calculate sample sizes for the logrank statistic under this restrictive constant hazards assumption (STOPP® software was used). The Markov approach for calculating sample size for the logrank statistic is based in part on the distribution of the logrank statistic derived by Schoenfeld [23].

For the Markov model approach, the actual time-dependent rates in Table 8.2 were used. For the constant hazards approach, the failure rates were calculated as follows. For the control group, the hazard is constant, so that hazard could be used directly. For the experimental treatment, for which the hazard appears at two levels, there is no "correct" way to arrive at a constant hazard for this arm. Two separate constant hazards were investigated. First, the smaller of the two levels was assumed to hold for the entire trial, resulting

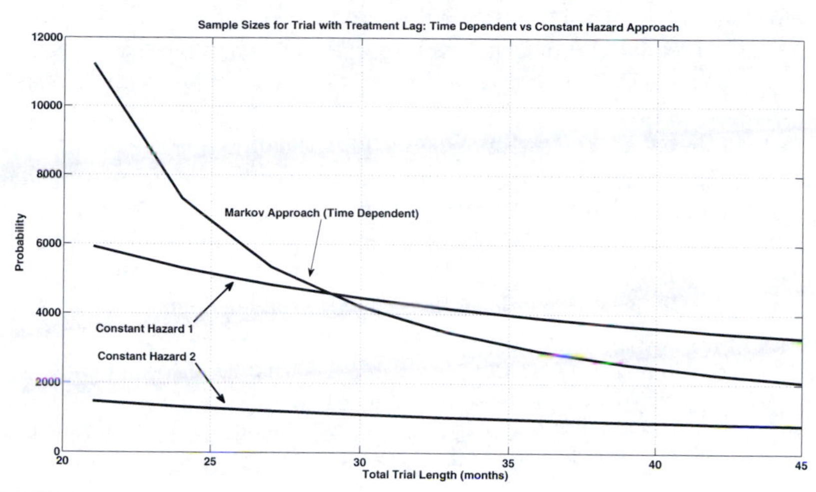

FIGURE 8.4: Treatment lag. Sample size by trial length. Time-dependent vs constant hazards.

in the largest constant treatment effect, and hence the smallest sample size that reasonably could be used. The second approach took the combined failure rate (based on the two levels) at the end of 30 months and calculated the corresponding constant hazard that would give that failure rate in 30 months.

During the design stage it is customary to explore various combinations of trial lengths and sample sizes to find a combination that best meets the needs of the sponsor. A comparison is now made between using the actual time-dependent rates versus assuming constant hazards to explore the relationship between trial length and sample size.

Figure 8.4 presents sample sizes for various lengths of trials when the underlying survival curves follow the treatment lag assumptions of Table 8.2.

With a threshold treatment lag, the control and experimental arm hazards are identical for some time period, here (Table 8.2) for the first 12 months. Any sample size calculation for a trial no longer than 12 months that recognizes this coincidence of the survival curves should return an infinite sample size. As the trial length increases beyond 12 months, the sample size gradually declines to approach more reasonable levels. For this reason, Figure 8.4 only shows trials of length at least 21 months. In contrast, the required number of events based on the exponential model will be constant for each of the two assumed hazards, independent of the trial length. (The number of events for the exponential or proportional hazards model depends only on the hazard ratio.) One can then calculate for any positive length trial, again using the exponential model, how many patients are needed to provide that number of events. So the exponential sample size calculation will provide finite sample sizes regardless of the length of trials, based on the assumed constant hazards, even for trials of length shorter than the treatment lag for which the treatment effect is zero (i.e., hazard ratio is 1). From Figure 8.4, sample sizes based on the questionable constant-hazards assumption rarely come close to those based on time-dependent rates.

Plots of the required number of events for the same Treatment Lag example result in a figure very similar to Figure 8.4. The primary difference is that the two lines labelled "Constant Hazards Approach I and II" would be replaced by straight horizontal lines. As with Figure 8.4, trials no longer than 12 months, in reality, require an infinite number of events. For the exponential model, the number of events depends only on the assumed control and treatment hazards. Arguably, one could calculate different constant hazards for every different trial length. (For example, Table 8.2 displays annual failure rates corresponding to a constant hazard derived from a trial 30 months long; one could also calculate the constant hazard derived from a trial 29 months long.) That was not done here. Part of the problem is that there is no obvious way to find a single hazard that represents survival with different hazards at different times. Further, the basic idea that the exponential model can be used because the assumption of a constant hazard is credible is undermined by the necessity for using different constant hazards depending on the length of the trial. For situations such as this, based on simulations, it should be noted that the Markov model provides sample sizes and numbers of events that are remarkably close to what is actually needed for the logrank statistic [12].

For the Markov approach, the reason for the decline in the required number of events as the length of trial increases is because the ratio of events after the lag ends to the number before the lag ends increases as the trial length increases beyond 12 months. Due to the treatment lag, events that occur prior to 12 months support the null hypothesis, whereas those that occur after 12 months support the alternative. The logrank statistic will combine evidence from all events, and as the trial length increases beyond 12 months, the balance becomes more and more favorable to the alternative, requiring fewer events overall. It is important to appreciate this fact during the design and interim analysis stages of the trial. For the constant hazard model, the failure rates are assumed constant, resulting in a fixed number of required events, independent of the length of the trial. This can lead to sub-optimal designs, or the sponsor's failure to fund the trial based on misleading sample size requirements.

The discussion and calculations above assume the length of recruitment is 0, i.e., simultaneous entry. This was to simplify the discussion and focus on the implications of modifying a single factor: the length of the trial.

Figure 8.5 shows how the sample size changes with the length of recruitment. A general rule of thumb is that, for a trial of fixed length, slower recruitment reduces the length of follow-up, leading to increased sample size. This is consistent with Figure 8.5. With treatment lag, the increased length of recruitment results in shorter average length of follow-up. With shorter length of follow-up, the early portion of the survival curves are "over-represented."

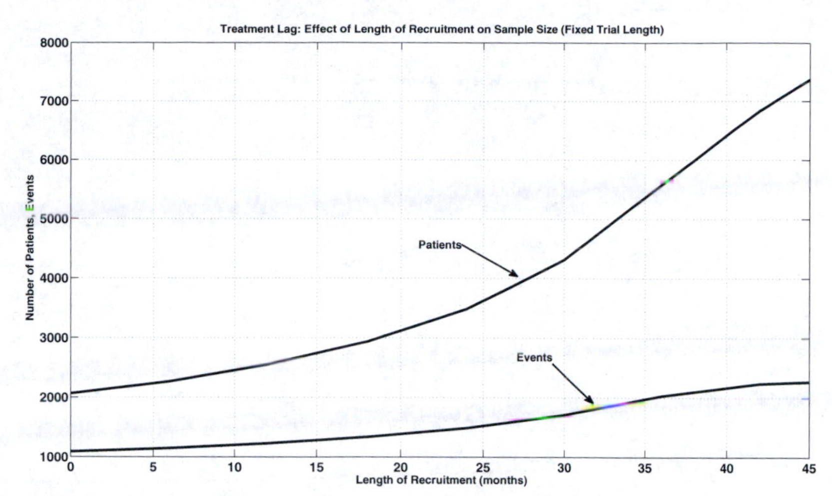

FIGURE 8.5: Threshold lag: Effect of length of recruitment on sample size (fixed-length trial).

Taken together with a treatment lag, the balance of events is shifted from the alternative to the null. This increases the required number of events. As before, if the hazards are assumed constant, the required number of events will also be constant. This can lead to poor trial design.

8.2.4.4 Treatment Anti-lag

This section focuses on the implications for sample size, power, length of the trial, and recruitment period, under the assumptions in the right two columns of Table 8.2, under the heading "Treatment Anti-lag."

Figure 8.6 compares the sample sizes obtained by varying the trial length for the Markov model using time-dependent hazards as compared to the constant hazards model. As discussed in detail in the Treatment Lag section above, two constant hazard rates were examined. And similar to the discussion of the exponential model for treatment lag, the exponential model for treatment anti-lag shows that the required number of patients declines as the length of the trial increases. The number of events required for the exponential model is constant, independent of the length of trial. The longer the follow-up, the greater the number of accumulating events, so the fewer the number of patients required.

But the Markov model with the actual time-dependent rates shows that the required number of patients increases as the length of the trial increases. What is going on here? As with treatment lag, this has to do with the balance of events prior to versus after the anti-lag period. It was assumed for this anti-lag example (Table 8.2 was constructed to have a strong treatment effect during the initial period, followed by a period of no treatment effect). Events

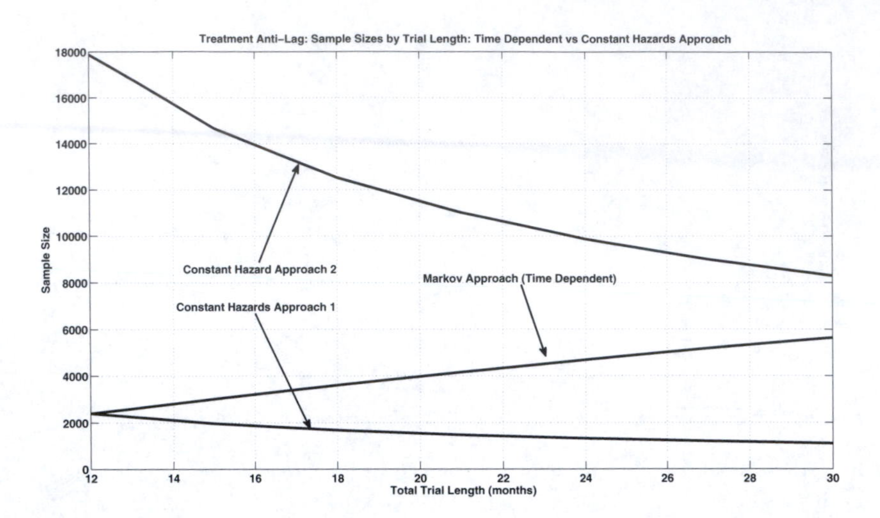

FIGURE 8.6: Treatment anti-lag: Sample size by trial length: Time-dependent versus constant hazards approach.

occurring during the initial period support the alternative, while events after support the null. Once a trial is longer than 12 months (the point at which the strong period of initial efficacy ends), the balance of events supporting the alternative gets less and less favorable, with increasing numbers of events favoring the null. The longer trials have a greater proportion and balance of events favoring the null.

Recognizing this characteristic of the anti-lag situation is very important. Figure 8.7 shows, for the anti-lag situation of Table 8.2, how the number of patients and events varies with the length of recruitment.

8.3 Two Paradigms for Which Conventional Wisdom Fails

8.3.1 Event-driven Trial

The basic principle of the event-driven trial is that for survival trials, the number of events rather than the number of patients drives the power. While that is true to some extent, the hazard ratio as a function of time plays a substantial role in the relationship of the number of events to the power. The

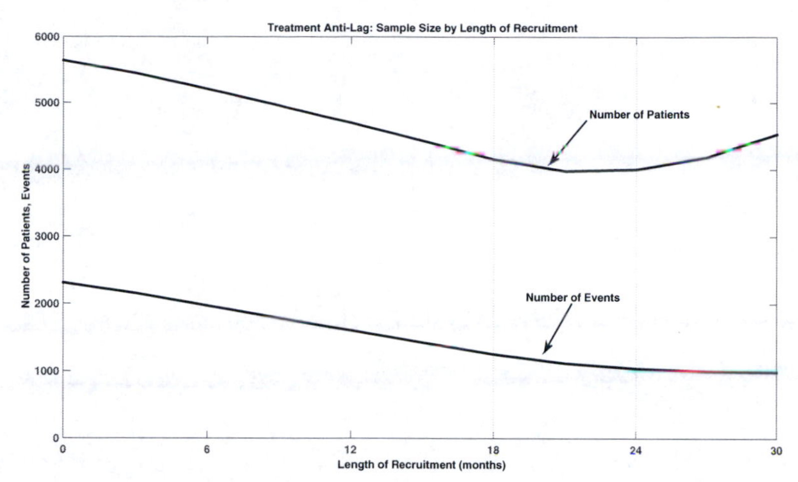

FIGURE 8.7: Threshold Anti-lag: Sample size by length of recruitment.

TABLE 8.3: Treatment Anti-lag Annual Failure Rates

	Period (Months from randomization)		
	0-3	3-10	10+
Control Group	0.1	0.1	0.1
Experimental Group	0.05	0.075	0.09

following example demonstrates what can go wrong if one assumes constant hazards when that is not justified.

Table 8.3 presents failure probabilities with treatment anti-lag properties. There is a substantial treatment effect (a 50% reduction in the annual failure rate) during months 1–3, a 25% reduction during months 3–10, and a 10% reduction starting a month 10.

Assume the time-dependent failure rates of Table 8.3 are in effect, and consider the design configurations presented in Table 8.4. STOPP® software was used for all calculations in Table 8.4.

In rows a–f, Table 8.4 presents results based on the constant hazards assumption. Time dependent results are presented in rows g–l. The basic idea of Table 8.4 is to design a trial assuming constant hazards (rows a–f). Rows g–l display the actual properties of the design, calculated using the actual time-dependent rates and the Markov model.

Rows a–c. Each column of rows a–c displays a trial configuration. The powers presented in row c assume constant hazards, with a 1-year failure rate of 10% control, 7.13% active; recruitment is uniform over months 1–18. Under these assumptions including exponential distributions, each configuration (column) has 84 events and provides about 90% power. Under the 48 month

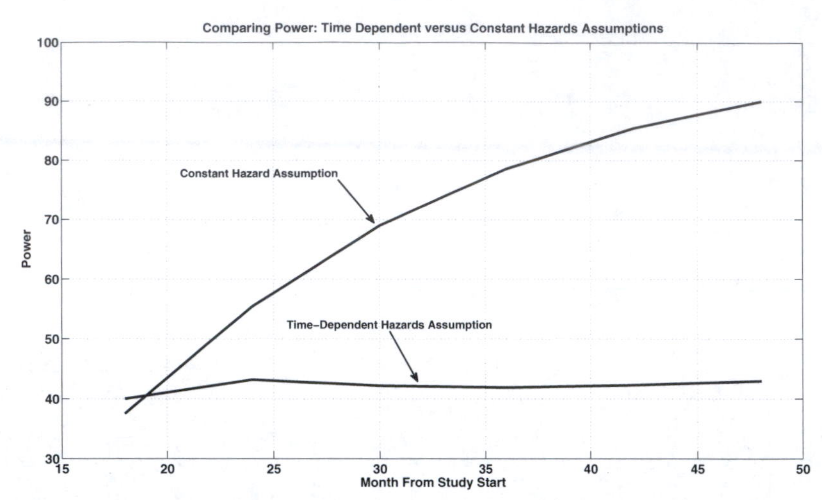

FIGURE 8.8: Comparing power derived under time-dependent versus constant hazards assumptions for the anti-lag example in Table 8.3.

column, 378 patients followed for 4 years will produce about 84 events and consequently provide 90% power. Under the 18 month column, still assuming an exponential model, it would take about 1446 patients to produce 84 events in 18 months. From a clinical operations perspective, enrolling 378 patients over 18 months and following them for a maximum of 4 years is generally the more cost effective and more easily managed approach (rows a–c also display intermediate options that could also be considered).

Rows d–f. Suppose the trial is sized at 378 patients, event driven at 84 events. Again assuming the same exponential model, rows d–f show how the events would accumulate and how the exponentially calculated power would increase as a trial with 378 patients progresses.

Rows g–i. Each column of rows g–i displays a trial configuration. Configurations in rows g-i are all based on 84 events (from the constant hazard design). The numbers of patients needed to produce those 84 events in their respective columns (row g) were determined using the Markov model and the actual underlying time-varying failure rates as given in Table 8.3. Comparing row i with row c shows that the exponential model overestimates the power. The effect is much more pronounced in the longer trials which include more and more periods of diminished treatment effect. At month 48, under the unjustified constant hazards assumption the power is 90%, whereas under the actual time-dependent hazards, the power is 34.4%.

Rows j–l. The configurations in rows j–l are similar to those in rows d–f, all examining the characteristics of a trial with 378 patients. Compared to row e, the events accrue slightly more rapidly in row k, because the treatment effect

TABLE 8.4: Design configurations and operating characteristics of trial based on Table 8.3, comparing operating characteristics when analysis uses time-dependent rates rather than assuming constant hazards.

		Month From Study Start					
		18	24	30	36	42	48
		Exponential Model					
a	Number of Patients	1446	897	656	522	437	378
b	Number of Events	84	84	84	84	84	84
c	Power	90	90.2	90.3	90.3	90.4	90.5
d	Number of Patients	378	378	378	378	378	378
e	Number of Events	22	35	48	61	73	84
f	Power	359	54.5	68.6	78.8	85.8	90.5
		Time-dependent Using Markov Model					
g	Number of Patients	1426	858	610	472	387	329
h	Number of Events	84	84	84	84	84	84
i	Power	85.1	54.5	64..1	78.8	41.6	34.4
j	Number of Patients	378	378	378	378	378	378
k	Number of Events	32	37	52	67	82	97
l	Power	22	41.8	44.2	43	40.8	38.7

diminishes over time. This causes the event rate to increase in the experimental arm.

It appears from the exponential model that if one waits until 84 events occur, the power (row f) will be 90%. But using the Markov model with time-dependent rates shows that 84 events will provide, at most, only about 41% power (row l).

The example above shows that if one ignores the non-proportionality of the hazards, the resultant design could end in a failed trial. Specifically, with the non-proportional hazards of Table 8.3, and the number of events designed to provide 90% power using the constant hazards assumption, the maximum power the trial will actually achieve will not exceed 41%, no matter how long the trial is continued.

Row i shows that the earlier the trial reaches 84 events, the greater the power. However, the relationships are complex. Using the Markov model calculations, better strategies would aim to enroll far more patients (compared with 378) quickly. However, it may be difficult to enroll so many patients in such a short time frame. Finding an optimal strategy also depends heavily on logistics. But ignoring time-dependent hazards and hazard ratios can produce very misleading results.

8.3.2 Group-sequential Sample Size Inflation Factor

Jennison and Turnbull [4] (p.26) state that "the maximum sample size that the group sequential test may need depends on" the number of looks K, the Type I and II errors α and β, and is proportional to σ^2/δ^2 where σ^2 is the

TABLE 8.5: Group-sequential deflation and inflation factors: Two trials of the same length with the same control and experimental group failure rates.

DESIGN		Annual Failure Rates During Specified Months		
		1-12	13+	Overall
Trial 1	Control	.1	.1	.2908
	Experimental	.05	.09	.2325
Trial 2	Control	.1	.1	.2908
	Experimental	.09	.0728	.2325

SAMPLE SIZES	Fixed Design		O'Brien-Fleming		Pocock	
	Events	Patients	Events	Patients	Events	Patients
Trial 1	538	2055	481	1839	405	1546
Trial 2	652	2492	690	2632	833	3182

variance and δ is the treatment effect. In other words, "it is sufficient to specify the ratio $R_P(K, \alpha, \beta)$ of the group sequential test's maximum sample size to the fixed sample size, and this ratio will apply for all δ and σ^2." The following example shows that this is generally not true for survival trials with non-proportional hazards. The ratio $R_P(K, \alpha, \beta)$ is often called an inflation factor. Consider two trials with piecewise exponential failure rates ("Annual Failure Rates") as presented in Table 8.5.

The Kaplan-Meier survival curves for these two trials from simulated data are presented in Figures 8.9 and 8.10.

The two trials in Table 8.5 were constructed to have identical overall failure probabilities in their corresponding treatment arms. Consequently, the same inflation factors should apply to both trials. Alternatively stated, there is nothing in the inflation factor $R_P(K, \alpha, \beta)$ that represents departure from proportional hazards. However, taking into account the non-proportional hazards assumptions, both the required number of events and patients deflate rather than inflate the sample sizes for Trial 1. The opposite happens in Trial 2.

The deflation can be explained as follows. As discussed earlier, including a period during which the treatment effect is much smaller than during other periods will reduce the overall size of the logrank statistic. If there is no treatment effect during some period, that portion of the survival experience contributes noise, but not signal, to the overall statistic, reducing its size. The early analyses of the group-sequential design of Trial 1 involve only the portion of the curve prior to the "no treatment effect" period. Those analyses will have greater power than the fixed sample design which includes large portions of the survival experience during which there is no treatment effect. As the time of the interim analysis increases, the ratio of the periods of strong treatment effect to no treatment effect diminishes, but still provide more power compared with the fixed sample design. Consequently, the group-sequential

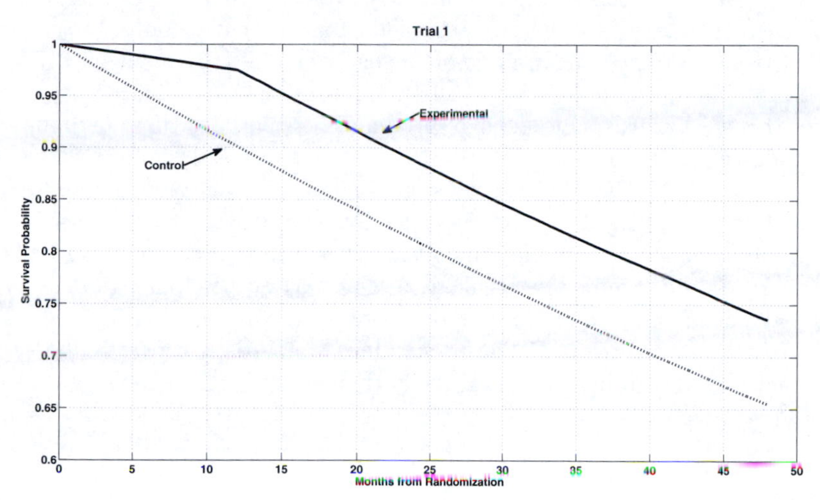

FIGURE 8.9: Group-sequential deflation factor: Kaplan-Meier curves from Trial 1 of Table 8.5.

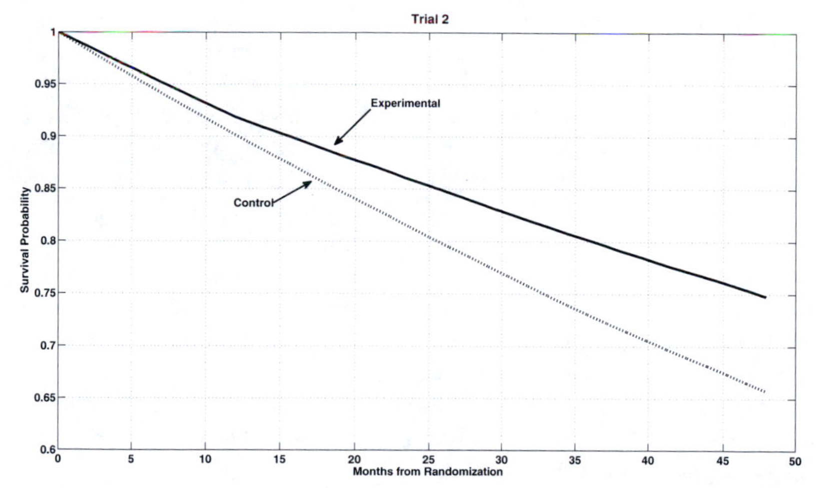

FIGURE 8.10: Group-sequential deflation factor: Kaplan-Meier curves from Trial 2 of Table 8.5.

design requires less sample size to achieve the same power as the fixed sample design. Comparing the Pocock boundary [18] to the O'Brien-Fleming [15], Pocock's boundary is easier to exceed during the early looks, so it is in a better position to take advantage of the early strong treatment effect.

This simple example was constructed to illustrate the fact that non-proportional hazards can have a profound impact on the maximum size of group-sequential trials relative to the fixed-sample design. But the message is somewhat different. Most survival trials have some degree of non-proportionality of hazards. This is certainly true if patients discontinue their randomly assigned treatment. And although one should not consider deflation of the maximum sample size as likely, it is important to challenge the concept that, given a group-sequential design, there exists an inflation factor that applies to all survival trials. If non-proportional hazards is a possibility, sample size methods for group-sequential trials that address the non-proportionality should be used [10].

8.4 Sample Size Re-estimation and Futility

This chapter thus far has dealt with some of the many issues that arise with sample size and power estimation for survival trials during the design stage. Methods for calculating power versus sample size for a particular situation are essentially the same. Sample size re-estimation and futility have much in common with power calculations. Since the advent of sample size re-estimation, the assessment of futility must be viewed in a different light. A trial can be declared futile at some interim if the probability of success, i.e., the conditional power, is deemed to be too low. However, sample size re-estimation can often be used to increase that probability of success. The question of futility must now additionally ask the question: "If a larger sample size is needed to provide adequate power, will the sponsor support such an increase?"

A large portion of the sample size re-estimation literature uses the interim estimate of the treatment effect to estimate the conditional power of (end-trial) success. In order to maintain the Type I error when sample sizes are re-estimated, weighting is often used. Jennison and Turnbull [5] provide a nice review of re-estimation using weighted statistics (But note that their approach to optimal design via the Average Sample Number (ASN) [18] conflicts with that of this author [11]. In particular, as discussed below, the "starting small" strategy generally should be avoided.

Typically, issues regarding sample size estimation at the design stage, such as those discussed in this chapter, carry over to sample size re-estimation. Importantly, there are additional concerns for sample size re-estimation, particularly with respect to nonproportional hazards. Some of these additional concerns are now discussed.

8.4.1 Estimating the Treatment Effect in a Trial with a Threshold Treatment Lag

For a gentle introduction to interim estimation in the presence of nonproportional hazards, consider the case of a treatment lag. For simplicity, restrict attention to the threshold lag, for which there is no treatment effect for some period, after which the treatment is fully effective. It is much easier to distinguish whether a threshold lag exists and the length of the lag, compared to doing so with a gradually increasing treatment effect. Further restrict attention to sample size re-estimation based on an interim estimate of the treatment effect. It is assumed that the significance level will be maintained by using a weighted statistic [5]. Weighted methods are less efficient compared with getting the sample size "right" at the design stage [2]. The impact of weighting is a large topic that is beyond the scope of this discussion (see also comments of the discussants of [2]).

Suppose we have a 5-year trial of experimental treatment versus placebo control of a drug with a possible 2-year threshold lag, followed by an assumed 20% treatment effect. The existence of, and/or exact length of, the treatment lag or the treatment effect is not known. As in many trials, we do not even know if there is any treatment effect, or, if the drug is effective, the size of the treatment effect. That is why the trial is being performed.

If we estimate the hazard ratio at any time up to 2 years after study start, and there is a true 2-year threshold lag, by definition of the threshold lag, the expected hazard ratio will be 1, i.e., no treatment effect. Equally obvious is the fact that the expected hazard ratio at 2 years + 1 day will essentially be 1 as well. There simply is not enough data after the lag has ended to influence the estimate. The typical approach to estimating the treatment effect is to assume proportional hazards, even if that assumption is clearly violated. The medical literature is replete with hazard ratio estimates from data for which non-proportionality of the hazards is clearly evident from the corresponding Kaplan-Meier curves. Alternately stated, the actual hazard ratio is time-dependent, but the estimate assumes that it is constant. Assuming proportional hazards, how does the hazard ratio estimate produced from repeated interim analyses change as time progresses, for example, during the 5-year course of the trial? (The discussion here is not about preserving the significance level, but rather is confined to the ability to obtain a reasonable estimate of the treatment effect.) This depends heavily on the rate of recruitment. To see this, consider Figure 8.11, a common enrollment pattern for a large trial.

The cumulative of this enrollment pattern in Figure 8.11 is presented in Figure 8.12. Note that the times in the x-axis for both Figures 8.11 and 8.12 are calendar times. In general, when Kaplan-Meier curves are plotted, the numbers of patients at risk are often provided at the bottom of the graph. Those numbers at risk decline as time from randomization increases. And those numbers at risk always depend on the calendar time of the interim anal-

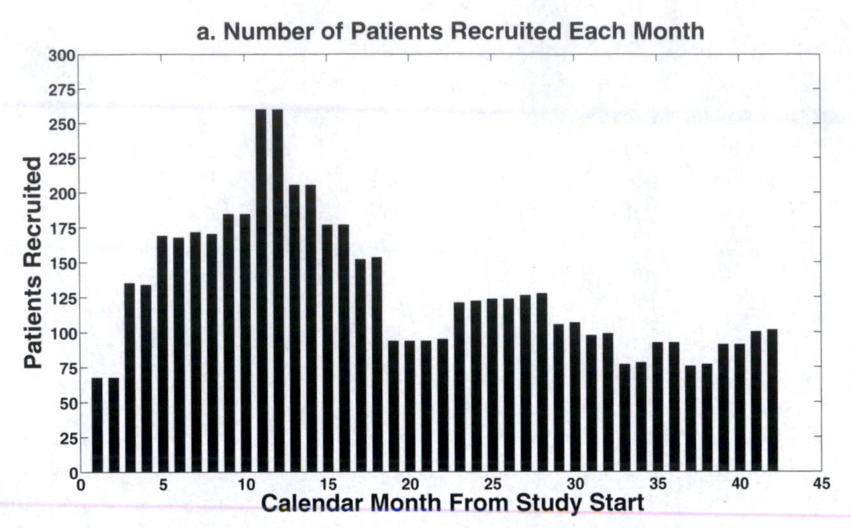

FIGURE 8.11: Example of a typical recruitment pattern formed from a composite of several actual large trials.

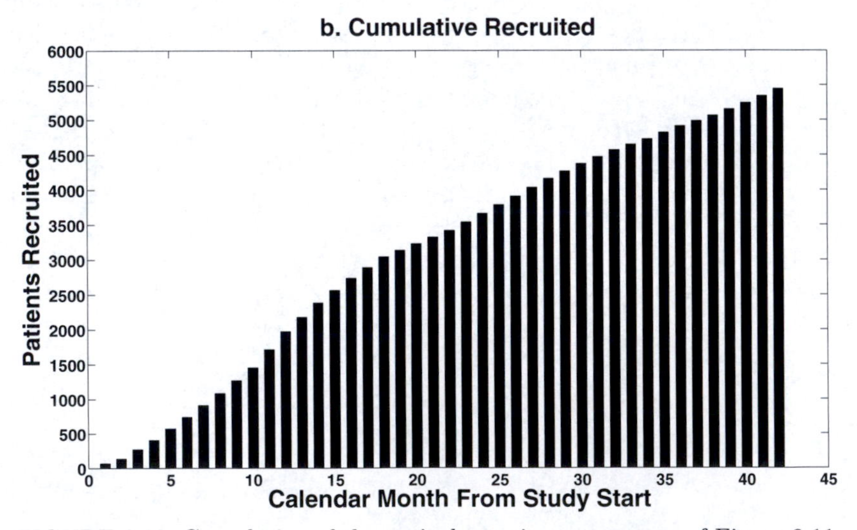

FIGURE 8.12: Cumulative of the typical recruitment pattern of Figure 8.11.

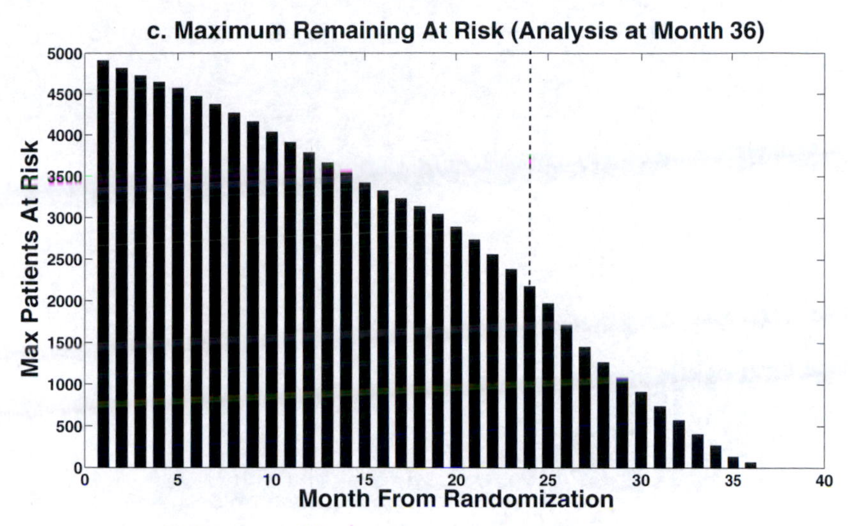

FIGURE 8.13: Maximum at risk at 36-month interim.

ysis. At a particular interim, all patients who were randomized up to the time of the interim are usually at risk in the Kaplan-Meier plots at time 0 (randomization time). As time from randomization increases, the number still at risk declines. This may happen because some of those patients will experience the primary event, while others may be lost to follow-up or competing risks. But it also happens because of staggered entry, i.e., the calendar time it takes to recruit patients. In this example, we only examine the decline in patients due to staggered entry. Thus the decline represents the maximum at risk, as it does not adjust for events or other losses.

From this cumulative distribution in Figure 8.12, the distribution of the maximum at risk can easily be calculated for any given interim analysis time (both Figures 8.13 and 8.14) as follows.

Note that the bar charts in Figures 8.13 and 8.14, like Kaplan-Meier plots, are based on time from randomization (RT). Consider an analysis performed 36 months after study start (cf. Figure 8.13). The patients recruited during the very first month after study start (Calendar Time (CT)) are the only ones who could still be at risk 36 months after randomization (RT). It is helpful to think of "exposure time" at the time of the analysis (RT). Only those enrolled at study start will have been exposed to randomized treatment for 36 months at the time of the 36-month analysis. Some of those patients may be lost to follow-up or competing risks, or even experience the endpoint of interest. As such, for the 36-month analysis, the number recruited during that first month (CT) is the maximum that could still be at risk 36 months (RT) after randomization. Similarly, those recruited during the first two months after study start represent the maximum who could still be at risk 35 months after random-

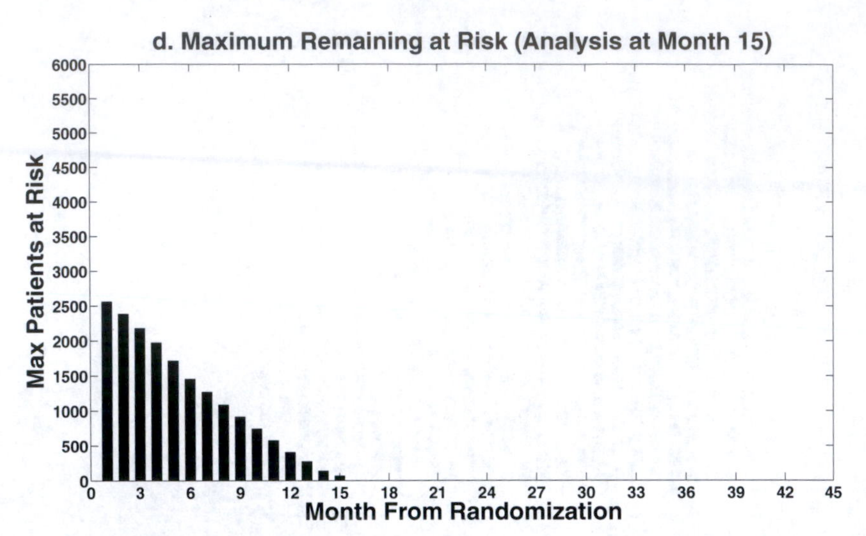

FIGURE 8.14: Maximum at risk at 15-month interim.

ization (for the 36-month analysis). Continuing, the entire distribution of the maximum at-risk for the 36-month analysis can be derived from the (cumulative) recruitment pattern. Similarly, the entire distribution of the maximum at risk for a 15-month interim can be derived from the numbers of patients enrolled during each of the 15 months after study start (Figure 8.14). While the numbers actually remaining at risk will also reflect losses and events, it is essential to appreciate the critical role of the recruitment pattern in limiting the maximum at risk. Note that the bars in Figure 8.14 are identical to the corresponding bars in Figure 8.13 to the right of month 22. The maximum number of patients at risk during the last 15 months leading up to the interim is limited by the recruitment pattern of the first 15 months, regardless of whether the interim takes place at month 15, month 36, or for any interim later than month 15.

What is depicted in Figures 8.13 and 8.14, the declining maximum number of patients at risk at the interim, is consistent with the number of patients at risk in typical published Kaplan-Meier plots. The focus on the maximum at risk derived in this way is simply to provide insight into the shape of the distribution of maximum number of patients remaining at risk during an interim.

The information for survival analyses is proportional to the number of events available for that analysis. For the 36-month analysis, only the events generated during the 36th month after randomization can provide information on the treatment effect during that 36th month. The expected number of events is the number of patients enrolled during the first month after study start (CT) multiplied by the one month failure rate during the 36th month

(RT), both groups combined. (All of the distributions displayed reflect both groups combined). In an actual trial, that number is smaller due to losses, etc. If there is a 24-month treatment lag, only the area under the curve to the right of 24 months (see vertical line at month 24 in Figure 8.13) will generate events that can be helpful in detecting whether there is a treatment effect. As discussed below, the much larger area to the left will generally be detrimental to detecting such an effect. If the 36-month interim was timed to occur at a specified fraction of information, only a small fraction of that fraction will actually be useful to detect a treatment effect. In other words, at best the interim is effectively occurring at a much smaller fraction of information than planned, since the only information supporting the alternative is collected after the period of treatment lag has ended.

Now consider the impact of the at-risk pattern on estimating the treatment effect in the presence of a treatment lag. If there is a potential threshold lag of about 24 months, estimating, or even detecting whether there is a treatment effect, even at a 36-month interim is likely to be exceedingly difficult.

First, what analysis should be used? Typically, even if non-proportionality is expected, the proportional hazards model is assumed. If there is a treatment effect and a 24-month lag, the area under the curve to the left of month 24 represents patients who are at risk, and who have been generating events during the period of no treatment effect. Only the small area under the curve to the right of month 24 could contribute to events at the time the treatment effect is emerging. The area under the curve to the right of month 24 is less than 5% of the entire area of both portions. The mountain of events generated when there is no treatment effect (95%) will overwhelm those generated during a possible treatment effect (5%). Consequently, the proportional hazards model will grossly underestimate the after-lag treatment effect. This is a very biased estimate of what the treatment effect will be for the remainder of the trial and will lead to very poor projections for sample size re-estimation or futility.

To avoid this problem, one could concentrate the analysis on the post-lag period (i.e., during the 24–36-month period). First note that the number of events during that period is a small fraction of the events on which the interim was planned. That is, if the interim was scheduled to occur at say 50% of the events, then restricting to the 24–36 month period will provide only a small fraction of that 50%, in this case, less than 5% of that 50%, i.e., less than 2.5%. With such a small number of events, such an analysis is of virtually no use. For example, suppose the trial was event-driven designed to terminate at a maximum of 1000 events, and a 50% interim was planned at 500 events. Then the actual number of events supporting the alternative would be $2.5\% \times 500 =$ 12.5 events, about 7 in each arm (and 487 events supporting the null). But further, what would the justification be for performing an analysis restricted to 24–36 months? Perhaps the lag is 30 months long. If so, then even this grossly underpowered analysis will be biased by including the no-treatment-effect period 24–30 months. And again, the number of events generated during the no treatment effect period will be larger than those generated after the actual lag. No matter what time we think the lag will end and the treatment will begin to show effectiveness, the possibility of gross bias of the estimate will still exist.

The above discussion is even more important for futility as compared to sample size re-estimation. When there is a treatment lag, an interim estimate of the treatment effect is likely to be a gross underestimate of the true post-lag treatment effect. No matter how good the drug, this underestimate can lead to terminating the trial for futility. And in oncology, treatment lags can last for many years. Futility assessment should be avoided when there is a possibility of treatment lag.

8.4.2 Increasing the Sample Size When There Is a Treatment Lag

Suppose, based on an interim, we perceive the trial as underpowered and decide to increase the sample size. Continue with the example of a 5-year trial and a likely 24-month treatment lag. Assume that the decision is to begin recruiting patients immediately after the 36-month interim. All such additional patients will be at risk and generating events during the lag period when there is no treatment effect. For these additional patients, their lag periods (RT) will begin no earlier than 36 months (CT) after study start (since they are recruited after that interim), and continue until the study concludes at 5 years. Consequently, all additional patients will contribute events only during their no-treatment effect period, so the events they contribute will only serve to diminish the power of the study. Although each situation should be carefully evaluated, if treatment lags are possible, one should avoid an initial small sample size combined with a possible increase through sample size re-estimation.

8.4.3 Interaction between Weighted Statistics and Non-proportional Hazards

Suppose through sample size re-estimation the sample size is increased, and the data collected after the interim at which the increase was determined down-weighted for the final statistic [5]. Down-weighting is relative, since the down-weighting of one portion of the data results in an up-weighting of the remaining data. In the presence of a threshold lag, down-weighting the post increase data will be down-weighting the portion of the data collected when the treatment was showing its greatest efficacy, while simultaneously up-weighting the "no treatment effect" portion. The issue is made more complex because treatment lag is a time-from-randomization phenomenon (RT), whereas re-weighting is performed on segments of the data identified as "pre" and "post" the calendar time of the interim (CT). The pre- and post-portions of the data will contain a mix of survival experience from various portions of time-from-randomization defined treatment effects.

8.4.4 Estimating the Treatment Effect in a Trial with a Threshold Treatment Anti-lag

For mid-course corrections, there are some similarities between the threshold treatment lag and anti-lag situations. Potentially the most important issue for mid-course correction is the ability to predict the treatment effect, or, more specifically, the hazard ratio function for the remainder of the trial. Recall that the hazard ratio function is a time from randomization concept. In the above discussion of treatment lag, the difficulty of obtaining even a reasonable estimate of the post-lag treatment effect was explained. With a substantially biased estimate, decisions regarding mid-course corrections may be seriously compromised. Certainly the same issue exists with treatment anti-lags. The consequences however, are somewhat different. In general, with the treatment lag, since the interim estimate is likely to be badly biased towards no treatment effect, erroneous decisions such as futility are likely.

For threshold anti-lags, there are two zones. The hazard ratio is greater than 1 in the initial, or alternative zone, supporting the alternative. The null zone begins at the time the treatment effect ends.

Just as an interim estimate of the treatment effect for a lag is likely to substantially underestimate the treatment effect after the interim, the interim estimate for an anti-lag is likely to substantially overestimate the treatment effect after the interim. As a result, for anti-lags, analysts and decision makers are more likely to believe that the power of the trial is adequate when in fact it is not. Although the situation depicted in Figure 8.8 does not exactly translate to the current discussion (Figure 8.8 reflects design issues rather than mid-course corrections), similar issues arise. In particular, an over-estimate of interim efficacy can lead one to believe that a curve similar to the upper curve of Figure 8.8 is applicable, when in fact the lower curve is more representative.

If, for example, based on interim data, one believes a curve like the upper curve in Figure 8.8 is in force, the conclusion mostly likely would be to stay the course. But if there is a realization that the bottom curve is more plausible, then it should be clear that staying the course is likely to lead to a failed trial. Consequently, some modification, such as a sample increase, may be in order. It should however be recognized that the situation is complex. To accommodate a sample size increase, extending the length of the trial is often required. But extending the length of the trial will extend the follow-up of patients who already have transitioned from the alternative zone and now reside in the null zone. And some patients in the alternative zone will migrate into the null zone. So part of the increase in power due to the increase in sample size will be offset by the increase of events occurring in the null zone. Staggered entry increases the complexity.

Further, there may be a narrow time window for the sample size re-estimation surge in patients to accomplish the desired goal. In particular, as more patients are added, initially they enter into the alternative zone, contributing to the power. But at the same time, some patients in the alternative zone are migrating into the null zone having the opposite effect. Once most of the patients have migrated out of the alternative zone, the power will diminish more quickly. The best approach in this situation is to size the trial as large as possible at the outset, to complete with as little overflow into the null zone as possible. Again, recruitment patterns, both before and after the sample size adjustment, must be considered. Had the protocol-specified sample size been sufficient at the outset, this problem would have been reduced substantially.

8.4.5 Sample Size Re-estimation in the Presence of Treatment Lag or Anti-lag: Concluding Remark

Interestingly, with both the treatment lag and anti-lag, the start small strategy is contraindicated. The best strategy is, as much as possible, to size the trial appropriately at the outset. Sample size adjustment should be used when it appears that this best effort needs adjustment.

8.4.6 Conditional Power, Current Trends, and Non-proportional Hazards

Conditional power is power calculated at the time of an interim, conditional on the observed data as well as assumptions about the data that will be collected for the remainder of the trial. Recall that the "remainder of the trial" is a calendar-time concept, which contrasts with the time from randomization concept of non-proportional hazards. The issues regarding conditional power when non-proportional hazards is possible are beyond the scope of this chapter. A few will be briefly mentioned here. The most common assumption for future data is that it follows the "current trend." How should the current trend be defined with possibly non-proportional hazards? Take for example a 2-year threshold treatment lag in a 5-year trial. Assume simultaneous entry for simplicity (CT=RT). Define the null zone as the initial 2-year period and the alternative zone as the remainder of the trial. If an interim is performed during the null zone, the expected hazard ratio is 1 and will remain 1 up to the junction of the two zones. If conditional power is calculated at this junction, the estimate will be based entirely on null zone events, while the remainder will be based entirely on the alternative. Conditional power based on the current trend at this point is worse than useless. As the time of the interim progresses into the alternative zone, the ratio of alternative to total events will gradually improve. In spite of the fact that events during the remainder of the trial will be generated solely from the alternative zone, at no point will the estimate of the hazard ratio for the remainder of the trial be based purely on alternative events. The expected size of the treatment effect will always be underestimated, with the size of the bias being a function of the time of the interim. For threshold anti-lags, the situation is reversed, with the expected size of the treatment effect always an overestimate. In general, the situation is worse for staggered entry. If mid-course corrections are contemplated, it should be approached very cautiously, and inflexible correction methods should be avoided.

8.5 How the Markov Model Works

8.5.1 Introduction

In a phase III placebo-controlled clinical trial [22], the efficacy of bevacizumab in combination with bolus-IFL chemotherapy (bolus irinotecan/5-FU/leucovorin) or 5-FU/leucovorin chemotherapy was evaluated as first-line therapy for previously untreated metastatic colorectal cancer (FDA Statistical Review: Avastin (2003)). Eligible patients were randomized to Bolus-IFL + placebo (Group 1) or bolus-IFL + bevacizumab (Group 2) or a third arm which is not of interest for this discussion. Median survival was increased from 15.6 months to 20.3.

8.5.2 The Exponential Model for Calculating Cumulative Survival Probabilities

In carrying out clinical trials, there are two time frames. One is calendar time (CT), the other, randomization time (RT). All times and/or dates are initially recorded as calendar times. For analyses such as the logrank statistic, Kaplan-Meier estimates, and the Markov model, the time frame is time from randomization. At this point in the discussion, the assumed timescale for this section is time from randomization. The discussion here begins with the assumption that failure rates are exponentially distributed; generalization to time-dependent hazards will be discussed later. Consider the placebo arm. Since it is assumed that survival is exponential, cumulative survival is given by $S(t) = e^{-\lambda t}$, where λ is constant. Solving for λ when $t = 15.6$ and $S(t) = .5$ gives $\lambda = 0.4443$ as the hazard in months. Using the same formula, the probabilities of surviving for any 1-, 6-, 12-, 24-, or 36-month period are given in Table 8.6.

8.5.3 The Life-table Approach to Calculating Cumulative Survival Probabilities

The description here will be for the control arm only; the experimental arm is similar. Simultaneous entry is assumed to facilitate comprehension. Assume the time line for survival (time is 0 for randomization, to the maximum follow-

TABLE 8.6: Bevacizumab registration study: Cumulative failure rates based on simple exponential model.

	Control		Bevacizumab	
Month	$S(t) = e^{-0.04443t}$	Failure	$S(t) = e^{-0.03415t}$	Failure
1	.95654	.04346	.96643	.03357
6	.76600	.23400	.81473	.18527
12	.58675	.41325	.66378	.33622
24	.34427	.65573	.44061	.55939
36	.20200	.79800	.29247	.70753

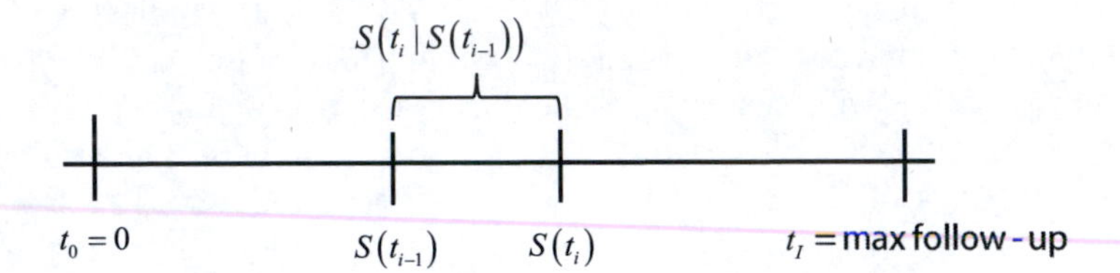

FIGURE 8.15: Calculating cumulative survival.

up) has been subdivided into 1-month intervals. The cumulative probability of surviving to the end of any 1-month interval is the product of the cumulative probability of surviving to the end of the previous interval times the conditional probability of surviving the current interval given at risk at the end of the previous interval:

$$S(t_i) = S(t_{i-1})\, S(t_i | S(t_{i-1})) \tag{8.1}$$

Since we are temporarily assuming an exponential model, the conditional probability of surviving any 1-month interval, given a patient is at risk at the beginning of that interval, is 0.95654 ($St_i | S(t_{i-1}) = .95654$ for all i) (first row of Table 8.6). Table 8.7 gives the results of successively applying (8.1) (rows 15–28 have been suppressed for space considerations). For example (focusing on the control group), at time 0, all patients are still at risk, with none failed and the at-risk probability of 1. Take the product of those still at risk at time 0 multiplied by the conditional probability of surviving one month ($1 \times .95654$) to get the cumulative probability of surviving to the end of the 1st month

TABLE 8.7: Bevacizumab registration study: cumulative failure rates based on life table and Markov methods

	Control		Bevacizumab	
Month	Failed	At Risk	Failed	At Risk
0	0.0000	1.0000	0.0000	1.0000
1	0.0435	0.9565	0.0336	0.9664
2	0.0850	0.9150	0.0660	0.9340
3	0.1248	0.8752	0.0974	0.9026
4	0.1628	0.8372	0.1277	0.8723
5	0.1992	0.8008	0.1570	0.8430
6	0.2340	0.7660	0.1853	0.8147
7	0.2673	0.7327	0.2126	0.7874
8	0.2991	0.7009	0.2390	0.7610
9	0.3296	0.6704	0.2646	0.7354
10	0.3587	0.6413	0.2893	0.7107
11	0.3866	0.6134	0.3131	0.6869
12	0.4132	0.5868	0.3362	0.6638
13	0.4387	0.5613	0.3585	0.6415
14	0.4631	0.5369	0.3800	0.6200
29	0.7243	0.2757	0.6285	0.3715
30	0.7363	0.2637	0.6410	0.3590
31	0.7477	0.2523	0.6531	0.3469
32	0.7587	0.2413	0.6647	0.3353
33	0.7692	0.2308	0.6760	0.3240
34	0.7792	0.2208	0.6868	0.3132
35	0.7888	0.2112	0.6973	0.3027
36	0.7980	0.2020	0.7075	0.2925

(.95654). Here, the cumulative survival probability is the probability of being at risk. Similarly, to get the cumulative probability of surviving to the end of month 6, multiply the cumulative survival at the end of the fifth month (.8008) by the conditional probability of surviving one month (.95654) to get the cumulative probability of surviving to the end of the sixth month ($.8008 \times .95654 = .7660$). Note that .7660 (Table 8.7) matches the survival probability calculated directly using the exponential formula (Table 8.6).

Each row of the "failed" columns can be calculated from the corresponding row of the same treatment arm of the "at-risk" columns by subtracting the latter from 1. If the final analysis will compare proportions failing, the sample size can be calculated using a standard sample size formula for comparing proportions. Using probabilities from the last row of Table 8.7, the sample size for a 36-month trial with a control group probability of failing of .7980 and .7075 for the bevacizumab group is 952 (PASS®, 90% power, 2-sided .05 significance level) for a binomial comparison of proportions. The entire table is used in calculating the sample size, 624, for the logrank statistic (STOPP®, Markov approach, same Type I and II errors).

8.5.4 The Markov Model Approach to Calculating Cumulative Survival Probabilities

The discrete Markov model for survival trials [8, 9] can be considered an extension of the Life Table approach. The Life Table approach to calculating cumulative survival probabilities, as in Table 8.7, considered a single process — the failure process. In clinical trials, failure processes rarely take place in isolation. Some other important processes are the loss process, the noncompliance (or Off Drug-In Study (ODIS)) process, and the recruitment process. Non-compliance is used here to refer to patients who are still in the trial but have discontinued randomized therapy. Patients may become non-compliant in a prevention trial as they decide to no longer adhere to a randomized diet, or in an in-hospital trial due to adverse events. The term ODIS refers to a more general concept than non-compliance, because it may include patients who have dropped out of the trial but who are still being followed for the endpoint of interest. In Table 8.7, the multiplications governed by (8.1) "transferred" patients from the at-risk columns to the failed columns. The "transfers" are in probabilities rather than numbers of patients. For a trial with a given number of patients per arm, the expected number of patients for each transfer can be obtained by multiplying by the total number of patients in that arm (under staggered entry, a different approach is needed). The loss process is similar to the failure process, and it could be modeled by a Life Table exactly as was just done for the failure process. The two processes take patients from the at-risk population. A table (not shown) similar to Table 8.7 could be created for losses.

The failure (respectively, loss) process transfers patients from the at-risk to the failed (respectively, loss) column at a specific rate. While the Life Table can only handle one process at a time, the Markov model is designed to handle simultaneous processes. Both the loss and failure processes are survival-type processes. At each time point (time from randomization) during a trial, at-risk patients can either be lost or can fail. It is very important to understand that from the viewpoint of survival processes, there is no difference between the loss process and the failure process. Typical analyses, such as the Kaplan-Meier or logrank statistics treat the failure process as the process of interest, while the loss process is viewed as censoring the failure process, a nuisance process which is not itself of interest. Table 8.7 is the result of using Life Table methods (8.1) to project cumulative failure/survival probabilities. Those probabilities can then be used to calculate sample size. Often, cumulative loss probabilities are used to adjust sample sizes. However, both processes, failure and loss, have an equal footing in nature — the Markov model is consistent with this phenomenon. The contrast between adjusting the sample size for loss as opposed to first calculating projections in which loss and failure are treated as simultaneous, co-equal, interdependent processes and then calculating sample sizes will be apparent shortly.

As was done in Table 8.7 for the Life Table approach, the Markov approach models each treatment arm of the trial separately. One of the fundamental concepts of discrete-state Markov models is the concept of "states" . These are mutually exclusive and exhaustive categories to which patients belong at any given time during the trial. In the simplest of Markov models for survival trials, there are two states: "Failed" and "At-Risk" (see Table 8.7). And these two states suffice for calculating sample size for the logrank statistic as well as a comparison of proportions. The original Markov model [8], which handles most clinical trial designs, includes four states:

I. Lost to Follow-up
II. Event
III. At-Risk (Complier)
IV. At-Risk (Noncomplier or ODIS)

Similar to the Kaplan-Meier and logrank statistics, and Cox proportional hazards model, it is a time from randomization model. At any time, the trial population has distribution $D_t = \left[P_L(t), P_E(t), P_{A_C(t)}, P_{A_O(t)}\right]'$ among these four states, where D_t is a column vector, $P_L(t)$ is the probability of being in the loss state at time t , etc. The Markov model also defines a transition matrix T for which $T_{t_{i-1},t_i}(i,j)$ is the conditional probability of going from state i to state j during the period $[t_{i-1}, t_i]$. The distribution at time t_i is given by

$$D_{t_i} = T_{t_{i-1},t_i} D_{t_{i-1}} \tag{8.2}$$

Thus, at any time t_j, the distribution is given by

$$\mathbf{D}_{t_i} = \left\{ \prod_{i=1}^{i=j} \mathbf{T}_{t_{i-1},t_i} \right\} \mathbf{D}_{t_0} \tag{8.3}$$

where

$$\mathbf{D}_0 = \mathbf{D}_{t_0} = \left[\begin{array}{cccc} 0 & 0 & 1 & 0 \end{array}\right]' \tag{8.4}$$

is the initial distribution at the time of randomization. The initial distribution has this form because at randomization, every patient is assumed at risk and compliant (i.e., adhering to randomly assigned therapy).

8.5.4.1 2-State Markov Model: At Risk, Failure

Restrict this 4-state model to the failed (or event) and at-risk states, with distributions similar to (8.3) and initial distribution similar to (8.4). The last two columns of Table 8.7 can be viewed as an implementation of this two-state model for the bevacizumab arm, with the rows representing successive distributions obtained from the products as in (8.2) (in the Life Table approach, this was handled by (8.1)). Although each distribution is a column vector, each is transposed for easy display in Table 8.7. Similarly, columns 2 and 3 display the successive control arm distributions. Although the discussion above of the calculations that gave rise to Table 8.7 was based on Life-Table methods, the actual table was generated using the Markov model. The results are the same.

The Transition Matrices. To derive the entries in Table 8.7 using the Life Table approach, the one-month conditional survival probabilities for the control and bevacizumab treatment arms were first calculated, based on the exponential assumption and their median survival times (1-month conditional survival probabilities: .95654 and .96643, respectively). For example, from above, "to get the cumulative probability of surviving to the end of month 6, multiply the cumulative survival at the end of the fifth month (.8008) by the conditional probability of surviving a month (.95654) to get the cumulative probability of surviving to the end of the sixth month ($.8008 \times .95654 = .7660$)." The conditional probability .95654 of surviving one month also determines the probability of failing in that same month for this simple 2-state model. In the Markov model, that conditional failure probability is referred to as the probability of "transitioning" from the At-Risk state to the failed (Event) state, conditional on being at risk just before that time period. The Markov model for calculating the distribution at month 6 from the distribution at month 5 is

$$\mathbf{D_{t_i}} = \mathbf{T_{t_{i-1},t_i}} * \mathbf{D_{t_{i-1}}} \tag{8.5}$$

$$\mathbf{D_6} = \mathbf{T_{5,6}} * \mathbf{D_5} \tag{8.6}$$

$$= \begin{bmatrix} a & b \\ c & d \end{bmatrix} * \mathbf{D_5} \tag{8.7}$$

$$= \begin{bmatrix} 1 & .04346 \\ 0 & .95654 \end{bmatrix} * \begin{bmatrix} .1992 \\ .8008 \end{bmatrix} \tag{8.8}$$

$$= \begin{bmatrix} .2340 \\ .7660 \end{bmatrix} \tag{8.9}$$

In (8.7), a–d are the (conditional) transition probabilities governing the transitions from month 5 to month 6:

- a is the conditional probability of an event remaining an event, which is assumed to be 1.
- b is the conditional probability of an at-risk patient having an event.
- c is the conditional probability of a patient who has had an event going back into the at-risk population, assumed to be 0.
- d is the conditional probability of an at-risk patient remaining at risk, which is 1 minus the probability of an at-risk patient failing.

Because an exponential model was assumed for the failure/survival probabilities, those failure probabilities will be the same for each transition matrix $\mathbf{T_{t_{i-1},t_i}}$, independent of i. Time-dependent probabilities will be discussed shortly.

8.5.4.2 3-State Markov Model: At Risk, Failure, Loss

Adding loss to follow-up to the two-state Markov model.

The Markov model approach provides a rich class of models for clinical trials. A working assumption in all of the models presented in this chapter is that once a patient has failed, that patient cannot transition out of the failed state. This is called an "absorbing' state. An example of the richness of the Markov model is that one need not require the failed state to be absorbing, and, as such, the Markov model can accommodate recurrent events.

Below, the two-state Markov model ("failed" and "at-risk") used to generate Table 8.7 will be expanded to three- and four-state models. First a "lost to follow-up" state is added. After that, the model adds an ODIS (Off Drug In Study) or "non-compliant" state. While the actual Markov models (8.2)–(8.4) were presented in equation form, only tables similar to Table 8.7 are used below; they present the results of applying the Markov models, i.e., the successive distributions obtained from successive applications of (8.2).

Although the general 4-state Markov model was introduced above (8.2)-(8.4), a 3-state Markov model which adds loss to the 2-state model will now be discussed.

A three state model ("At-Risk", "Failed", and "Lost to Follow-up" states).

Losses can arise for a variety of reasons: patients may die from competing risks, may move out of the area and lose contact with the clinic, etc. One of the most important reasons for loss is "administrative censoring." Patients who are still at-risk at the time of an analysis are "administratively censored" from that analysis because they have not yet had the primary event. All that is known is that the event can happen sometime in the future. If such an analysis is at an interim time point, any still-at-risk patient will generally continue participation in the trial. If that patient fails by the time of the next analysis, that patient will not be administratively censored from later analyses. Because none of these loss categories is used in calculating the logrank statistic, all such losses can be merged into a single loss state. Here we assume that the loss state is absorbing: once a patient is lost, that patient cannot return to the at-risk state. For the bevacizumab example, assume that the loss rate is 15%/year. Using the survival formula $S(t) = e^{-\lambda t}$ again, but with 15% at one year, the probability of surviving this loss process in one month is 0.98655, with corresponding 1-month loss probability of 0.01345, as seen in the month 1 row of Table 8.8. (There is a slight difference between the 0.01330 in the table and the .01345 calculated here. It is due to the fact that the program that generated this table performs the multiplications every half-month. The .0433 in the month 1 row of the Control Failed column differs from the .0435 of Table 8.7 for the same reason. The explanation for this phenomenon should become clear shortly.) So the losses during the first month decrement the "at-risk" probability of 1 by .0133, while the failures decrement the "at-risk" probability by .0433. The probability of remaining at risk declines faster in Table 8.8 compared with Table 8.7.

TABLE 8.8: Bevacizumab registration study: Cumulative failure rates based on Markov model with loss to follow-up added to model.

	Control			Bevacizumab		
Month	Loss	Failed	At Risk	Lost	Failed	At Risk
1	0.0133	0.0433	0.9434	0.0133	0.0335	0.9532
2	0.0259	0.0842	0.8900	0.0261	0.0654	0.9086
3	0.0377	0.1227	0.8396	0.0382	0.0958	0.8661
4	0.0489	0.1591	0.7921	0.0497	0.1247	0.8255
5	0.0594	0.1934	0.7472	0.0607	0.1524	0.7869
6	0.0693	0.2257	0.7049	0.0712	0.1787	0.7501
7	0.0787	0.2563	0.6650	0.0812	0.2038	0.7150
8	0.0876	0.2851	0.6274	0.0908	0.2277	0.6815
9	0.0959	0.3122	0.5918	0.0999	0.2505	0.6496
10	0.1038	0.3379	0.5583	0.1085	0.2722	0.6192
11	0.1112	0.3621	0.5267	0.1168	0.2930	0.5903
12	0.1182	0.3849	0.4969	0.1247	0.3127	0.5626
13	0.1248	0.4064	0.4688	0.1322	0.3315	0.5363
14	0.1311	0.4267	0.4422	0.1393	0.3495	0.5112
29	0.1916	0.6239	0.1845	0.2140	0.5369	0.2491
30	0.1941	0.6318	0.1741	0.2173	0.5452	0.2374
31	0.1964	0.6394	0.1642	0.2205	0.5532	0.2263
32	0.1986	0.6465	0.1549	0.2235	0.5607	0.2157
33	0.2007	0.6532	0.1461	0.2264	0.5680	0.2056
34	0.2026	0.6595	0.1379	0.2291	0.5748	0.1960
35	0.2044	0.6655	0.1301	0.2318	0.5814	0.1868
36	0.2062	0.6711	0.1227	0.2342	0.5876	0.1781

Using a sample size formula for comparing the proportions .6711 versus .5876 (PASS® 90% power, 2-sided significance level .05), the sample size accounting for loss using the Markov model corresponding to Table 8.8 is 1404 patients, compared with 952 patients ignoring loss (Table 8.7). Often, sample size is adjusted for loss by calculating what the 15% yearly loss probability would be over 3 years (this can be done using the exponential model, or simply taking $1 - (1 - .15)^3 = .386$), and increasing the 952 accordingly $(952/ (1 - .386) = 1550)$. This adjustment is about 146 patients larger than the one using the Markov model. The Markov model correctly models the two processes, failure and loss, as concurrent, interdependent processes. Take, for example, the loss column under bevacizumab in Table 8.8. The last row gives the cumulative probability of being lost after 36 months as .2342, much smaller than the .386 calculated just above, in isolation of the failure process. This happens because the proportion of patients remaining at risk declines much more quickly in Table 8.8 compared with that of Table 8.7. Similarly, Table 8.8 has fewer failures. And the reason is that both the loss and failure processes continually deplete the pool of patients remaining at risk. Going down the event column, the failure probabilities accumulate more slowly in Table 8.8 with the 36-month failure probability of .6711 of Table 8.8 as compared with .7980 of Table 8.7. That accumulation is slower because the loss process continually depletes the pool of at-risk patients, leaving fewer available to fail. In calculating the logrank statistic, the Markov model approach uses the entire column of failure and at-risk probabilities, not just the 36-month probability.

8.5.4.3 4-State Markov Model: At Risk, Failure, Loss, ODIS (Noncompliance)

Now consider the effects of ODIS (Off Drug, In Study) or, equivalently, noncompliance as compared to loss. Initially, the focus of ODIS will be on patients in the bevacizumab arm. This is modelled by including a new state, the ODIS state. The usual assumption for ODIS is that once patients stop taking their randomly assigned treatment, they no longer receive the benefits of that treatment. Other assumptions are possible, but for simplicity, this assumption will be in force here. The reason a separate at-risk state is needed is that the failure rate of ODIS patients is different from the other at-risk patients who are still taking their randomly assigned therapy. In contrast to the loss state, ODIS patients are still being followed for the primary endpoint, but have a worse failure rate (the control group rate) since they are no longer taking their assigned therapy. Lost patients deplete the remaining at-risk patients; ODIS patients do not deplete the at-risk pool, but rather change the "average" failure rate of the at-risk mixture. The results of applying this Markov model are presented in Table 8.9. One of the fundamental Markov properties is that the probability of failure depends only on the state in which a patient resides at a given time, and not on how that patient arrived in that state. If both

TABLE 8.9: Bevacizumab registration study: Cumulative failure rates based on Markov model with loss to follow-up and ODIS/non-compliance added to model

	Control				Bevacizumab			
			At Risk				At Risk	
Month	Loss	Event	ODIS	On Rx	Loss	Event	ODIS	On Rx
0	0.0000	0.0000	0.0000	1.0000	0.0000	0.0000	0.0000	1.0000
1	0.0133	0.0433	0.0000	0.9434	0.0000	0.0336	0.0132	0.9532
2	0.0259	0.0842	0.0000	0.8900	0.0000	0.0662	0.0252	0.9086
3	0.0377	0.1227	0.0000	0.8396	0.0000	0.0978	0.0361	0.8661
4	0.0489	0.1591	0.0000	0.7921	0.0000	0.1285	0.0459	0.8255
5	0.0594	0.1934	0.0000	0.7472	0.0000	0.1583	0.0548	0.7869
6	0.0693	0.2257	0.0000	0.7049	0.0000	0.1871	0.0628	0.7501
7	0.0787	0.2563	0.0000	0.6650	0.0000	0.2150	0.0700	0.7150
8	0.0876	0.2851	0.0000	0.6274	0.0000	0.2421	0.0764	0.6815
9	0.0959	0.3122	0.0000	0.5918	0.0000	0.2683	0.0820	0.6496
10	0.1038	0.3379	0.0000	0.5583	0.0000	0.2937	0.0870	0.6192
11	0.1112	0.3621	0.0000	0.5267	0.0000	0.3183	0.0914	0.5903
12	0.1182	0.3849	0.0000	0.4969	0.0000	0.3421	0.0952	0.5626
13	0.1248	0.4064	0.0000	0.4688	0.0000	0.3652	0.0985	0.5363
14	0.1311	0.4267	0.0000	0.4422	0.0000	0.3875	0.1013	0.5112
29	0.1916	0.6239	0.0000	0.1845	0.0000	0.6459	0.1050	0.2491
30	0.1941	0.6318	0.0000	0.1741	0.0000	0.6588	0.1037	0.2374
31	0.1964	0.6394	0.0000	0.1642	0.0000	0.6713	0.1024	0.2263
32	0.1986	0.6465	0.0000	0.1549	0.0000	0.6834	0.1009	0.2157
33	0.2007	0.6532	0.0000	0.1461	0.0000	0.6950	0.0994	0.2056
34	0.2026	0.6595	0.0000	0.1379	0.0000	0.7062	0.0978	0.1960
35	0.2044	0.6655	0.0000	0.1301	0.0000	0.7171	0.0961	0.1868
36	0.2062	0.6711	0.0000	0.1227	0.0000	0.7275	0.0944	0.1781

non-compliant and compliant patients resided in the same state, their failure probabilities would depend on whether a given patient had transitioned into noncompliance.

To understand how the ODIS model works, consider columns 6–9 under bevacizumab. Recall that Table 8.9 displays the successive distributions among the 4 states. These are the results of applying the model, not the model itself. What is displayed in this table can be considered an extension of the Life Table procedure. There are now two "at-risk" columns under bevacizumab in Table 8.9 compared with one in the previous tables. At randomization, all patients are assumed to be On Therapy (a "1" at month 0). As time progresses, patients gradually transition from the At-Risk On Therapy state to the At-Risk ODIS state. They do so at the assumed rate of 15% per year which can be converted to a monthly rate using the exponential model as was done earlier. This gradual migration of patients from on-therapy to ODIS is witnessed as the At-Risk patients migrate from the On-Therapy column to the ODIS column (all under bevacizumab). Again, the assumption is that a

TABLE 8.10: Sample sizes using the Markov model comparing loss to follow-up with ODIS/non-compliance

	Control		Bevacizumab		Sample Size	Log Rank
Design	Loss	ODIS	Loss	ODIS	Patients	Events
1	0	0	0	0	800	608
2	.15	0	.15	0	960	608
3	.15	0	0	.15	1248	879
					Failure Probability	
					Control	Bevacizumab
1	0	0	0	0	.7980	.7075
2	.15	0	.15	0	.6711	.5876
3	.15	0	0	.15	.6711	.7275

given patient will stop taking bevacizumab at some point, rather than reduce the quantity of therapy (the latter can also be modeled within the Markov framework). The difference in the two At-Risk columns is that the failure rate for On-Therapy patients remains at the original assumed bevacizumab rate (.0336 per month), while the failure rate for ODIS is that of the control group (.0434 per month). The events column now receives events from both At-Risk columns, each according to its assumed failure rate.

Table 8.10 summarizes several sample size results for the bevacizumab example. The number of patients and events required for the logrank statistic with no loss and no ODIS is 800 patients, 608 events. Including loss at 15% for both treatment arms increases the sample size to 960 patients; the number of events, 608, remains the same.

Changing the bevacizumab arm from 15% loss to 15% ODIS increases the required number of events by 44% from 608 to 879. The sample size is also increased by about 30%, from 960 to 1248.

The inclusion of loss (Table 8.9 Control Group) reduces the number of patients at risk, so more patients will be required to produce the 608 events. The required number of events is not affected.

In contrast, the inclusion of ODIS creates a mixture distribution of At-Risk patients in the bevacizumab arm, some with the bevacizumab failure rate of .0366 per month and others at the control rate of .0434 per month. The treatment effect "averaged" over the two At-Risk categories is thus diminished, which requires more events. In trials with ODIS, there is a mixture distribution that is constantly changing as the trial progresses. In turn, the failure rate for that mixture is continually changing. It is important to note that the Markov model, which is designed to handle multiple concurrent processes, can easily model this situation. In contrast, an exponentially based approach, (see [7] for example) models constant hazards. As mentioned above, ODIS results in a constantly changing hazard ratio. To address this issue, Lachin and Foulkes (who use the term "noncompliance" which in this instance is equivalent to ODIS) assume that all non-compliance takes place at the time of randomization. This is a conservative assumption, but how conservative is difficult to assess.

The commercial software package PASS® offers the Markov approach. To the best of the author's knowledge, non-compliance/ODIS has only been addressed in commercial software packages using either the Lachin and Foulkes or the Lakatos Markov approach. Commercially available simulation programs do not appear to address ODIS. The most likely reason for this is that simulations require assumptions about the values of the parameters. For ODIS, the failure rate is constantly changing in a very complex way, because the at-risk distribution is a constantly changing mixture of patients on and off drug. While patients are transitioning from On Drug to ODIS, they are also failing from both parts of the mixture, and at different failure rates from each part of the mixture.

In purchasing commercial software, caution is advised if the term "dropout" is used. "Dropout" is typically used to refer to loss to follow-up, not ODIS. The example just discussed shows that these two concepts are associated with dramatically different consequences.

The Markov Model including ODIS used to generate Table 8.9 modeled ODIS for the bevacizumab arm, but only loss for the control arm. The rationale for this is that patients may discontinue bevacizumab due to adverse events directly related to bevacizumab, and this is not likely to happen for the control arm, who are receiving placebo in addition to backbone therapy. If a patient discontinues bevacizumab, she is not likely to receive any further benefit of bevacizumab, and so is assumed to transition to the control group rate. A patient discontinuing control therapy is not likely, however, to begin taking bevacizumab and thus transition to the bevacizumab failure rate. However, the real world is never simple. Patients may discontinue any and all portions of their randomly assigned therapy.

Appropriate modeling must carefully consider all aspects of a particular trial setting. In a dietary cancer prevention trial, patients randomized to the experimental diet may stop adhering to that diet and in turn transition to the control group rate. Patients in the control group could read about the purported benefits of the experimental diet and begin adhering to that diet on their own. Such patients would then transition from the control failure rate to the experimental failure rate. This phenomenon is referred to as "drop-in." Another consideration is whether the discontinuation of therapy might be associated with a gradual decline in the treatment effect. If an estimate of a treatment effect is derived from a prior study, it is important to understand whether that estimate already includes some degree of ODIS. This issue is complicated by the fact that treatment effects assumed for sample size calculation often are based on a balance between cost considerations and what is termed the "smallest clinically meaningful difference."

The summary presented in Table 8.10 presents an interesting contrast. The two upper configurations of Table 8.10, without ODIS, have 36-month failure rates favoring bevacizumab. The 36-month failure rates of the bottom configuration favor control. The middle configuration includes loss of 15% in each treatment arm which reduces the at-risk populations, and which in turn reduces the 36-month event rates. The reduction is similar in both treatment arms resulting in both failure rates being reduced by a similar amount. ODIS does not reduce the 36-month event rate, but rather increases it since patients who transition to the ODIS state have a higher failure rate than those who remain on therapy. This results in a reversal of failure rates (the two upper configurations favor bevacizumab; the third favors control). The sample size based on a comparison of proportions or on an exponential model based on comparing hazards derived from the 36-month failure rates is fooled by this reversal. The differential failure rate of the mixture distribution of the two at-risk populations favors bevacizumab compared with control at every time point during the trial. This is due to the fact that the mixture is a combination of the part of the population experiencing no treatment effect (the ODIS population) with those who are still at risk and on therapy which has a favorable treatment effect. The failure rate mixture is always more favorable than the control. Thus the logrank will not be fooled. What is going wrong here for the proportions and exponential tests is that the sizes of the populations (control and bevacizumab) remaining at risk are changing in an unusual way. The control group is experiencing loss to follow-up and shrinking, generating fewer events, but still at the higher control group failure rate. The bevacizumab group has no loss to follow-up, and thus is not contracting the way the control group is. In contrast, the corresponding 15% of the at-risk population in the bevacizumab group that is transitioning to the higher failure rate is generating more events at an increased rate. At every event, the logrank statistic compares the observed to the expected, and that expected is always adjusted to the current balance of patients in the control and treatment groups. The Markov model works analogously.

Table 8.9 was intended to contrast the effect of replacing the 15% per year loss assumption (Table 8.8) in the bevacizumab group with a 15% per year ODIS assumption. The control group maintained the 15% per year loss assumption. This is what led to the changing balance of patients in the two groups as the trial progressed. This strong imbalance is not likely to occur in an actual clinical trial. But depending on the trial, forces unique to the active versus control group can result in differential censoring of the two groups. The above example shows that such imbalances are not a problem for sample sizes based on the Markov model and the logrank statistic, but could create chaos for sample sizes based on the proportions or exponential tests.

Time-dependent Rates. In cancer trials, the conditional survival/failure rates of (8.1) for the Life Table approach can and usually do change over time. Time dependent rates enter the Markov model through the transition matrices in (8.2). Consider for example, the time-dependent rates of Table 8.2, presented again here (Table 8.11) for convenience.

In the 2-state Markov model for the experimental group, the basic equation (8.10) is

TABLE 8.11: Time-dependent annual failure rates

	Annual Failure Rates		
	Period*		
	0-3	3-10	10+
Control	.1	.1	.1
Experimental	.05	.075	.09
*Months from randomization			

TABLE 8.12: Calculating time-dependent transition matrix entries for the experimental arm from time-dependent annual failure rates

	Annual Failure Rates		
	Period*		
	0-3	3-10	10+
Experimental	.05	.075	.09
$T_{t_{i-1},t_i}(A_C,E)$	$1-(1-.05)^{1/12}$	$1-(1-.075)^{1/12}$	$1-(1-.1)^{1/12}$
$T_{t_{i-1},t_i}(A_C,A_C)$	$(1-.05)^{1/12}$	$(1-.075)^{1/12}$	$(1-.1)^{1/12}$
*Months from randomization			

$$\mathbf{D_i} = \begin{bmatrix} 1 & T_{t_{i-1},t_i}(A_C,E) \\ 0 & T_{t_{i-1},t_i}(A_C,A_C) \end{bmatrix} * \mathbf{D_{i-1}} \tag{8.10}$$

for which $T_{t_{i-1},t_i}(j_1,j_2)$ is the conditional probability of going from state j_1 to state j_2 during the period $[t_{i-1},t_i]$.

The values of $T_{t_{i-1},t_i}(A_C,E)$ in (8.10) for the experimental group are defined in Table 8.12, since the failure rates in the table are annual rates, while the transitions are monthly. The entry in the right bottom of (8.10) is given by $T_{t_{i-1},t_i}(A_C,A_C) = 1 - T_{t_{i-1},t_i}(A_C,E)$. This approach can be used to model time-dependent rates for any of the processes being considered: failure, loss-to-follow-up, noncompliance/ODIS, and accrual.

Non-uniform Accrual. Treatment of accrual is beyond the scope of this chapter. It is handled in detail by Lakatos [10].

8.5.5 Using the Markov Model to Calculate Sample Sizes for the Log-rank Statistic

This section presents a heuristic discussion of how any of Tables 8.7–8.9 can be used to calculate sample sizes for the logrank statistic. For a formal mathematical presentation, see Lakatos [9]. In the original formulation of the logrank statistic by Mantel [14], event times were sorted, and at each unique event time, a 2 x 2 table was formed. Each such table was analyzed in the usual way, comparing the observed minus expected. This is very similar to how the typical comparison of proportions statistic is calculated; however, that statistic is based on a single 2×2 table including all data, whereas the logrank statistic forms a conditional 2×2 table at every distinct event time. By doing so, the logrank statistic is able to adjust to the sizes of the groups remaining at risk at each event time. Further, the hazards need not be proportional. As such, it is a censored-data statistic, in contrast to the comparison of proportions test.

Using the distribution of the logrank statistic Schoenfeld [23] and Lakatos [9] derived a sample size formula for the logrank statistic for use with the Markov model. Heuristically, the derivation is as follows. Just as in the Mantel formulation of the logrank statistic, 2×2 tables are formed at each distinct event time, and so the Markov model can be used to form a 2×2 from each row of Table 8.7. The observed minus the expected for Mantel's logrank statistic is calculated based on the 2×2 at each given event time. Similarly, the expected value of the logrank statistic is calculated based on the 2×2 at each given row of the table. The calculations for each of those 2 x 2 tables involve calculating the observed minus expected, and depends only on the conditional failure and at-risk probabilities for that 2×2 table. The loss state added to the model allows modeling of the loss process simultaneously with the failure process. The lost state is not used in the Markov approach for calculating the expected value of the logrank statistic, or, in turn, sample sizes. However, the loss process continually updates the remaining at risk probabilities, which in turn modifies the observed minus expected. The expected depends on the at-risk ratio of the two groups, while the "observed" is calculated from the between-group change in failure probability from the preceding row. So the "observed" is actually an expected observed.

Because the Markov approach evaluates each successive row of tables like Tables 8.7–8.9, it can accommodate time-dependent rates of all associated processes (failure, loss, ODIS/noncompliance, accrual).

8.5.6 Speed and Accuracy

Markov model calculations are exceedingly fast, with most computations taking only a small fraction of a second.

Precision. Precision is governed by how fine the subdivisions of the timeline are, i.e., how many multiplications of (8.2) are used. Early programs implementing the Markov approach allowed the user to specify how fine the subdivisions would be. Current programs use 2 subdivisions per month. Small gains can be obtained by using smaller subdivisions, but 2 per month appears more than adequate for most situations.

Accuracy. Lakatos and Lan [12] performed simulation studies comparing the accuracy of three approaches designed to calculate sample size for the logrank statistic: the Markov approach, exponentially based approaches, and proportional hazards based approaches. Formulas representative of the latter two were obtained from Rubinstein et al. [21] for the exponential, and Schoenfeld [23] for proportional hazards. It was not a surprise that the Markov approach did far better when proportional hazards was violated. However, the

Markov approach was also more accurate than either of the other two approaches when the hazards were exponential or proportional.

The better accuracy of the Markov approach compared to the proportional hazards approach of Schoenfeld when the hazards are proportional can be explained as follows. Although both Schoenfeld and Lakatos use the distribution of the logrank as derived by Schoenfeld [23], Schoenfeld assumes that the at-risk ratio is constant for his derivation of the sample size formula. As discussed above, the logrank statistic calculates the observed minus the expected at each distinct event time. A critical value in estimating the expected is the at-risk ratio (cf. any test of association using the chi-square statistic). Whenever there is a treatment effect, the at-risk ratio will change over the course of the trial. Using the bevacizumab versus control trial as an example, the at-risk ratio at randomization as given in the first row of Table 8.7 is 1/1 = 1. By going down the two at-risk columns, it is easy to see how this ratio is expected to change as the trial progresses. At the end of the trial, the last row shows that the ratio is no longer 1 but rather .2020/.2925 = .69. And as mentioned earlier, the Markov model calculates the expected value of the observed minus expected at each row of Table 8.7, similar to the way the actual logrank forms the observed minus expected at each distinct event time.

8.6 Discussion and Conclusions

Survival trials in oncology often exhibit non-constant and/or non-proportional hazards. In contrast, most methods for sample size calculation and sample size re-estimation assume constant or proportional hazards. Throughout this chapter, it has been shown that making such simplistic assumptions, when those assumptions are not warranted, can lead to sample size estimates that are far off the mark. For example, if the trial length is chosen based on an exponential model when the hazards are non-proportional, the power may be well off the mark.

The implications go well beyond sample size. Depending on the form of the non-proportionality, the required number of events to provide a desired power may increase as the length of trial increases. This is very problematic for the concept of the event-driven trial, since the concept relies on the power to be independent of the trial length. For this reason, the use of inappropriate assumptions such as constant hazards could lead to failed trials.

For group-sequential designs, the sample size "adjustment" for using a group-sequential boundary compared to a fixed design depends not only on that boundary, but also on the non-proportionality. Since ODIS or non-compliance results in non-proportionality, the "inflation factor" concept will not provide the correct adjustment for a trial with non-compliance.

For sample size re-estimation, if the non-proportionality is not carefully addressed, increases in sample size through sample size re-estimation may actually reduce power. The implications of sample size re-estimation in the presence of non-proportional hazards can be very complex, and currently is not well understood. Further, interim estimation of the treatment effect in the presence of a treatment lag is likely to be extremely biased.

Non-compliance/ODIS results in a mixture distribution whose mixture is constantly changing as the trial progresses. In turn, the failure probability of the experimental group is also constantly changing. The Markov model addresses this changing failure rate by modeling the mixture distribution in separate at-risk states. Exponentially based models, such as that proposed by Lachin and Foulkes (1986)[7], do not model the changing failure rate. Most simulation programs use the term "dropout", but generally mean "loss to follow-up", which is easy to model, but does not address non-compliance/ODIS.

The Markov model approach provides a means of dealing with complex situations including non-proportional hazards, time-dependent rates of loss, non-compliance, ODIS, and non-uniform patient entry. It was also shown that the typical approach to adjusting for loss to follow-up can lead to excessive sample sizes, because those approaches treat the failure and loss processes as independent processes. The Markov approach correctly treats all the processes as simultaneous and interdependent, and has been shown through simulations to provide very good results.

Non-compliance/ODIS is a fact of life in oncology clinical trials. It is always a problem in free-living trial populations. It is also a problem for trials in which toxic side-effects can lead to discontinuation of therapy. Non-proportional hazards are more common than may be recognized, because non-compliance/ODIS results in non-proportional hazards.

Bibliography

[1] J. Bernier, C. Domenge, M. Ozsahin, K. Matuszewska, J. Lefèbvre, R. H. Greiner, J. Giralt, P. Maingon, F. Rolland, M. Bolla, et al. Postoperative irradiation with or without concomitant chemotherapy for locally advanced head and neck cancer. *New England Journal of Medicine*, 350(19):1945–1952, 2004.

[2] C. Burman and C. Sonesson. Are flexible designs sound? *Biometrics*, 62(3):664–669, 2006.

[3] J. S. Cooper, T. F. Pajak, A. A. Forastiere, J. Jacobs, B. H. Campbell, S. B. Saxman, J. A. Kish, H. E. Kim, A. J. Cmelak, M. Rotman, et al. Postoperative concurrent radiotherapy and chemotherapy for high-risk

squamous-cell carcinoma of the head and neck. *New England Journal of Medicine*, 350(19):1937–1944, 2004.

[4] C. Jennison and B. W. Turnbull. *Group Sequential Methods with Applications to Clinical Trials.* CRC Press, 1999.

[5] C. Jennison and B. W. Turnbull. Mid-course sample size modification in clinical trials based on the observed treatment effect. *Statistics in Medicine*, 22(6):971–993, 2003.

[6] E. L. Kaplan and P. Meier. Nonparametric estimation from incomplete observations. *Journal of the American Statistical Association*, 53(282):457–481, 1958.

[7] J. M. Lachin and M. A. Foulkes. Evaluation of sample size and power for analyses of survival with allowance for nonuniform patient entry, losses to follow-up, noncompliance, and stratification. *Biometrics*, pages 507–519, 1986.

[8] E. Lakatos. Sample size determination in clinical trials with time-dependent rates of losses and noncompliance. *Controlled Clinical Trials*, 7(3):189–199, 1986.

[9] E. Lakatos. Sample sizes based on the log-rank statistic in complex clinical trials. *Biometrics*, pages 229–241, 1988.

[10] E. Lakatos. Designing complex group sequential survival trials. *Statistics in Medicine*, 21(14):1969–1989, 2002.

[11] E. Lakatos. Optimizing group-sequential designs with focus on adaptability: implications of nonproportional hazards in clinical trials. In W. Young and D. Chen, editors, *Clinical Trial Biostatistics and Biopharmaceutical Applications*, pages 137–178. Chapman & Hall/ CRC Press, Boca Raton, FL, 2014.

[12] E. Lakatos and K. K. Lan. A comparison of sample size methods for the logrank statistic. *Statistics in Medicine*, 11(2):179–191, 1992.

[13] J. Lu and T. F. Pajak. Statistical power for a long-term survival trial with a time-dependent treatment effect. *Controlled Clinical Trials*, 21(6):561–573, 2000.

[14] N. Mantel. Evaluation of survival data and two new rank order statistics arising in its consideration. *Cancer Chemotherapy Reports. Part 1*, 50(3):163–170, 1966.

[15] P. C. O'Brien and T. R. Fleming. A multiple testing procedure for clinical trials. *Biometrics*, pages 549–556, 1979.

[16] T. J. Perren, A. M. Swart, J. Pfisterer, J. A. Ledermann, E. Pujade-Lauraine, G. Kristensen, M. S. Carey, P. Beale, A. Cervantes, C. Kurzeder, et al. A phase 3 trial of bevacizumab in ovarian cancer. *New England Journal of Medicine*, 365(26):2484–2496, 2011.

[17] R. Peto and J. Peto. Asymptotically efficient rank invariant test procedures. *Journal of the Royal Statistical Society: Series A*, pages 185–207, 1972.

[18] S. J. Pocock. Group sequential methods in the design and analysis of clinical trials. *Biometrika*, 64(2):191–199, 1977.

[19] E. Pujade-Lauraine, F. Hilpert, B. Weber, A. Reuss, A. Poveda, G. Kristensen, R. Sorio, I. Vergote, P. Witteveen, A. Bamias, et al. Bevacizumab combined with chemotherapy for platinum-resistant recurrent ovarian cancer: the AURELIA open-label randomized phase III trial. *Journal of Clinical Oncology*, 32(13):1302–1308, 2014.

[20] M. Roach, K. Bae, J. Speight, H. B. Wolkov, P. Rubin, R. J. Lee, C. Lawton, R. Valicenti, D. Grignon, and M. V. Pilepich. Short-term neoadjuvant androgen deprivation therapy and external-beam radiotherapy for locally advanced prostate cancer: long-term results of rtog 8610. *Journal of Clinical Oncology*, 26(4):585–591, 2008.

[21] L. V. Rubinstein, M. H. Gail, and T. J. Santner. Planning the duration of a comparative clinical trial with loss to follow-up and a period of continued observation. *Journal of Chronic Diseases*, 34(9):469–479, 1981.

[22] A. Sandler, R. Gray, M. C. Perry, J. Brahmer, J. H. Schiller, A. Dowlati, R. Lilenbaum, and D. H. Johnson. Paclitaxel-carboplatin alone or with bevacizumab for non-small cell lung cancer. *New England Journal of Medicine*, 355(24):2542–2550, 2006.

[23] D. Schoenfeld. The asymptotic properties of nonparametric tests for comparing survival distributions. *Biometrika*, 68(1):316–319, 1981.

[24] D. M. Zucker and E. Lakatos. Weighted log rank type statistics for comparing survival curves when there is a time lag in the effectiveness of treatment. *Biometrika*, 77(4):853–864, 1990.

9

Non-inferiority Trials

Rajeshwari Sridhara

Thomas Gwise

CONTENTS

9.1 Introduction

Randomized clinical trials help us in evaluating the treatment effect of a therapy compared to a control treatment.In these trials, efficacy can be established by testing for superiority, non-inferiority, or equivalence. In a superiority trial, the aim is to demonstrate that the treatment effect of an experimental product (T) is superior to the treatment effect of a control where the control may be a placebo (P), best supportive care (BSC), or an active control (C). In a non-inferiority trial, the aim is to demonstrate that the treatment effect of an experimental product T is not inferior to an active control C by more than a prespecified quantity (δ) where δ is small enough so that it does not matter clinically. The aim in an equivalence trial is to demonstrate the treatment effect of T compared to an active control C is neither inferior nor superior by a prespecified margin of error. The null and alternative hypotheses in each of these scenarios are different and captured in the following formulations and Figure 9.1. Let Δ denote the difference in treatment effect between T and C.

In a superiority trial the null and alternative hypotheses are:

$$\begin{aligned} H_0 : \Delta &= 0 \\ H_1 : \Delta &> \delta, \text{ where } \delta > 0 \end{aligned} \tag{9.1}$$

In a non-inferiority trial, the null and alternative hypotheses are:

$$\begin{aligned} H_0 : \Delta &> \delta \\ H_1 : \Delta &\leq \delta, \text{ where } \delta > 0 \end{aligned} \tag{9.2}$$

In an equivalence trial the null and alternative hypotheses are:

$$\begin{aligned} H_0 : \Delta &\leq \delta_L \text{ or } \Delta \geq \delta_U \\ H_1 : \delta_L &< \Delta < \delta_U \end{aligned} \tag{9.3}$$

δ_L and δ_U are prespecified margins such that if the treatment effect lies within the two limits, then T and C are considered equivalent, as illustrated in Figure 9.1.

In this chapter we will focus on testing hypotheses and inference in a non-inferiority trial, referred to as an NI trial hereafter. The fundamental assumption in this type of trial is that the comparator active control C has an established, measurable treatment effect compared to a placebo P and that this effect has not changed over time (also known as the constancy assumption) and is detectable (also known as assay sensitivity). In other words in an NI trial we establish efficacy indirectly without actually comparing T to a placebo. The specific hypothesis and the selection of the margin δ are dependent on the primary endpoint based on which the treatment effect needs to be established. Note that an NI hypothesis can be considered while comparing combination therapies with substitution; for example, if the study is designed to compare the combination treatment $A + T$ with $A + C$, then one can evaluate if T is non-inferior to C. However, only a superiority hypothesis may be considered if the study is designed to compare $A + T$ vs. $A + P$.

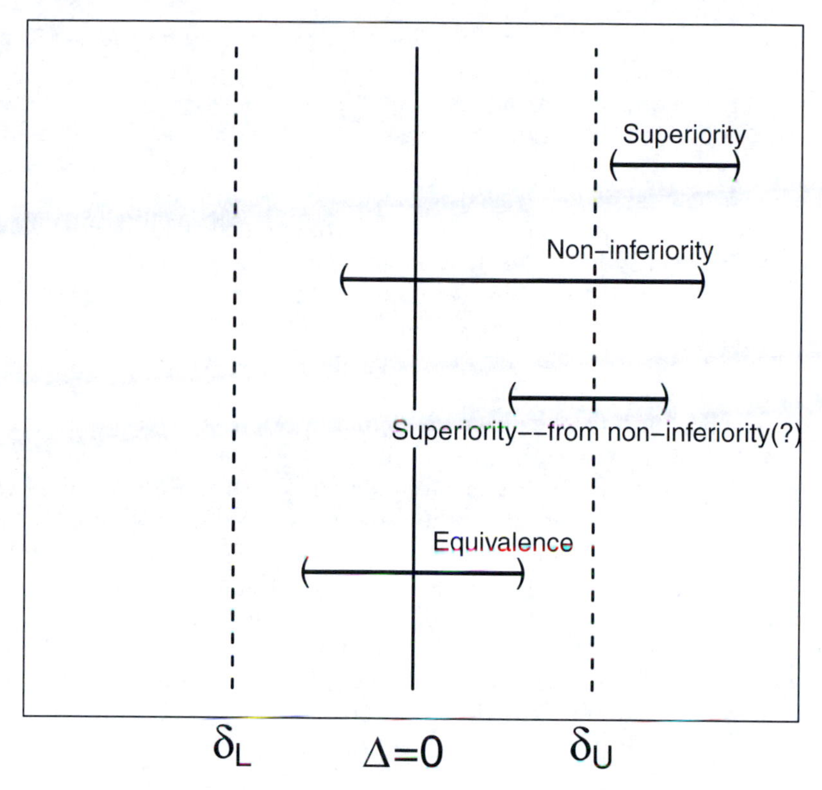

FIGURE 9.1: Confidence intervals for Δ showing superiority, non-inferiority and equivalence.

9.2 Endpoint Selection

Outcomes or endpoints most commonly used in oncology/hematology trials are those endpoints that are based either on disease burden, e.g., objective response rate (ORR) or progression-free survival (PFS), or the overall clinical benefit, e.g., overall survival (OS) or results of a clinical outcome assessment (COA, formerly referred to as a patient-reported outcome). In the adjuvant treatment setting, disease-free survival (DFS) is commonly used as an endpoint and considered to represent clinical benefit. ORR in a given treatment arm is defined as the ratio of the number of patients who respond to the number of patients randomized to that treatment. PFS is defined as time from randomization to either disease progression or death, whichever occurs first. OS is defined as time from randomization to death and DFS is defined as time from randomization to recurrence of disease or death. Both ORR and PFS measurements depend on frequency of assessment, criteria for defining response or progression, and the mode of measurement used (e.g., CT scan vs. MRI). However, if documentation of an objective response is missed in one assessment, it is likely to be observed in the next assessment, and the ORR endpoint does not have a time component. On the other hand, PFS may be overestimated if the frequency of assessment is longer in one treatment arm, or an assessment is missed. It is also difficult to verify the constancy assumption as frequency of assessment may vary from trial to trial, and the mode of measurement may also change over time. For these reasons, NI trials with PFS as the primary endpoint are generally discouraged. The subjective nature of COA endpoints can add to the challenges in estimating the active control effect and verifying the constancy assumption. Therefore, COAs are not often considered as primary endpoints in NI trials.

For the purposes of setting up the hypotheses and testing procedure, we can broadly classify the endpoints as binomial, continuous, or time-to-event (TTE) endpoints, where TTE includes endpoints such as PFS, OS, and DFS. In general, endpoint selection for the NI trial is based on the endpoint that was evaluated in establishing the treatment effect of the active control. If ORR is selected as the primary endpoint for evaluating the new treatment T versus the active control C, then the test of hypothesis can be based on either the risk ratio (RR, Δ = RR) or the absolute difference in ORR. For a time-to-event primary endpoint such as OS, the test of hypothesis is commonly based on the hazard ratio (HR, Δ = HR).

9.3 Methods for Evaluating the Active Control Effect and Selecting the Non-inferiority Margin

Drug development is an important motivator of NI trials. For example, a pharmaceutical company may wish to market a drug for a condition for which there is already an effective treatment. In such a situation, ethical considerations could preclude randomizing patients to a placebo control arm. Demonstrating the experimental treatment to be as efficacious as or perhaps slightly less efficacious than the current treatment becomes an attractive option, especially if the experimental treatment promises improvement in other dimensions, such as fewer adverse side effects than the current treatment. In drug development, NI trials are used as indirect comparisons to placebo controls. Choosing the NI margin δ for clinical trials is therefore often done through a combination of statistically estimating the effect size of the active control compared to a placebo control, and subjectively assessing what might be a clinically tolerable loss of efficacy in comparison with the treatment effect of the active control.

Setting the NI margin with the goal of indirectly demonstrating the efficacy of the experimental treatment, that is demonstrating T is more efficacious than a placebo, requires the investigator to have an understanding of the relationship of the active control to a placebo. This understanding is often addressed through meta-analysis of available studies comparing the active control to placebo. A common approach discussed in the FDA guidance for industry [9], as well by D'Agostino et al. [6], Rothmann et al. [26], and others is to estimate the active control effect and consider what fraction of that effect could be forfeited without risking untenable clinical consequences. The indirect inference that T is effective therefore depends on the meta-analysis, and thus all of the usual concerns as to the validity of these analyses, e.g., selection, publication, and search biases, are raised [32]. Furthermore, component studies of a meta-analysis deserve careful scrutiny to ensure all studies are applicable to the situation for which the NI trial is designed. Also, the best estimator of effect size from a meta-analysis may not be representative of the subset of the population being considered in the NI trial. The appropriate meta-analytic approach, a fixed effects model or a random effects model, will depend on the setting in which the NI study is being planned, as well as the available data. Often, researchers will have access to only published results and not the underlying data of each component trial. Meta-analyses can still be done in such situations, but the added uncertainty of not observing the component study data quality should be recognized. Details of performing meta-analysis will not be discussed here, but methods and software have been described in numerous publications. Borenstein et al. contains a thorough introduction to the subject with references to software packages including one developed by the authors [3].

Margin selection is the most controversial and important part of NI testing. To better comprehend the importance and the role of the NI margin, we first heuristically consider the logic of using NI tests. Conceptually, showing T superior to C is easy to grasp. We can set up a test of a null hypothesis that the difference between T and C is zero. There is no ambiguity concerning the objective of such a test. On the other hand, what if the goal is to show treatment T is just as efficacious as treatment C? An equivalence test can be constructed as is done in bioequivalence trials described by Berger and Hsu [2]. In designing the study, the need to consider variability in the data and selection of a tolerable difference between the treatments would mean realizing a difference near zero would be a relatively low probability outcome. A pragmatic solution is to translate the test so that it rejects the null hypothesis for a difference Δ that is negative, but not so negative that the implications would be materially untenable. This is the problem of choosing the NI margin. Choosing an NI margin in the context of drug development is a multi-dimensional problem. The margin must be chosen such that it is not so large that it could permit unacceptable levels of inferiority, including failing to rule out the possibility that the experimental treatment T is no more effective than placebo, while also being large enough to preclude a prohibitive sample size. Approaches to NI testing can be broadly categorized as fixed margin, synthesis, Bayesian, and placebo-controlled.

9.3.1 Fixed Margin

The preceding discussion has focused on the notion that an NI test can be thought of as a superiority test translated by some margin δ in order to permit some negligible degree of inferiority. In the fixed margin approach, δ is selected through evaluation of historical clinical trials as discussed above, subjective clinical consideration, or a combination of the two. Once chosen, the margin is considered to be fixed. The null and alternative hypotheses are then constructed as above. While we have considered the difference as the metric of comparison for the sake of simplicity in (9.2), it may vary according to clinical application. The fixed margin approach can be implemented using risk ratio (RR), odds ratio (OR), or hazard ratio (HR) to compare T and C.

The null and alternative hypotheses for a NI test considering risk ratio and odds ratio as the comparison measures could be written, respectively, as follows:

$$\begin{aligned} H_0 : \text{RR} &\geq 1 + \delta \qquad (9.4) \\ H_1 : \text{RR} &< 1 + \delta \end{aligned}$$

and

$$\begin{aligned} H_0 : \text{OR} &\geq 1 + \delta \qquad (9.5) \\ H_1 : \text{OR} &< 1 + \delta \end{aligned}$$

Similarly, the null and alternative hypotheses for an NI test considering the hazard ratio as the measure can be written as follows:

$$\begin{aligned} H_0 : \text{HR(T/C)} &\geq 1 + \delta \qquad (9.6) \\ H_1 : \text{HR(T/C)} &< 1 + \delta \end{aligned}$$

As with superiority tests there is a duality with confidence intervals in NI tests. The procedure can be summarized as observing whether or not a confidence interval about the parameter Δ at the desired level lies entirely above δ as illustrated in Figure 9.1. When approaching NI with a fixed margin, using confidence intervals allows the researcher to easily consider the treatment comparison independently of the margin. This has the advantage of permitting the researcher, if necessary, to focus on the data taken in the current study and to separately consider any concerns with δ, such as the validity of the constancy assumption or uncertainty related to meta-analysis or subjective judgment.

9.3.2 Synthesis Approach

The synthesis approach is the name given to NI trials designed to incorporate historical information on the active control in the NI test, permitting one to draw inference on the efficacy of T with respect to placebo. Holmgren [16] describes the approach in terms of relative risk and writes the comparison as

$$\frac{p_T}{p_C} < 1 + (1 - f)\left(\frac{p_P}{p_C} - 1\right) \tag{9.7}$$

where f is the percent of the active control effect to be retained. and p_T, p_P,and p_C are the probabilities of events for T, P, and C, respectively. Note that one does not observe results obtained from the current study data in isolation using this method.

A similar formulation can be constructed for a TTE endpoint, assuming that $HR(P_2/C_2) = HR(P_1/C_1)$, where C_1 and C_2 are active control arms in the historical trial and NI trial, respectively, and P_1 and P_2 are placebo arms in the historical trial and NI trial, respectively, recognizing that P_2 is unlikely to be included as a third arm in the NI study. The null and alternative hypotheses can then be written as

$$\begin{aligned} H_0 : log\left(HR\left(\frac{T}{C_2}\right)\right) &\geq (1-f)log\left(HR\left(\frac{P_1}{C_1}\right)\right) \\ H_1 : log\left(HR\left(\frac{T}{C_2}\right)\right) &< (1-f)log\left(HR\left(\frac{P_1}{C_1}\right)\right) \end{aligned} \tag{9.8}$$

where $0 < f < 1$ is the fraction of the active control effect to be retained [26]. Thus, in the synthesis approach both the estimate of active control effect from the historical studies and the clinically relevant fraction of treatment effect to be retained are required to set up the hypotheses. For example, $f = 0.5$ would imply that T should retain at least 50% of the effect of C and $f = 1$ will lead to a superiority hypothesis. An estimate of effect of C obtained from the meta-analysis of historical studies could be chosen as the point estimate of HR, the lower (or upper) 95% confidence limit of HR, or a value in between the point estimate and the lower (or upper) 95% confidence limit as shown in Figure 9.2. It can be shown that using the point estimate as the active control effect in the hypotheses stated in (9.8) results in inflation of type I error rate, and that using the worst case of least effect, i.e., lower 95% confidence limit as the estimate of control effect, results in a one-sided type I error rate that is much less than 0.025.

Rothmann et al. [26] have proposed a method to find a lower γ% confidence limit that would approximately control the one-sided type I error rate at 0.025 using the following equation:

$$\gamma = \frac{2\Phi\left(1.96\sqrt{(1+y^2)} - 1.96\right)}{y - 1} \tag{9.9}$$

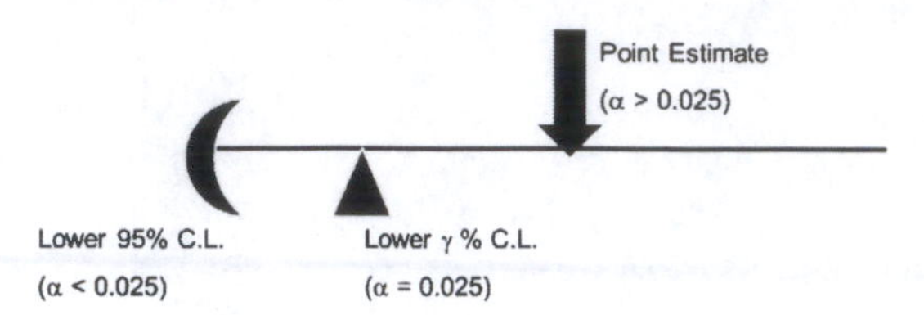

FIGURE 9.2: Estimate of effect C obtained historical studies

Here Φ denotes the standard normal distribution function, $y = (1-f)(s_2/s_1)$, s_1 = the estimate of standard error of $log(HR(T/C_2))$, and s_2 = the estimate of standard error of $log(HR(P_1/C_1))$. Note that in the calculation of the sample size it is assumed that $s_1 = s_2$.

The synthesis test method does not have a fixed NI margin to be excluded, as the margin depends on both historical and current NI study data (Guidance for Industry NI Trials 2010) [9]. On the other hand, the fixed margin method controls a type I error rate within the NI study that is conditioned on the prespecified fixed NI margin, separately estimated from the historical active comparator data. In general the fixed margin approach is desirable as the margin can be agreed to before start of the trial and separately from conducting the NI test.

9.3.3 Bayesian Approach

Bayesian methods that incorporate historical information appear to be a natural choice for the investigator wishing to draw inference about T with respect to placebo not included in the current study. Simon [29] proposed a method through which a posterior probability that T will be no more inferior than a specified fraction of C can be calculated. The comparison of C to P can be incorporated in the model through the prior distribution provided in part by a meta-analysis of placebo-controlled trials and assuming a non-informative prior for the comparison of T to P. Gamalo et al. [10–12] discuss a method in which the NI margin is provided using the credible interval about $C-P$ and inference is made using the posterior probability of $T-C$ in comparison. They developed the Bayesian approaches for establishing NI of T with respect to C that parallel the fixed margin and synthesis approaches described above by incorporating the historical data on C using 'power priors' and meta-analyses approaches. Ghosh et al. [13] considered Bayesian approaches in three-arm trials. We note these methods will also depend in some respect on the constancy assumption, as frequentist approaches do.

A Bayesian design was implemented in a clinical trial comparing capecitabine to standard chemotherapy as an adjuvant chemotherapy in women with breast cancer who were 65 years or older with the primary endpoint of relapse-free survival [25]. Enrollment was halted at 600 patients when it was determined that the probability that capecitabine therapy was highly likely to be inferior to standard chemotherapy, based on a prespecified probability level.

9.3.4 Placebo-controlled Approach

One way to compare an experimental treatment to placebo and a current standard of care treatment is to design a clinical trial which includes treatment arms for each. This has been referred to as the "Gold Standard" NI study design. Koch and Rohmel [21] discuss a hierarchical approach for such a trial that conserves the type I error probability. The two steps of this approach are testing the hypothesis that T is less than or equal to P, where P represents the placebo effect, and testing the hypothesis that the difference between T and C is less than or equal to some preselected non-inferiority margin. Rejecting both hypotheses at levels conserving the overall type I error probability is sufficient to declare T non-inferior to C. Because there are situations in which a reference treatment's superiority to placebo may be in question [31], Hauschke and Pigeot [15] point out that assay sensitivity may be questionable without demonstrating that T is greater than C and C is greater than P.

***Example 1*: Differences in margin selection using the same historical data**

We will consider selected examples of oncology clinical trials from the literature or which were discussed in FDA Advisory Committee meetings. In the first example we will consider two NI studies to illustrate how interpretation of historical data can influence the choice of margin and thus the inference drawn through NI studies. Two NI studies were designed to show non-inferiority of their respective investigative treatments to docetaxel in the population of patients having non-small cell lung cancer and having already received some treatment. Both studies calculated estimates of the active control effect of docetaxel based on the study results reported in Shepherd et al. [28].

The study by Kim et al. [20] was designed to show NI of gefitinib to docetaxel. The margin of 1.154 was intended to preserve 50% of the docetaxel treatment effect, which was based on the estimated HR determined from the results of Shepherd et al. [28]. The HR was estimated as the ratio of median overall survival estimates (4.6 months/ 7.5 months = .61). The study showed a gefitinib:docetaxel HR of 1.020, 96% CI [0.905, 1.150]. Because the upper bound of 1.15 is less than 1.154, the authors concluded NI of gefitinib. Although the study included a multiple testing procedure that dictated using a 96% CI for inference, that procedure does not affect the margin selection.

The NI study by Hanna et al. [14] was designed to demonstrate NI of pemetrexed to docetaxel. The authors stated that the HR of docetaxel compared to best supportive care was estimated as 0.56 from the study by Shepherd et al. [28]. The margin was then set at 1.21 to preserve 50% of the effect of docetaxel. The HR of pemetrexed to docetaxel estimated in Hanna et al. [14] was reported as 0.99, 95% CI [0.8, 1.20]. It is to be noted that the FDA's position was that in both of these cases, the effect of the active control effect size could not be reliably estimated due to inadequate historical data (Oncologic Drugs Advisory Meeting, 2004).

***Example 2*: Margin selection using synthesis approach**

Two randomized studies comparing capecitabine to 5-flurouracel (5-FU) in combination with leucovorin (LV) as first-line chemotherapy in patients with advanced and/or metastatic colorectal carcinoma were conducted [9]. The protocol-specified NI margin for both studies was set at 1.25, i.e., if the upper 95% limit of the HR for overall survival did not exceed 1.25 while testing at the 0.025 significance level, NI would be concluded. There were 10 randomized studies reported in literature comparing 5-FU/LV to 5-FU. Based on these studies, a meta-analysis using random effects model was conducted and the HR was estimated to be 1.264, 95% CI [1.091, 1.464]. If the worst case scenario were used, described as the 95-95 method in FDA's Guidance on NI trials (2010) [9] then the margin would be 1.091. On the other hand, if lower limit of the 30% CI for HR (5-FU/5-FU+LV) were used (synthesis approach, Figure 9.2, equation 9.9), then with a margin of 1.114, 50% of active control effect would be retained while controlling one-sided type I error at 0.025.

The active control effect was also estimated based on eight published reports (and leaving out two outlier results) by conducting a meta-analysis using random effects model. The estimated HR for 5-FU to 5-FU/LV was 1.271, 95% CI [1.132, 1.428].

In study 1 the HR of capecitabine vs. 5FU/LV based on OS was estimated as 1.07, 95% CI [0.86, 1.33], in the per-protocol population and 1.13, [95% CI [0.92, 1.38], in the intent-to-treat population. In study 2 the HR for OS was estimated as 0.96, 95% CI [0.77, 1.19], in the per-protocol population and 0.98, 95% CI [0.80, 1.20], in intent-to-treat population.

9.4 Sample Size Determination

The size of a clinical trial is one of the central design questions, in part because cost is a function of sample size. Generally speaking, estimating sample size is dependent on assuming values for

- power i.e., 1-type II error probability $(1 - \beta)$,
- type I error probability (α),
- the difference to be detected by the hypothesis test (ω) and
- the variance of the test statistic $(\sigma^2_{teststat})$.

Then the sample size n is given by the following equation, assuming that the test statistic follows a normal distribution:

$$n = \frac{\left(Z_\alpha + Z_{1-\beta}\right)^2 \sigma_{teststat}^2}{\omega^2} \tag{9.10}$$

It is seen from the expression above (9.10) that the sample size increases as Z_α, $Z_{1-\beta}$, and/or $\sigma_{teststat}^2$ increases. Considering the definitions of these variables brings their influence into focus more clearly. Small α corresponds to large values of Z_α. Recall that the probability of making a type I error in the context of a drug efficacy trial is the probability of incorrectly concluding the experimental drug is efficacious. Sample size increase as α decreases makes sense intuitively: more information, thus a larger sample size, is required to lower the probability of making a false conclusion. Similar reasoning can be associated with power (1-β). Power, which is the probability of rejecting the null hypothesis when it is false, in other words the probability of concluding a new treatment is efficacious when it in fact is efficacious, increases as $Z_{1-\beta}$ increases. The other assumption to be set is the difference the investigator wishes the hypothesis test to detect (ω). It is intuitively obvious and easily seen by observing expression (9.10) that smaller differences will be more difficult to detect than larger ones, and thus their detection will require larger sample sizes. Sample size estimates for NI tests are slightly more complicated by the inclusion of the NI margin δ. As will be shown later δ will be combined in the denominator with the difference factor.

Sample sizes for continuous outcomes and for differences of proportions may be addressed in the usual way, noting that the difference to be detected must accommodate δ. Fleming [8] discusses the fact that NI study sample sizes do not necessarily need to be extremely large in comparison to superiority tests.

9.4.1 Ratio of Proportions

The approach of Dann and Koch [7] for estimating sample size in NI tests comparing proportions via a ratio is similar to the expression in (9.10) above. We will first examine the development of the variance estimator for a ratio of proportions, but omit the details of the sample size estimate derivation. We follow the conventions that when considering responses, the active control rate will be in the numerator, and that for a ratio of risks or failures, the active control rate will be in the denominator. While arbitrary, these rules are consistent in that the ratio of $C : T$ or $T : C$, respectively, will be smaller than unity when T is the treatment having a larger proportion of clinically preferable outcomes. Data originating in binary outcome clinical trial can be tabulated as in Table 9.1.

From the delta method we have $Var(log(RR)) = \frac{1}{a} - \frac{1}{n_1} + \frac{1}{c} - \frac{1}{n_2}$. After some manipulation and assuming equal allocation, the expression reduces to the smaller term in the following inequality:

TABLE 9.1: A typical tabulation of binary data

	Response to Treatment		
	(Response)	(No Response)	Totals
Treatment	a	b	a+b =n_1
Active Control	c	d	c+d =n_2
			N= a+b+c+d

$$Var(log(RR)) = \frac{1}{n}\left[\frac{n}{c}\left(\frac{c}{a}+1\right)-2\right] < \frac{1}{n}\left[\frac{n}{c}\left(\frac{c}{a}+1\right)\right] \tag{9.11}$$

Note that it is conservative and convenient for calculation to use the last term in expression (9.11) above. Letting $\pi_c = \frac{c}{n}$, the assumed response rate of the active control, and $\phi = \frac{a}{c} = \frac{a\pi_c}{n}$ be the effect ratio under the null hypothesis, we have:

$$n = \frac{(Z_\alpha + Z_{1-\beta})^2\left[\frac{1}{\pi_c}\left(\frac{1}{\phi}+1\right)\right]}{\left[log\left(\frac{\phi}{\phi_0}\right)\right]^2}. \tag{9.12}$$

This expression is the sample size estimate derived by Dann and Koch [7], who evaluate several interval estimation methods for ratios of proportions, noting that all of the methods apply when both proportions are less than 0.5. As sample size calculations are estimates, simulation studies are useful in verifying power and operational characteristics. In a non-inferiority setting, it might be reasonable to assume for sample size calculation purposes that the two treatments under consideration are equal. In that case, the postulated ratio is set to one. We tabulate several cases below under varying situations. We calculated sample size and then ran 10,000 simulated clinical trials (Appendix 1) to determine the proportion of simulations in which the null hypothesis was rejected. Our results show that the calculation method performs adequately for reasonable values of δ. Software packages such as East 6.3® provide menu options to calculate sample sizes for testing NI hypotheses.

9.4.2 Survival Endpoints

Sample size calculations for time to event outcomes also follow a pattern similar to (9.10). See Chapter 6 for more details. The estimate provided here is taken from Chow and Liu [4], where p_c is the fraction of the total sample size allocated to the active control treatment, d is the probability of observing an event, and HR_0 is often set to one.

TABLE 9.2: Simulation results

Planned Power	δ	Control Rate	N	Simulated Power
0.9	0.10	0.10	23134	0.9292
0.9	0.10	0.25	9254	0.9633
0.9	0.10	0.45	5141	0.9900
0.9	0.25	0.10	4220	0.9239
0.9	0.25	0.25	1688	0.9633
0.9	0.25	0.45	938	0.9910
0.9	0.50	0.10	1278	0.9267
0.9	0.50	0.25	511	0.9603
0.9	0.50	0.45	284	0.9907
0.8	0.10	0.10	17281	0.8393
0.8	0.10	0.25	6912	0.8988
0.8	0.10	0.45	3840	0.9660
0.8	0.25	0.10	3153	0.8416
0.8	0.25	0.25	1261	0.8974
0.8	0.25	0.45	701	0.9622
0.8	0.50	0.10	955	0.8360
0.8	0.50	0.25	382	0.8877
0.8	0.50	0.45	212	0.9582

$$n = \frac{\left(Z_{\alpha/2} + Z_{\beta}\right)^2}{\left(log\left(HR_0\right) - \delta\right)^2 p_c\left(1 - p_c\right) d} \tag{9.13}$$

Often, for simplicity, d is omitted from the calculation and estimated sample size is stated in terms of events. As with the other sample size calculations, one must consider consider the non-inferiority margin in the term for the difference to be detected. Here δ is log of the hazard ratio considering the non-inferiority margin.

***Example 3*: Computing sample size**

Statistical considerations that need to be examined in designing future clinical trials for first-line hormonal treatment of metastatic breast cancer were discussed at a 2001 meeting of FDA's Oncology Drug Advisory Committee [30]. The debate was whether future clinical trials should have tamoxifen or letrozole as the active control, because a recent study had demonstrated that letrozole was superior to tamoxifen with respect to ORR and time-to-progression (TTP).

For the purpose of illustration only, letrozole was considered as the active control comparator. In this case letrozole was assumed to be effective compared to placebo based on the observed response rate in one randomized clinical trial compared to tamoxifen, and the assumption that the ORR for placebo was 0%. It was also assumed that we can reliably estimate letrozole's effect size. If response rate is the endpoint under consideration, then all the effect can be attributed to the treatment. However, for the time to progression endpoint, the available comparison was to tamoxifen and not placebo. Thus, the tamoxifen effect size with respect to TTP could not be estimated. For the purpose of illustration the active control (tamoxifen) effect in the historical study was assumed to be carried over to the future study.

In the letrozole registration study, the point estimate of response rate was 30%, 95% CI [26%, 35%], and the point estimate of the HR of tamoxifen vs. letrozole with respect to TTP was 1.4, two-sided 95% CI [1.24, 1.56]. The question was which of these estimates should be used as the control effect size for computing sample sizes for the future studies. A decision would also need to be made regarding what proportion of the active control effect should be preserved so that there is no clinically meaningful decrease in benefit provided by the new drug.

As a first step, we need to estimate the size of the active control effect. From a given study or studies, we generally describe the effect by a point estimate and a two-sided 95% CI (Figure 9.2), i.e., we can say with 95% confidence that the true effect is between these two confidence limits. We can consider four methods to estimate the true control effect. If we choose the point estimate as the estimated active control effect, then this will inflate type I error. On the other hand, if we choose the other extreme, i.e., the lower 95% confidence limit as the estimated control effect, then the type I error will be very small. A compromise is to use a lower γ % limit as the estimated control effect which will ensure one-sided type I error to be 0.025 (Figure 9.2). Choosing a fixed margin approach such as $\leq$ 10% is quite arbitrary [26]. Whatever we choose as our estimate of the control effect, we have to then decide on how much of that effect we are willing to give up (or, alternatively, how much of that effect must be retained by the new drug).

The point estimate of the effect size of letrozole was 30% based on the single randomized study. The right column in Table 9.3 gives the sample sizes required retaining delta % of this value. For example, if 50% of the effect (15% RR) should be retained, then a sample size of 294 is necessary. When simulations of studies designed with the point estimates are conducted, it can be shown that the type I error, alpha, is always $>$ 0.025. This can also be proved mathematically. And therefore this is a less than optimum design and not recommended. The purpose of presenting this approach here is only to illustrate the concept and not to recommend its use in future trials.

If we consider the lower 95% confidence limit as the estimate of active control effect (worst case scenario), then in the letrozole-tamoxifen study the lower 2-sided 95% confidence limit of response rate was 26%. To retain 50% of this effect, a total sample size of 358 patients is required.

However, using a fixed margin with tamoxifen as the active control, i.e., the lower limit of the 95% confidence interval for the difference in response

TABLE 9.3: Sample size estimate based on ORR endpoint using point estimate of letrozole relative to placebo with one-sided $\alpha = 0.025$ and $\beta = 0.2$ (East 6®)

Response Estimate (letrozole)	Control Effect to be Retained	Sample Size (patients)
30%	25%	131
30%	50%	294
30%	75%	1173

TABLE 9.4: Sample size estimate based on ORR endpoint using effect size as lower confidence limit of letrozole relative to placebo with one-sided $\alpha = 0.025$ and $\beta = 0.2$ (East 6®)

Lower 95% Confidence Limit Response in Control (letrozole)	Control Effect to be Retained	Sample Size (patients)
26%	25%	159
26%	50%	358
26%	75%	1430

between Drug T and Letrozole must be $\leq 10\%$ (assuming placebo response is 0%), the sample size required is 660 patients.

Now let us consider TTP as the endpoint. Suppose the effect size used is the point estimate of the hazard ratio of tamoxifen to letrozole. (Note that this is not the placebo versus letrozole effect size.) The point estimate of the hazard ratio of tamoxifen to letrozole in the tamoxifen-letrozole study was 1.4. If, for example, we retain 50% of the letrozole effect over tamoxifen, then the total number of events required is 945 (Table 9.5). Using the point estimate is a sub-optimal approach and not recommended as it inflates type I error.

TABLE 9.5: Sample size based on TTE endpoint using point estimate with one-sided $\alpha = 0.025$ and $\beta = 0.2$ (East 6®)

Point Estimate of HR tamoxifen vs. letrozole	Control Effect to be Retained	Sample Size (events)
1.4	25%	457
1.4	50%	945
1.4	75%	3457

On the other hand if we consider the lower 95% confidence limit of the hazard ratio of tamoxifen to letrozole as the estimate of active control effect with time to progression as the endpoint, then to retain 50% of the letrozole effect over tamoxifen, a total of 2445 events (not patients) are required (Table

9.6). This is a conservative approach. Simulations of such designs show that type I error is much less than 0.025.

TABLE 9.6: Sample size estimate based on TTE endpoint using lower 95% confidence limit with one-sided $\alpha = 0.025$ and $\beta = 0.2$ (East 6®)

Lower 95% Confidence Limit of HR tamoxifen vs. letrozole	Control Effect to be Retained	Sample Size (events)
1.24	25%	1147
1.24	50%	2445
1.24	75%	9247

A less conservative approach, but one that preserves type I error at 0.025, is the synthesis approach. In this approach, to retain, for example, 50% of the letrozole effect over tamoxifen with respect to time to progression, and maintain type I error at 0.025, the number of events required is 1427 (Table 9.7). This translates to using a 55% lower confidence limit as an estimate of the control effect, instead of the conservative lower 95% confidence limit. Because of the fact that in this approach type I error is fixed, depending on the % effect retained, the % confidence limit varies as listed in this table.

TABLE 9.7: Sample size estimate based on TTE endpoint using synthesis approach with one-sided $\alpha = 0.025$ and $\beta = 0.2$ (East 6®)

Lower γ% Confidence Limit of HR tamoxifen vs. letrozole	Control Effect to be Retained	Sample Size (events)
53%	25%	665
55%	50%	1427
58%	75%	5465

9.5 Interim Monitoring and Analyses

It is common and helpful to conduct interim monitoring and analyses for efficient conduct of clinical trials. Such monitoring makes it possible to detect safety signals early, stop the study for futility, or stop the study early for demonstrated efficacy. This is described in greater detail in Chapter 10. Formal statistical methods for interim analyses avoid inflation of type I error, for example, using group sequential analyses using a spending function, stochastic curtailment, or repeated confidence interval approach. An ongoing trial may be stopped based on the interim analysis results when (a) the trial is still accruing subjects, (b) accrual is completed and treatment is still ongoing, or (c) the accrual and treatment are completed and the trial is in the follow-up phase. There are examples of superiority studies stopped for reasons of futility (example: Kelly et al. [19]) avoiding patients being assigned to an inferior treatment, or efficacy (example: Johnson & Johnson press release [17]), and stopping further assignment to inferior control treatment. This is particularly important when the control is a placebo where there are ethical concerns raised by denying access to an efficacious treatment. A group sequential design can also be employed in an NI trial by using an appropriate spending function to ensure control of family-wise type I error rate. However, stopping a NI study for efficacy is rare as this would mean that NI is established with a highly conservative margin. Regulators may also discourage stopping early for efficacy in a NI study because adequate safety data may not be available to evaluate the benefit-to-risk ratio of the new treatment, particularly because the new treatment is not deemed to have better efficacy than the active control treatment.

9.6 Multiple Comparisons

Multiplicity considerations are discussed in detail in Chapter 3. Without going into the details of each adjustment method, we will expose the readers to how multiplicity should be taken into consideration while designing NI trials. Multiple testing can occur if (1) one or more interim tests of the primary endpoint (E_1) hypothesis is conducted, and/or (2) if hypotheses of other secondary endpoints (E_2, E_3, ..., etc.) are tested, or (3) if both NI and superiority are tested with respect to the same endpoint (E_1). Examples of situations where multiplicity concerns may arise would be a group sequential design with one interim analysis-based ORR primary endpoint, a trial designed to test a hypothesis based on the primary endpoint of ORR, with OS as a secondary endpoint, or a study designed to test NI as well as superiority of T versus C with respect to the same endpoint.

The commonly used Hochberg procedure can control type I error rate if multiple endpoints are simultaneously tested without priority (Hochberg Y 1988). In all cases a closed testing procedure will ensure control of family-wise type I error rate. An example of an NI trial with interim analysis is reported by Lang et al. [23] in the randomized, open-label, NI, Phase 3 TURANDOT trial where Bevacizumab + paclitaxel was compared to Bevacizumab + capecitabine as first-line treatment for HER2-negative metastatic breast cancer. The primary endpoint of the trial was OS, and the objective was to establish Bevacizumab + capecitabine to be non-inferior to Bevacizumab + paclitaxel. One interim analysis was planned using the Lan-DeMets alpha spending method with an O'Brien-Fleming-type boundary with approximately 45% information controlling the overall one-sided type I error rate of 0.025. The authors report results of an interim analysis in which the criterion for NI was not met.

If NI is the primary objective based on endpoint E1 (primary endpoint), and superiority for E1 and superiority for E2 (secondary endpoint) are simultaneously tested, alpha adjustment is necessary as such a testing procedure will inflate type I error [18].

9.6.1 Testing of Non-inferiority to Superiority and Superiority to Non-inferiority

Non-inferiority and superiority hypotheses testing based on an endpoint E1 can be conducted within a randomized clinical trial. If superiority testing is conducted first and superiority is demonstrated, then NI testing is moot. If hierarchical testing of superiority is conducted after establishing NI based on an endpoint E1, then family-wise type I error is controlled as the rejection region for NI is a subset of the rejection region for superiority testing. However, if NI and superiority are tested simultaneously, the NI margin must be prespecified and careful consideration is needed so that the family-wise type I error is controlled. In this case efficacy of the treatment T compared to control C can be established either by demonstrating NI or superiority. This type of simultaneous testing can be conducted by dividing *alpha* allocation, for example, using the Bonferroni procedure, so that the overall type I error rate is controlled. If a group sequential design is used and interim analyses are planned within each of these hypotheses tests, then several approaches using closed testing procedure have been proposed to control family-wise type I error rate [22, 33]. Note that if the study is stopped due to demonstration of NI at the interim analysis, then the power for testing superiority will be low.

An example of testing sequentially of both non-inferiority and superiority testing in the same trial is the ATAC (arimidex, tamoxifen alone or in combination) trial, which was set up with the primary objective of establishing arimidex to be non-inferior to tamoxifen with respect to DFS as an adjuvant treatment for patients with early-stage breast cancer. After establishing NI, a superiority test was conducted and arimidex was demonstrated to be superior to tamoxifen. These results were based on final analyses although interim results did not cross the efficacy stopping criterion (ATAC Trialist Group [1]).

9.7 Missing Data and Non-compliance

Missing data, non-compliance, switching treatments (example: switching to experimental treatment in patients who receive active control initially), and use of concomitant medications can confound the results in an NI trial and introduce 'bias towards the null,' i.e., a true difference between T and C beyond the specified NI margin may not be detectable when these deficiencies exist. The assay sensitivity and constancy assumptions are also affected if there are missing data. The potential impact of missing data depends on the missing mechanism. The mechanisms as defined by Little and Rubin [24] are (1) missing completely at random (MCAR) where missingness is independent of both observed and unobserved data, (2) missing at random (MAR) where missingness is independent of unobserved data conditional on observed data, and (3) not missing at random (NMAR) where missingness is dependent on unobserved data. If the missing data are either MCAR or MAR, then the impact on type I error are marginal [35, 36]. However, most often missing data and/or non-compliance are related to the treatment, and it is important to evaluate the mechanism of missing or censoring data, especially because most statistical methods used in hypotheses testing assume that missing is MCAR or MAR. For example, while comparing two observed TTE curves using survival analysis methodology, if an observation is missing, then the observation is censored at the missing time, assuming that the TTE estimate of this observation is the same as another observation which has not reached an event at that time. However, this assumption will not be true if missing patterns differ between treatment and control arms, particularly in open-label studies. As recommended by the 'working group' [5], avoiding missing data is the best solution. It is important to plan at the clinical trial design stage how the missing data will be handled. After the trial is completed, the missing pattern and its impact on the outcome of the trial must be carefully evaluated, for example, using sensitivity analyses [5]. In NI trials inference is even more challenging, as a poorly conducted study can conclude that the treatment is non-inferior to control while in reality it may be worse than the control. In other words missing data and non-compliance can also inflate type I error rate.

9.8 Statistical Inference and Reporting

Failure to show statistical significance in superiority hypothesis testing does not imply NI. No inference can be drawn from a large p-value as it can be due to low study power or poor quality data. There are three main sources of uncertainty in NI trials: (1) the precision of the active control estimate, for example, active control effect size estimate based on single study vs. multiple studies, (2) the constancy assumption, for example, past studies may have shown bigger treatment effects which may not be replicable in the current study, and (3) type I error or the risk of wrong decision based on the NI hypothesis test. The inference in an NI trial is tied to the margin specified in the null hypothesis. Therefore, it is extremely important to estimate the active control effect at the NI trial design stage. Similar to testing a superiority hypothesis, in an NI hypothesis test, the observed p-value decreases with increasing sample size as can be seen from the equations (9.12) and (9.13) presented in Section 9.4. However, with a fixed sample size in a superiority test, the observed p-values decrease as the magnitude of difference in treatment effect increases. On the other hand, in an NI test one has to be cautious in interpreting an observed small p-value. Although a small observed p-value in a given NI trial demonstrates that the new treatment is non-inferior to the active control, it is specific to the margin specified in the null hypothesis. With a fixed sample size, as the margin is set tighter (i.e., the new treatment's effect closer to the active control effect), the observed p-values increase.

In a superiority trial, using intent-to-treat population avoids biases such as those associated with patients switching treatment, selection bias, and dropout/withdrawal patterns and is a conservative approach. However, in a NI trial, use of intent-to-treat population can lead to bias towards the null, particularly if the trial is conducted poorly and has missing data, treatment discontinuations, or misclassification of endpoints, as these can lead to the conclusion of no or minimal difference (success) between treatment arms. Although a per-protocol or as-treated population can be more conservative in an NI trial (ICH E10, CHMP, NI guidance), it cannot be assured that this will assure unbiased results. In general, analyses based on both intent-to-treat and per-protocol population should be reported. Apart from reporting results from the NI hypothesis testing, it is customary to report the percentage of active control effect retained by the experimental treatment as well as to report results from a superiority hypothesis. Note that the parameter estimates are the same whether it is NI or superiority testing and that the difference is in the calculation of p-values and interpretation.

9.9 Summary

In the oncology setting, non-inferiority trials play an important role in developing new products. In general, non-inferior products are expected to have a better or different safety profile and/or ease of administration of the drug. It may also not be feasible to conduct a superiority study if the active control has already established a remarkable efficacy (example: ORR of 90%). In such circumstances, acceptance of superiority may lead to no further drug development for that particular disease and could potentially lead to drug shortages. For these reasons testing for non-inferiority provides an alternative approach to establish efficacy.

In this chapter we have defined non-inferiority testing and given an overview of several approaches to the problem, including discussions of design and analysis. Non-inferiority trials necessarily depend on more subjective decisions in the design phase than do superiority trials. These decisions can include the selection of historical trials on which the NI margin is based and the determination of the fraction of the control treatment historical effect that can be discounted in declaring the experimental treatment efficacious. The choice of this fraction depends on the stage and severity of the disease and a clinical judgment on how much loss of efficacy can be tolerated so that the overall benefit to the patient is not compromised. Incorporating such decisions in the design of a clinical trial requires extra care in interpretation.

Generally, a limited number of historical placebo (or best supportive care) controlled oncology studies of the active control are conducted and reported in literature. This poses difficulty in estimating the active control effect size and in obtaining an NI margin. It is also possible that control effect is overestimated due to biased historical data. In many situations only one historical randomized study comparing control to placebo has been conducted. If there are deficiencies in this one study, or if the historical trial was stopped early due to efficacy, it would be difficult to assume assay sensitivity and constancy assumption. The NI study may also be undermined with the use of a less effective control. Caution should also be exercised in interpreting the results of an NI test as the calculated p-value is specific to one NI margin, and hence it is generally recommended to also report the p-value for the superiority test.

Finally there is the issue of "biocreep" [6], which is best understood by reexamining the term non-inferiority. Trials described as non-inferiority trials are often designed to indirectly show superiority to a placebo. This allows conclusions of efficacy even when a study treatment is slightly inferior to the active control. One can imagine a series of trials in which the NI study treatment becomes the active control for a subsequent NI study. If all the experimental treatments in such a sequence were slightly less effective than their predecessors, an incorrect conclusion of superiority to placebo would eventually occur. This is an extremely important issue to be aware of in designing NI trials.

The sample size calculation should always be based on a prespecified margin and this margin should also be justified on clinical grounds [9, 27]. A review of responses given by the European Medicines Agency (EMA) regarding NI trials for questions posed by applicants reported by Wangge et al. [34] suggests that the regulators are concerned a majority of the times about the choice of margin. Given the uncertainties in designing a NI trial, there should be a scientific rationale for using an NI hypothesis instead of a superiority hypothesis. Investigators should also be aware that a false NI conclusion may be reached due to poor conduct of the trial that biases the difference between T and C towards zero.

In this chapter we have defined and given examples of an NI hypothesis, and described how a trial with NI hypothesis can be designed, and analyzed. As we have discussed, there is an extra layer of complexity in these trials compared to superiority trials. Establishing superiority of a new treatment over existing treatment benefits the patient population and is the primary mechanism for moving the field forward. However, non-inferior treatments can provide alternative options to patients with potentially less toxicity or ease of administration (example, oral product vs. intravenous administration).

Acknowledgments

Lisa LaVange, Ram Tiwari, Thomas Permutt, and Division of Biometrics V Reviewers

Bibliography

[1] M. Baum, A. U. Budzar, J. Cuzick, J. Forbes, J. H. Houghton, J. G. Klijn, and T. Sahmoud. Anastrozole alone or in combination with tamoxifen versus tamoxifen alone for adjuvant treatment of postmenopausal women with early breast cancer: first results of the atac randomised trial. *Lancet*, 359(9324):2131–9, 2002.

[2] R. Berger and J. Hsu. Bioequivalence trials, intersection union tests and equivalence confidence sets. *Statistical Science*, 11(4):283–319, 1996.

[3] M. Borenstein, L. Hedges, J. Higgins, and H. Rothstein. *Introduction to Meta-analysis.* John Wiley & Sons, Ltd, Chichester, UK, 2009.

[4] S.C. Chow and J.P. Liu. *Design and Analysis of Clinical Trials: Concepts and Methodologies*, volume 507. John Wiley & Sons, 2008.

[5] Division of Behavioral Committee of National Statistics and Social Sciences & Education. *The Prevention and Treatment of Missing Data in clinical Trials. Panel on Handling Missing Data in Clinical Trials.* The National Academies Press, Washington DC, USA, 2010.

[6] R. D'Agostino, J. Massaro, and L. Sullivan. Non-inferiority trials: design concepts and issues - the encounters of academic consultants in statistics. *Statistics in Medicine*, 22:169–186, 2003.

[7] R. S. Dann and G. G. Koch. Review and evaluation of methods for computing confidence intervals for the ratio of two proportions and considerations for non-inferiority clinical trials. *Journal of Biopharmaceutical Statistics*, 15(1):85–107, 2005.

[8] T. R. Fleming. Current issues in non-inferiority trials. *Statistics in Medicine*, 27(3):317–32, 2008.

[9] U.S. Food and Drug Administration. Guidance for Industry Non-inferiority Clinical Trials, 2010.
http://www.fda.gov/downloads/Drugs/{\protect\newline}
GuidanceComplianceRegulatoryInformation/Guidances/UCM202140.pdf.

[10] M. A. Gamalo, R. C. Tiwari, and L. M. LaVange. Bayesian approach to the design and analysis of non-inferiority trials for anti-infective products. *Pharmaceutical Statistics*, 13(1):25–40, 2014.

[11] M. A. Gamalo, R. Wu, and R. C. Tiwari. Bayesian approach to non-inferiority trials for proportions. *Journal of Biopharmaceutical Statistics*, 21(5):902–19, 2011.

[12] M. A. Gamalo, R. Wu, and R. C. Tiwari. Bayesian approach to non-inferiority trials for normal means. *Statistical Methods in Medical Research*, 2012.

[13] P. Ghosh, F. Nathoo, M. Gonen, and R. C. Tiwari. Assessing non-inferiority in a three-arm trial using the Bayesian approach. *Statistics in Medicine*, 30(15):1795–808, 2011.

[14] N. Hanna, F. A. Shepherd, F. V. Fossella, J. R. Pereira, F. De Marinis, J. von Pawel, U. Gatzemeier, T. C.Y. Tsao, M. Pless, T. Muller, et al. Randomized phase III trial of pemetrexed versus docetaxel in patients with non-small cell lung cancer previously treated with chemotherapy. *Journal of Clinical Oncology*, 22(9):1589–97, 2004.

[15] D. Hauschke and I. Pigeot. Establishing efficacy of a new experimental treatment in the 'gold standard' design. *Biometrical Journal*, 47(6):782–6; discussion 787–98, 2005.

[16] E. B. Holmgren. Establishing equivalence by showing that a specified percentage of the effect of the active control over placebo is maintained. *Journal of Biopharmaceutical Statistics*, 9(4):651–9, 1999.

[17] Johnson & Johnson. Independent data monitoring committee recommends early stopping of phase 3 study of ibrutinib in relapsed/refractory CLL/SLL patients based on a planned interim analysis, January 7, 2014. http://www.investor.jnj.com/releasedetail.cfm?ReleaseID=817572.

[18] C. Ke, B. Ding, Q. Jiang, and S. M. Snapinn. The issue of multiplicity in non-inferiority studies. *Clinical Trials*, 9(6):730–5, 2012.

[19] K. Kelly, K. Chansky, L. E. Gaspar, K. S. Albain, J. Jett, Y. C. Ung, D. H. Lau, J. J. Crowley, and D. R. Gandara. Phase III trial of maintenance gefitinib or placebo after concurrent chemoradiotherapy and docetaxel consolidation in inoperable stage III non-small cell lung cancer: SWOG S0023. *Journal of Clinical Oncology*, 26(15):2450–6, 2008.

[20] E. S. Kim, V. Hirsh, T. Mok, M. A. Socinski, R. Gervais, Y. L. Wu, L. Y. Li, C. L. Watkins, M. V. Sellers, E. S. Lowe, Y. Sun, M. L. Liao, et al. Gefitinib versus docetaxel in previously treated non-small cell lung cancer (INTEREST): a randomised phase III trial. *Lancet*, 372(9652):1809–18, 2008.

[21] A. Koch and J. Rohmel. Hypothesis testing in the "gold standard" design for proving the efficacy of an experimental treatment relative to placebo and a reference. *Journal of Biopharmaceutical Statistics*, 14(2):315–25, 2004.

[22] K. S. Kwong, S. H. Cheung, and A. J. Hayter. Step-up procedures for non-inferiority tests with multiple experimental treatments. *Statistical Methods in Medical Research*, 2013.

[23] I. Lang, T. Brodowicz, L. Ryvo, Z. Kahan, R. Greil, S. Beslija, S. M. Stemmer, B. Kaufman, Z. Zvirbule, G. G. Steger, B. Melichar, et al. Bevacizumab plus paclitaxel versus bevacizumab plus capecitabine as first-line treatment for her2-negative metastatic breast cancer: interim efficacy results of the randomised, open-label, non-inferiority, phase 3 turandot trial. *Lancet Oncology*, 14(2):125–33, 2013.

[24] R. J. Little and D. B. Rubin. *Statistical Analysis with Missing Data*. John Wiley & Sons, 2014.

[25] H. B. Muss, D. A. Berry, C. T. Cirrincione, M. Theodoulou, A. M. Mauer, A. B. Kornblith, A. H. Partridge, L. G. Dressler, H. J. Cohen, et al. Adjuvant chemotherapy in older women with early-stage breast cancer. *New England Journal of Medicine*, 360(20):2055–65, 2009.

[26] M. Rothmann, N. Li, G. Chen, G. Y. Chi, R. Temple, and H. H. Tsou. Design and analysis of non-inferiority mortality trials in oncology. *Statistics in Medicine*, 22(2):239–64, 2003.

[27] E. D. Saad and M. Buyse. Non-inferiority trials in breast and non-small cell lung cancer: choice of non-inferiority margins and other statistical aspects. *Acta Oncologica*, 51(7):890–6, 2012.

[28] F. A. Shepherd, J. Dancey, R. Ramlau, K. Mattson, R. Gralla, M. O'Rourke, N. Levitan, L. Gressot, M. Vincent, R. Burkes, S. Coughlin, Y. Kim, and J. Berille. Prospective randomized trial of docetaxel versus best supportive care in patients with non-small cell lung cancer previously treated with platinum-based chemotherapy. *Journal of Clinical Oncology*, 18(10):2095–103, 2000.

[29] R. Simon. Bayesian design and analysis of active control clinical trials. *Biometrics*, 55(2):484–7, 1999.

[30] R. Sridhara. Statistical considerations in clinical trial designs for first-line hormonal treatment of metastatic breast cancer - Oncologic Drug Advisory Committee Meeting, 2001. http://www.fda.gov/ohrms/dockets/ac/01/slides/3782s1.htm.

[31] R. Temple and S. S. Ellenberg. Placebo-controlled trials and active-control trials in the evaluation of new treatments. part 1: ethical and scientific issues. *Annals of Internal Medicine*, 133(6):455–63, 2000.

[32] E. Walker, A. V. Hernandez, and M. W. Kattan. Meta-analysis: its strengths and limitations. *Cleveland Clinic Journal of Medicine*, 75(6):431–9, 2008.

[33] S. J. Wang, H. M. Hung, Y. Tsong, and L. Cui. Group sequential test strategies for superiority and non-inferiority hypotheses in active controlled clinical trials. *Statistics in Medicine*, 20(13):1903–12, 2001.

[34] G. Wangge, M. Putzeist, M. J. Knol, O. H. Klungel, C. C. Gispen-De Wied, A. de Boer, A. W. Hoes, H. G. Leufkens, and A. K. Mantel-Teeuwisse. Regulatory scientific advice on non-inferiority drug trials. *PLoS One*, 8(9):e74818, 2013.

[35] B. Weins and G. Rosenkranz. Missing data in non-inferiority trials. *Biopharmaceutical Research*, 5(4):383–393, 2013.

[36] B. Yoo. Impact of missing data on type 1 error rates in non-inferiority trials. *Pharmaceutical Statistics*, 9(2):87–99, 2010.

10

Quality of Life

Diane Fairclough

CONTENTS

10.1 Introduction

Traditionally, clinical trials have focused on endpoints that are physical or laboratory measures of response. Therapies for cancer are typically evaluated on the basis of disease progression and survival. Although traditional biomedical measures are often the primary endpoints in clinical trials, they do not reflect how the patient feels and functions in daily activities. Yet these perceptions reflect whether or not the patient believes he or she has benefited from the treatment. The patient's perception of his or her well-being may be the most important health outcome [41]. More recently, clinical trials have included endpoints that reflect the patient's perception of his or her well-being and satisfaction with therapy. The term Quality of Life (QOL) is used in a variety of ways. In this chapter, I will use it as a surrogate for measures of health-related quality-of-life (HRQoL) as well as other patient reported outcomes such as health status and symptoms.

There are a number of issues surrounding the use of QOL measures in oncology trials. The first is the role of the QOL assessments given that survival or disease progression is the primary endpoint in most oncology trials. The second issue is how the potential multiplicity of endpoints will be handled. This includes both all primary and secondary endpoints as well as the multiplicity generated by the longitudinal assessments (multiple time points) on multiple scales (e.g., physical well-being, emotional well-being, or multiple symptoms). The final issue is missing data due to morbidity and mortality, especially the latter. In this chapter, I will attempt to address all of these issues.

10.2 Measures of HRQoL

There are two general types of measures, often referred to as *health status* and *patient preference* [48]. These two forms of assessment have developed as a result of the differences between the perspectives of two different disciplines: psychometrics and econometrics, respectively. In the health status assessment measures, aspects of the patient's perceived well-being (physical, functional, emotional, social, symptoms, etc.) are self-assessed using multiple questions. A score is derived from the responses, typically by summing or averaging the responses and rescaling so that the possible range is 0 to 100. This score reflects the patient's relative HRQoL as compared to other patients and to the HRQoL of the same patient at other times. The assessments range from a single global question asking patients to rate their current quality of life to a series of questions about specific aspects of their daily life during a recent period of time. These instruments generally take 5 to 10 minutes to complete. Well-known examples of these measures are the cancer-specific FACIT [5, 46] and EORTC [1] measures and the generic Medical Outcomes Survey Short-Form or SF-36 [45]. Among these measures, there is considerable variation in the context of the questions with some measures focusing more on the perceived impact of the disease and therapy (How much are you bothered by hair loss?) and other measures focusing on the frequency and severity of symptoms (How often do you experience pain?). These measures are primarily designed to compare groups of patients receiving different treatments or to identify change over time within groups of patients. As a result, health status has most often been used in clinical trials to facilitate the comparisons of therapeutic regimens.

Measures of patient preference are influenced strongly by the concept of *utility*, borrowed from econometrics, that reflects individual decision-making under uncertainty. These preference assessment measures are primarily used to evaluate the tradeoff between the quality and quantity of life. Values of utilities are generally between 0 and 1 with 0 generally associated with death and 1 with perfect health. These preference measures may be elicited directly from patients or indirectly from the general public depending on the intended use. Utilities have traditionally been used in the calculation of quality-adjusted life years for cost-effectiveness analyses and in analytic approaches such as Q-TWiST [19, 20] described in Section 10.5.5.

The choice between the two types of measures depends on the objectives of the trial. Choices within the classes of measures tend to depend on the audience, the domains (e.g., physical well-being, fatigue), and potentially on the available language translations. In cancer trials, options include but are not limited to the cancer-specific FACIT [5] and EORTC [1] measures, and symptom-specific PROMIS [18, 49] and patient reported versions of the common toxicity criteria (CTC) measures [2].

10.3 QOL as an Endpoint in Cancer Trials

Given that most cancer clinical trials are designed to identify new drugs or combinations that improve survival, the role of QOL measures is often questioned. There are, however, important roles for QOL measures depending on the setting and the nature of the treatments. At the two extremes of the cancer trajectory, adjuvant therapy and stage IV disease, most experimental treatments relative to the active control intervention have minimal if any impact on survival. In the context of adjuvant therapy, any side effect profile such as fatigue or bone pain is likely to impact compliance and thus the potential benefits. At the other extreme, therapies for advanced stage disease typically have a modest impact on survival and their benefits are thus typically palliative as measured by QOL endpoints.

Even in the evaluation of interventions likely to change survival there are lessons to be learned from QOL outcomes. Sometimes clinical investigators assume that a change in a biomedical outcome will also improve the patient's quality of life. While in many cases this may be true, sometimes surprising results are obtained when the patient is asked directly. One classic example of this occurred with a study by [42] comparing two therapeutic approaches for soft-tissue sarcoma, limb-sparing surgery followed by radiation with full amputation. The investigator hypothesized "Sparing a limb, as opposed to amputating it, offers a quality of life advantage." Most would have agreed with this conjecture. But the trial results did not confirm the expectations; subjects receiving the limb-sparing procedures reported limitations in mobility and sexual functioning. These observations were confirmed with physical assessments of mobility and endocrine function. As a result of these studies, radiation therapy was modified and physical rehabilitation was added to the limb-sparing therapeutic approach [21].

An example where there were no survival differences and the QOL measures were critical in determining the value of the intervention is a trial in metastatic prostate cancer that evaluated the effects of flutamide versus placebo. There were no statistically significant differences in survival. However, the patient in the flutamide arm experienced more symptoms of diarrhea at 3 months and poorer emotional functioning at 3 and 6 months [33].

Identifying the role of QOL as an endpoint is a critical step in the design of a trial. Roles differ from aims and could range from the primary measure that demonstrates efficacy or safety in a registration trial to solely exploratory for the purpose of hypothesis generation. The exact nature of the role will obviously guide the analysis plan, but will also determine the resources that will be employed to ensure compliance with assessments.

10.4 Multiple Endpoints

It is well known that performing multiple hypothesis tests and basing inference on unadjusted p-values increase the overall probability of false positive results (Type I errors). Multiple hypothesis tests in trials assessing HRQoL arise from three sources: 1) multiple HRQoL measures (scales or subscales), 2) repeated post-randomization assessments, and 3) multiple treatment arms. As a result, multiple testing is one of the major analytic challenges in these trials [26]. Not only does this create concerns about type I error, but reports containing large numbers of statistical tests generally result in a confusing picture of HRQoL that is hard to interpret.

Although widely used in the analysis of HRQoL in clinical trials [40], univariate tests of each HRQoL domain or scale and time point can seriously inflate the type I (false positive) error rate for the overall trial such that the researcher is unable to distinguish between the true and false positive differences. Post hoc adjustment is often infeasible because, at the end of analysis, it is impossible to determine the number of tests performed. This approach also makes the strongest assumptions about missing data, an issue that will be discussed later.

So what are the options? The first is to limit hypothesis tests to a limited number of measures that have been prespecified in the trial design. The second is to consider summary measures or statistics across time or across subscales. And the third is to utilize multiple comparisons adjustments or gate-keeping strategies.

10.4.1 Summary Measures and Statistics

There are two dimensions of measurement that lend themselves to summary measures and statistics. The first is the assessment over time and the second is the multiple scales that measure the general and disease-specific domains of HRQoL. Developing composite measures from multiple scales is the more controversial as it leads to endpoints that are a combination of different aspects of QOL. If, in fact, all of the components are affected in the same direction and to a comparable extent, the composite is interpretable and clinically useful. However, if the components are impacted in different directions the use of the composite may miss the detection of treatment-related differences. Or if only one of the components drives the observed differences, the results may be misinterpreted [17].

Summary statistics across time are a very useful way of minimizing the impact of multiple comparisons procedures as well as facilitating the interpretation of results. Examples of summary statistics are area under the curve (AUC), average of post intervention measurements minus baseline, and slope. The choice depends on the trial design and usefulness to clinical practice. For example, if the intervention has a limited duration, two statistics might be proposed: one reflecting the impact of treatment while on therapy and the other post-therapy. Depending on the impact of the intervention on disease control and survival, either may be clinically useful. For example, if the more toxic intervention has better disease control and equivalent post-intervention QOL, poor QOL during therapy could be used to provide patient education and thus compliance. When therapy does not have a defined time line (e.g., is continued in the absence of disease progression) a summary measure such as the AUC may be more useful.

There are two approaches to summarizing longitudinal data. The first is to develop a strategy to compute a measure within each individual and then to perform univariate analysis. This sounds very attractive, but in practice creating rules â priori that cover all the contingencies is very difficult. The more practical approach is to select a method of analysis that addresses missing data as described in Section 10.5 and then to compute summary statistics as linear combinations of the estimated parameters [14].

10.4.2 Multiple Comparisons Adjustments and Gate-keeping Strategies

There are numerous multiple comparison adjustment procedures. The most well known and most conservative is the Bonferonni adjustment which divides alpha by the number of tests to be performed. Alternatives that are slightly less conservative include Holm's step-down procedure [24], Hochberg's step-up procedure [22], and the False Discovery Rate (FDR) procedure. However, all of these procedures will reduce the power to detect meaningful differences unless the trial is very large. Summary measures when appropriate in the clinical context vastly improve the situation primarily by reducing the number of comparisons.

The critical decision is whether to control the type I error solely at the level of the primary endpoints with no adjustments for secondary endpoints. Alternatives include controlling the type I error for both primary and secondary endpoints. An innovative procedure not often used is a gate-keeping strategy. It requires a very clear specification of the roles of each of the outcomes (e.g., survival, disease progression, and QOL). In some settings, there is a prespecifed sequence of testing families of hypotheses. Trial designs can include those with a single primary and multiple secondary endpoints (if the primary is non-significant, all other endpoints are irrelevant), multiple co-primary endpoints (significance of any of the endpoints is meaningful), and joint co-primary endpoints (tests of all endpoints need to be significant). In all of these designs, the two families of hypotheses are tested sequentially with the first family acting as a gatekeeper for the second family. Ideally the gate-keeping strategy is based on a mechanistic model in which the first family consists of measures of a proximal effect of the intervention on outcomes and the second family consists of more distal outcomes. For example, the first family could consist of biological and physiological factors and the second would consist of measures of symptom status. Alternatively, the first family could consist of symptom status and the second family of measures of the perceived impact of those symptoms.

Typically, HRQoL endpoints are poorly integrated into clinical trials. However, a gatekeeping procedure with sequential families provides one strategy for better integration. As an illustration, consider a trial with hypotheses A, B, and C testing treatment differences in disease response, survival, and QOL. Let's assume hypothetically that the unadjusted (marginal) p-values are $p_A = 0.08$, $p_B = 0.02$, and $p_C = 0.03$ as indicated in Table 10.1. We will consider four scenarios (three of which consist of sequential families of hypotheses) to illustrate the methods. The closed-testing procedure proposed by Marcus [32] provides a theoretical basis for controlling the experiment-wise type I error in a wide variety of settings. Dmitrienko et al. [11] present a formal way of displaying the procedure. The concepts are presented here; details are illustrated by Fairclough [14].

TABLE 10.1: Reported p-values for multiple hypotheses using gatekeeping strategies

Endpoint	Unadjusted p-value	All Primary	Single Primary	Co-Primary	Joint Co-Primary
A: Disease Control	0.08	0.24	0.08	0.16	0.16
B: Survival	0.02	0.06	0.08	0.04	0.04
C: QOL	0.03	0.09	0.08	0.04	0.16

Design 1. All primary with Bonferroni Corrections

If all three endpoints are considered primary endpoints and the Bonferroni procedure is used for the multiple comparisons adjustment, the null hypothesis for none of the comparisons would be rejected and the reported p-values would be 0.24, 0.06, and 0.09, respectively. In this scenario, the results for the Holms and Hochberg procedures would be qualitatively the same, though the p-values would differ.

Design 2. Single Primary Endpoint

In the second design, assume that disease response (H_A) was designated as the primary endpoint and both survival (H_B) and HRQoL (H_C) as the secondary endpoint. The first family consists of H_A and the second family of H_B and H_C. In this design, if the null hypothesis for the primary endpoint (A) is not rejected, all of the secondary null hypotheses must be accepted. If we apply this design using the unadjusted p-values from the previous example, the adjusted p-values are 0.08, 0.08, and 0.08. Thus, none of the three hypotheses are rejected and the (adjusted) results are negative for all three endpoints. If our trial design had designated survival as the primary endpoint, both the hypotheses for survival and QOL would have been rejected.

Design 3. Co-primary Endpoints

In the third design, disease control and survival are the co-primary endpoints and HRQoL the secondary endpoint. If either hypothesis in the first family (H_A or H_B) is rejected, then the second family of hypotheses will be considered. The hypotheses in the first family are tested as if the Holm procedure was applied to two endpoints. The adjusted p-values are 0.16 and 0.04. The adjusted p-value for the second family can not be smaller than the smallest in the first family because the gatekeeping procedure requires that H_C can not be rejected unless one of the hypotheses in the first family is rejected. Thus $\tilde{p}_B = 0.04$. With design 3, we would reject the null hypotheses associated with one of the primary endpoints, survival, and for the secondary endpoint, QoL.

Design 4. Joint Co-primary Endpoints

In the final design, disease control and survival are joint co-primary endpoints. This design differs from the previous one as it requires both H_A and H_B to be rejected before considering the second family of hypotheses. The adjusted p-values for the first family of hypotheses are identical to those in Design 3. Because the gatekeeping procedure requires that H_C can not be rejected unless both of the hypotheses in the first family are rejected, the adjusted p-value can not be smaller than the largest in the first family and thus $\tilde{p}_C = 0.16$. Thus in design 4, only the survival hypotheses is rejected.

10.5 Informative Missing Data Due to Dropout

Missing data due to morbidity or mortality is a common occurrence in oncology trials. Table 10.2 summarizes the classes of missing data. Missing assessments are very rarely completely random that are unrelated to the current status of the individual at the time of the planned assessment or other assessments (e.g., missing completely at random (MCAR)). In an advanced non-small cell lung cancer (NSCLC) trial [3], Figure 10.1 illustrates the average trajectories as function of the last observed assessment. If the missing data were MCAR, then the lines would overlap. A formal test for MCAR vs. MAR is described by Little [28]. The roughly fan-shaped trajectories also suggest that dropout depends on both the initial value and slope. A second example comes from a renal cell carcinoma trial [34]; the trajectories are non-linear but also suggest that dropout is related to the previously observed values and thus not MCAR (Figure 10.2).

TABLE 10.2: Simple overview of missing data mechanisms.

		Dependent on ...	Independent of ...
Missing Completely at Random	MCAR†	Covariates	Observed Outcome Missing Outcome
Missing at Random	MAR	Covariates Observed Outcome	Missing Outcome
Missing Not at Random	MNAR	Missing Outcome	

† and Covariate-dependent Dropout

10.5.1 Methods to Be Avoided

Methods that assume the data are MCAR, particularly those that do not utilize all the available data, will typically be biased. Limiting the analysis to those who have completed all assessments (complete case analyses) is the most well known example and is rarely used anymore. However, repeated univariate

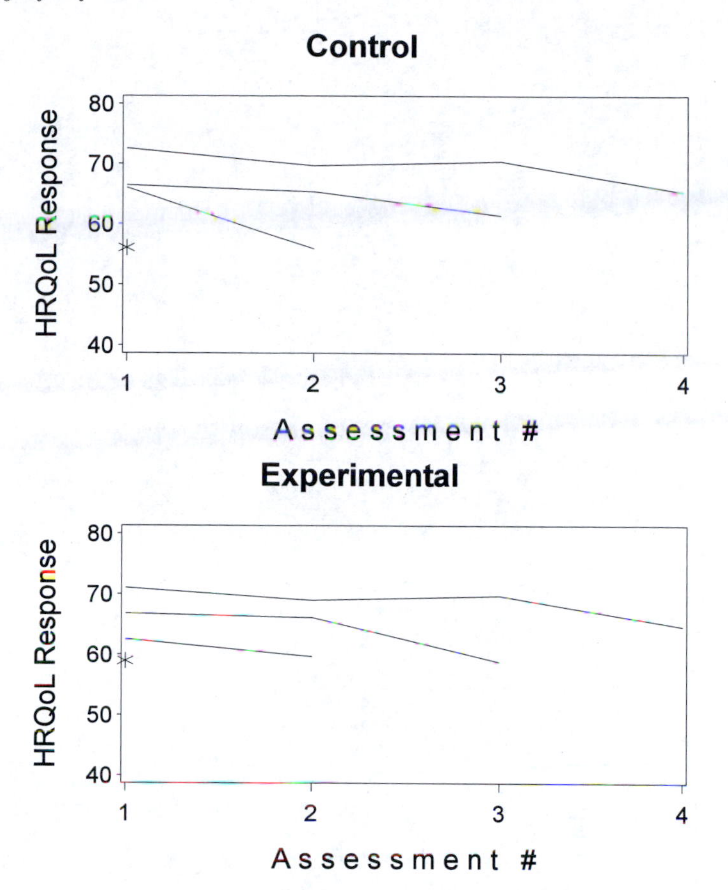

FIGURE 10.1: Average FACT-Lung TOI (A composite of Physical, Functional, and Disease-specific symptoms) scores for the control (top) and experimental (bottom) arms stratified by time of last assessment.

analyses of each endpoint at each time point is still frequently employed. As it does not utilize information from assessments at other time points it assumes that assessments are MCAR and thus is biased in most oncology trials. Generalized estimating equations (GEEs) [23, 38] also assume the data are MCAR. While these methods have been extended using re-weighting techniques, they assume that there are subjects with data that are similar to those without. This is typically not true in oncology trials.

10.5.2 Recommended Approach

In most oncology trials, missing data are associated with toxicity, disease progression, or death and thus are likely to be non-ignorable (e.g., MNAR).

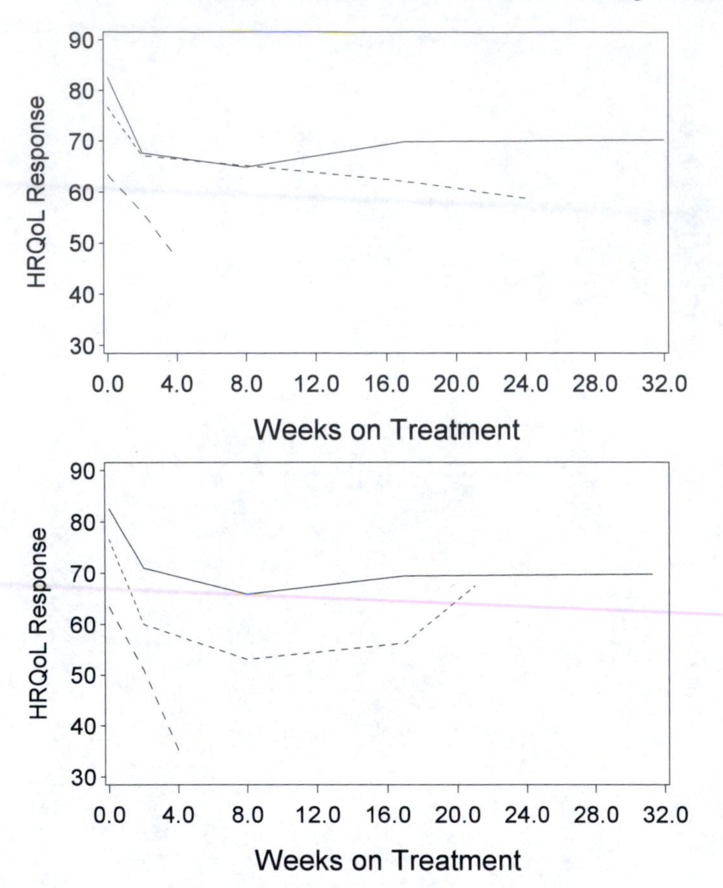

FIGURE 10.2: Average FACT-BRM TOI scores for control (top) and experimental (bottom) arms stratified by time of last assessment. Patients with 25+ weeks of follow-up are represented by the solid line, with between 5 and 25 weeks with the short dashed lines, and with less than 5 weeks with the long dashed lines.

Most experts recommend a likelihood-based approach using all available data supplemented by a sensitivity analysis [4, 14, 23]. The choice between growth curve mixed models (GCMM) [8] and repeated measures mixed models (RMMM) [25] will depend on the timing and number of assessments. Trials with a limited number of assessments (2–5) that can be thought of as ordered categories (e.g., Pre-, Early, Late and Post-Therapy) and where all assessments can be uniquely classified are typically analyzed using a repeated measures model: $Y_i = X_i\beta + \epsilon_i$ for the i-th subject where the variance Σ_i is unstructured. These trials are typical for interventions of limited duration. Trials with larger number of assessments or where the timing of assessments becomes more varied over time are typically analyzed using the growth curve models that incorporate random effects: $Y_i = X_i\beta + Z_id_i + \varepsilon_i$. The random effects, Z_id_i, typically allow variation of the subject-specific intercepts and slope relative to the predicted trajectory. The variance is structured, $\Sigma_i = Z_i' D Z_i + \sigma^2 I$.

10.5.3 Sensitivity Analyses

In most oncology trials, non-ignorable missing data should be suspected. Unfortunately, any test of MAR versus MNAR would require the data that are missing. Similarly, determining the dropout mechanism also would require the data that are missing. It is possible to find evidence that data are not MAR assuming a particular model [10, 39, 47], but the lack of evidence under a particular model does not confirm the data are MAR. These issues are the basis for the recommendations to plan for a sensitivity analysis and the use of the term 'sensitivity'.

There are a number of methods for sensitivity analyses that are popular. All require strong assumptions and are difficult to prespecify prior to data collection. The common theme among them is that they attempt to convert the problem to one that is conditionally MAR. For example, the assumption underlying pattern mixture models is that the data are MAR within each pattern [14].

Mixture Models

The basic concept of mixture models is the true distribution of the measures of HRQoL for the entire group of patients is a mixture of the distributions from each of the P groups of patients [29–31]. The distribution of the responses, Y_i, may differ across the P strata with different parameters, $\beta^{\{p\}}$, and variance, $\Sigma^{\{p\}}$:

$$Y_i|M^{\{p\}} \sim N\left(X_i\beta^{\{p\}}, \Sigma_i^{\{p\}}\right),\ p = 1, \ldots, P. \tag{10.1}$$

The complete data, $f(Y)$, are characterized as a mixture (weighted average) of the conditional distribution, $f(Y|M)$, over the distribution of dropout times, the patterns of missing data, or the random coefficients. The specific form of M distinguishes the various mixture models where M is either dropout time, $\mathcal{T}_i^D$, the pattern of missing data, R_i, or a random coefficient, d_i.

$$\text{Pattern mixture} \quad f(Y_i|R_i) \tag{10.2}$$

$$\text{Time-to-event mixture} \quad f(Y_i|\mathcal{T}_i^D) \tag{10.3}$$

$$\text{Random effects mixture} \quad f(Y_i|d_i) \tag{10.4}$$

Pattern mixture models are a special case of the mixture models. When $M_i = R_i$, the missingness can be classified into patterns.

Pattern mixture models are attractive because they are amenable to plots displaying the observed data as in Figures 10.1 and 10.2. The strong assumptions center around the extrapolation of the curves past the time of dropout. When the trajectories are linear (Figure 10.1), it may be very reasonable to extend the slopes for patterns with at least two assessments. The slope for the pattern with only baseline data will require an additional assumption, possibly using the slope from the pattern with two assessments. But when the trajectories are non-linear (Figure 10.2) it can be very difficult to identify a procedure even after the results are plotted. Pre-specifying the methods for extrapolation is almost impossible. One strategy that is used is to pool the strata so that all the model parameters are estimable. Pauler et al. [35] illustrate this in a trial of patients with advanced stage colorectal cancer where they did not form the strata based on the patterns of observed data but on a combination of survival and completion of the last assessment. First they defined two strata based on whether the patient survived to the end of the study (21 weeks), then they split the patients who survived 21 weeks based on whether they completed the last assessment. They assumed that the trajectory within each strata was linear. The assumption is that the missing data are ignorable within each strata. This assumption implies that within the group of patients who did not survive 21 weeks, there are no systematic differences between those who die early versus later, and within those who survived, there are no differences between those who drop out early versus later.

Joint Models with Shared Parameters

In this class of models, we are jointly estimating the longitudinal trajectories of the QOL outcomes with another process, typically time to dropout, disease progression, or survival. The underlying assumption is that the data are MAR conditional on the time to the event. The concept is that the random effects of the model for the QOL outcomes are correlated with the time to the event. Specifically, the individuals who experience an earlier event will tend to start with lower QOL scores and will decline more rapidly. This is illustrated in the NSCLC example (Figure 10.1), where those with early dropout tend to have poorer QOL scores at baseline and decline more rapidly. When applied to this study, estimates of the decline over time roughly double in both treatment groups (Table 10.3). This illustrates the sensitivity of within group estimates of change, but relative stability of the differences when studying two active interventions with similar survival and toxicity.

TABLE 10.3: NSCLC Trial: Joint Model for FACT-Lung TOI and various measures of the time to dropout ($\mathcal{T}^D$). Parameter estimates of intercept (β_0), slopes for control group (β_1) and experimental group (β_2), and the difference in slopes ($\beta_2 - \beta_1$).

	Estimates (s.e.)			
Dropout Event	$\hat{\beta}_0$	$\hat{\beta}_1$	$\hat{\beta}_2$	$\hat{\beta}_2 - \hat{\beta}_1$
None (MLE)	65.9 (0.66)	-1.18 (0.29)	-0.58 (0.19)	0.60 (0.31)
ln(Survival)	65.7 (0.66)	-1.85 (0.30)	-1.43 (0.24)	0.47 (0.31)
Last assessment	66.1 (0.66)	-2.15 (0.39)	-1.53 (0.31)	0.62 (0.32)

The most critical characteristic for the implementation of these models is that there is variation in the random effect, particularly associated with change over time. There are a wide variety of parametric and non-parametric models [37, 39, 43] that have been proposed. Vonesh et al. [44] extended the model by relaxing the assumptions of normality allowing distributions of the random effects from the quadratic exponential family and event-time models from accelerated failure-time models (e.g., Weibull, exponential extreme values, and piece-wise exponential). Numerous investigators have joined proportional hazard models with the longitudinal models. Other extensions include multiple reasons for dropout [6, 12] and the possibility that some subjects would not eventually experience the dropout event and could stay on the intervention indefinitely [6, 27, 50].

Multiple Imputation

As software for multiple imputation (MI) has become extremely accessible, it is being proposed more often to address missing data issues. Most MI techniques assume the missing data are MAR conditional on the variables included in the imputation procedure. If the imputation procedure only includes the available information that will be used in the analysis (previous assessments, treatment assignment and baseline covariates) the results will be very similar to those obtained from the likelihood-based methods previously described. Thus, there is a danger of believing that any bias due to missing data has been eliminated when in fact it has not. In the context of oncology trials, if surrogate measures for the QOL response were available and were incorporated into the imputation scheme, the missing data would be MAR conditional on those measures. However, those surrogate measures are typically both unmeasured and unknown, limiting the usefulness of MI techniques.

10.5.4 QOL after Death

One of the most controversial areas of research involving QOL is the analysis of trials with significant morbidity. The controversy occurs because of philosophical issues about imputing a value for measures of QOL or other patient reported measures. What is often ignored is that even if explicit imputation is avoided, most methods of analysis implicitly impute a value. This is most obvious when using the EM algorithm for likelihood-based methods. In the E-step, the conditional expectations of the missing assessments given the observed data are used to compute the sufficient statistics. One class of measures referred to as patient preference or utility measures (e.g., EQ-5D or HUI) explicitly defines death as value of zero and is typically used in health economics.

Analyses that Avoid Imputation

There are a limited number of approaches that avoid imputation and are primarily descriptive. The first is to examine the trajectory as a function of the time prior to death (Figure 10.3). This is useful when trying to determine if and when there are changes prior to death. For example, in the NSCLC trial patient, the decline in the FACT-TOI measure tends to be quite gradual until approximately a week before death. A second approach also relies on graphical presentation, where subjects are stratified by the time of death in a manner similar to Figures 10.1 or 10.2. While it is possible to construct strata-specific contrasts of these trajectories across treatment groups [7], the interpretation is limited to just that and can not be used as a overall comparison of the outcome under the intent-to-treat concept.

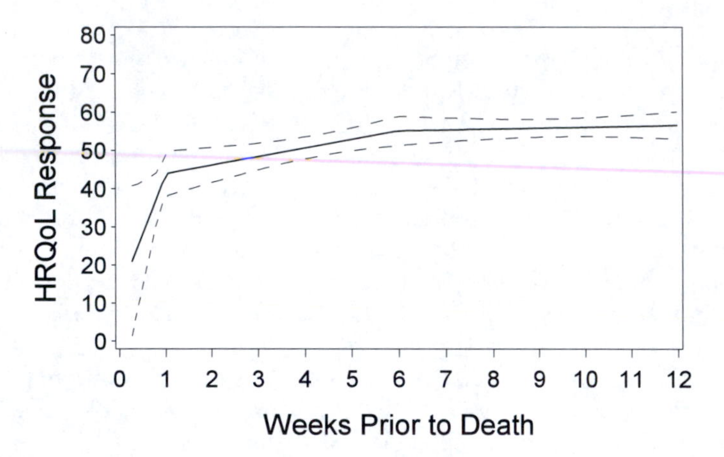

FIGURE 10.3: Change in FACT-Lung TOI prior to death.

Explicit Imputation Methods

A number of simple imputation techniques have been described, but none have attained widespread use. An example of simple imputation is the substitution of an arbitrary low (or high) value for the assessments that occur after death [13, 36]. Values of 0 as well as a value just below the minimum of all observed scores have been suggested. Both approaches can be partially justified, but neither can be completely defended. It also should be noted that when a large proportion of the subjects expire then distribution of scores will tend to become bimodal, approximating a binary indicator for death, and the analysis becomes an approximation to the analysis of survival rather than QOL.

Diehr et al. [9] describe a variation on a last value carried forward (LVCF) procedure. In this procedure a value δ is subtracted from (or added to) the last value observed. If this value can be justified, this approach could be a useful option in a sensitivity analysis. In Diehr's example, a value of 15 points on the SF-36 physical function scale was proposed, where 15 points was justified as the difference in scores between individuals reporting their health as unchanged vs. those reporting worsening.

It is possible to utilize multiple imputation methods in this setting. A variation of Diehr's approach could utilize multiply imputed values with varying values of δ as a sensitivity analysis to see if the results of treatment comparisons are robust to a range of values of δ. Alternatively, models similar to the one displayed in Figure 10.3 could be used as the basis for imputation of values at the time of death and beyond.

Implicit Imputation Methods

Joint models with shared parameters previously described in Section 10.5.3 comprise a wide class of models that can be used in trials with dropout due to death. As these are likelihood-based methods, they use implicit imputation of the missing data or the random effects in the estimation procedures, conditioning on both the previously observed measures and the time to death.

10.5.5 QALYs and Q-TWiST

Quality-adjusted life years (QALYs) and Q-TWiST measures integrate quality and quantity of life; these measures may be useful when there are tradeoffs associated with the interventions being assessed in the clinical trial. Questions of this nature are particularly relevant in diseases that have relatively short expected survival and the intent of treatment is palliative such as advanced-stage cancer. In contrast to the above analyses, in which the outcomes are expressed in the metric of the QOL scale, QALYs and Q-TWiST measures are expressed in the metric of time.

There are two approaches that might be encountered in a clinical trial. In the first, measures of patient preferences are measured repeatedly over time and the outcome is QALYs. In the second approach, the average time in various health states is measured and weighted using preference measures that are specific to each of the health states generating Q-TWiST estimates.

QALYs

In some trials patient preferences are measured repeatedly over time often using multi-attribute measures (e.g., HUI, EQ-5D, QWB) or transformations health status scales (e.g., SF-36) to utility measures [15, 16]. The basis for all of the methods is estimation of the area under a curve (AUC) generated by plotting the utility measure versus time. There are two approaches. The first strategy estimates the average trajectory in each treatment group using a longitudinal model and then calculates AUC as a function of the parameter estimates in the same manner as described above for health status measures.

The difference is that since the preference measure is measured on a unit-less scale from 1 (perfect health) to 0 (death) the estimate can be interpreted as an estimate of QALYs.

The second strategy starts with the calculation of a value for each individual, $QALY_i$, that is a function of the utility scores and time. These values will then be subsequently analyzed as univariate measures. The calculation of $QALY_I$ will depend on a rule for estimating the measure between assessments, possibly extrapolation back in time, or using a trapezoidal function as illustrated in Figure 10.4.

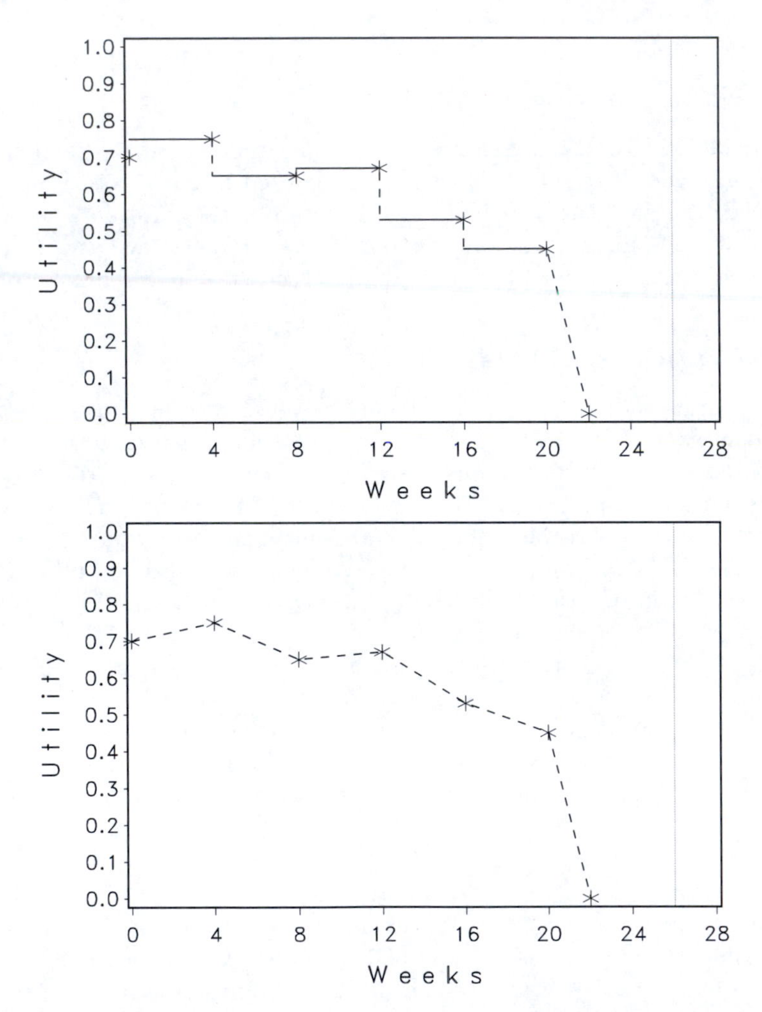

FIGURE 10.4: Illustration of two techniques to estimate $QALY_i$ when time between assessments (4 weeks) equals the period of recall using horizontal (left) and trapezoidal (right) extrapolation. Observations are indicated by $\star$. Periods using trapezoidal approximation are indicated by a dashed line.

The major limitation for both of these approaches is that all patients are rarely followed until death and thus the estimates are limited to a fixed time period.

Q-TWiST

A second method to integrate quality and quantity of life is Q-TWiST. A fundamental requirement for this approach is that we can define distinct health-states. In the original application of this method [19] in breast cancer patients, four health states were defined:

TOX	the period during which the patients were receiving therapy and presumably experiencing toxicity;
TWiST	the period after therapy during which the patients were without symptoms of the disease or treatment;
REL	the period between relapse (recurrence of disease) and death;
DEATH	the period following death.

The second assumption is that each health state is associated with a weight or value of the health state relative to perfect health that is representative of the entire time the subject is in that health state. The assumption that the utility for each health state does not vary with time has been termed *utility independence* [19].

A third assumption is that there is a natural progression from one health state to another. In the above example, it was assumed that patients would progress from TOX to TWiST to REL to DEATH. The possibility of skipping health states, but not going backwards, is allowed. Thus, a patient might progression from TOX directly to REL or DEATH, but not from TWiST back to TOX or REL back to TWiST. Obviously, exceptions could occur, and if very rare they might be ignored. The quantity Q-TWiST is a weighted score of the average time spent in each of these health sates, where the weights are based on preference scores. Typically the weight for the period of time without symptoms U_{TWiST} is fixed at a value of 1 implying no loss of QALYs and for the period after death U_{DEATH} is fixed at a value of 0. Thus, for this example, there are only two potentially unknown weights, U_{TOX} and U_{REL}.

$$\begin{aligned} Q-TWiST &= T_{TOX} * U_{TOX} + T_{TWiST} * \underbrace{U_{TWiST}}_{=1} \\ &+ T_{REL} * U_{REL} + T_{DEATH} * \underbrace{U_{DEATH}}_{=0} \end{aligned} \tag{10.5}$$

If all of the patients in the study have been followed to death, finding the average time in each health state is quite easy as the time for each is known for every patient. But when there is censoring, we need to use methods developed for survival analyses. Figure 10.5 illustrates Kaplan-Meier estimates for the time to the end of treatment (TOX), the end of the disease-free survival (DFS), and the end of survival (SURV) for the patients in an adjuvant breast cancer trial with up to 60 months of follow-up. The average time in TOX is equal to the AUC for the time to the end of treatment. The health state TWiST is defined as the time between the end of TOX and DFS. The average time spent in TWiST is equal to the area between the two curves. Similarly, the health state REL is defined as the time between the end of DFS and SURV. The average time in REL is again the area between the curves. When follow-up is incomplete, we must estimate restricted means which estimate the average times in each health state up to a set limit. At first glance it might appear that 60 months (5 years) would be a good choice. However, for practical reasons related to estimation of the variance of the estimates, it is more appropriate to pick a time where follow-up is complete for 50–75% of the subjects who are still being followed.

10.5.6 How Much Data Can Be Missing?

There are no magic rules about how much missing data are acceptable in a clinical trial. When the proportion of missing assessments is very small (<5%), the potential bias or impact on power may be very minor. In some cases, 10–20% missing data will have little or no effect on the results of the study. In other studies, 10–20% may matter. As the proportion of missing data increases to 30–50%, the conclusions one is willing to draw will be restricted. The seriousness of the problem depends on the reasons for the missing data, the objectives of the study, and the intended use of the results.

10.6 Sample Size or Power Estimation

Sample size estimation for longitudinal studies of continuous outcomes utilizes standard methods. There are issues that are specific to assessment of QOL in cancer, but the steps are the same as in any trials. The first step is to determine the endpoint, which can be as simple as the difference in scores at a particular time point or the area between the curves for the longitudinal assessments. The second step is determining the size of the effect that would be clinically meaningful. This might be based on a minimally important difference (MID) that has been determined in previous research, a rule of thumb argument for 0.5 SD, or a difference that is typical of a certain type of intervention (e.g., 0.3 SD). The third step is to predict the drop-out rate. The final assumption is the correlation of the repeated assessments. For measures of QOL, these are typically between 0.5 and 0.8. Making the assumption that the correlation is 0.5 is conservative with respect to the detectable difference or the power and my personal recommendation.

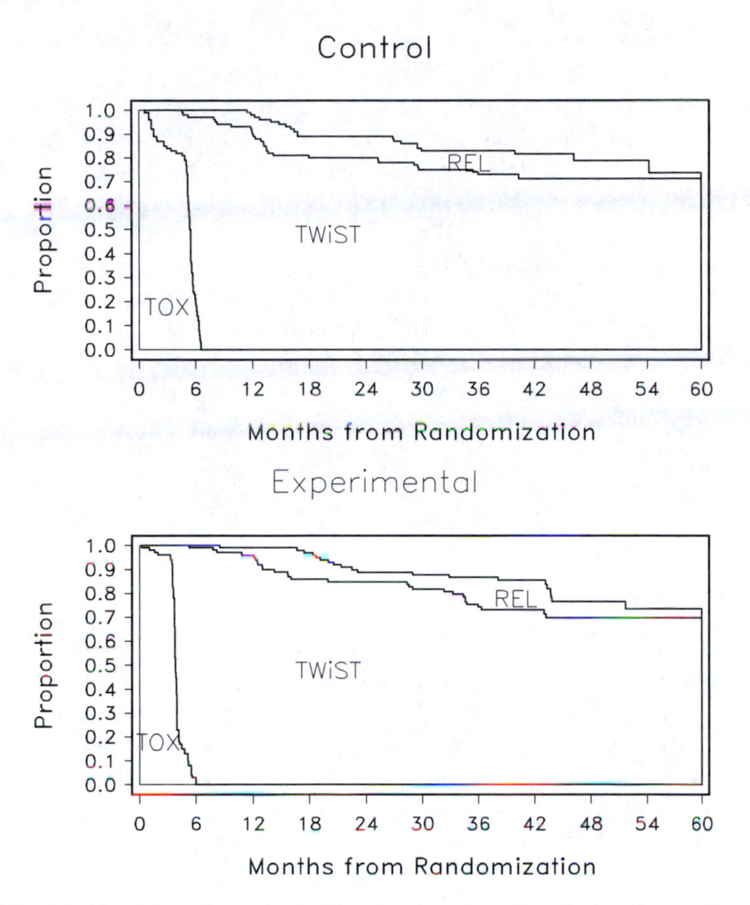

FIGURE 10.5: Partitioned survival plots for the control and experimental groups of the breast cancer trial. Each plot shows the estimated curves for TOX, DFS, and Surv. Areas between the curves correspond to time spent in the TOX, TWiST, and REL health states.

For the first example, consider a very simple example where the endpoint is the difference at a particular point in time. The planned sample size for the trial is 200 in each of two arms and we will have 20% dropout at that point in time. A simple sample size calculation assuming 160 subjects per group and $\alpha = 0.05$ would have 90% power ($\beta = 0.1$) to detect a difference of 0.36 SD. If we were comparing change from baseline and assumed the correlation between baseline and the follow-up was 0.5, the results would be identical; higher correlations between baseline and follow-up would result in increased power or a decreased effect size.

For the second example, consider the same trial but with a more complex endpoint, the average difference between the curves (e.g., AUC) when assessment were taken every 3 months over 1 year. For the purpose of estimating sample size, assume β_g represents the mean at each point in time for one of the groups, then $\theta = C'\beta_g$ where $C = (1.5\ 3\ 3\ 3\ 1.5)/12$. Then the variance is estimated using $Var(C\beta_g) = CVar(\beta_g)C'$. The two elements that change in the sample size estimation are the difference in this summary statistic and its standard deviation, which can be calculated using any matrix software (e.g., SAS Proc IML or R). Suppose we specify the expected difference at each point in time as $\delta = (0\ .3\ .3\ .3\ .3)'$ representing no difference at baseline and an effect of 0.5 SD at all subsequent follow-ups, then $\delta_\theta = C\delta = 0.2625$. If we assume that the correlation of measures is 0.5, then $SD(Y_\theta) = \sqrt{C(.5 * I(5) + .5 * J(5,5))C'} = 0.7806$. Then using these values in standard equations (any sample size program) for the two-sided t-test of difference in two independent means, we have 85% power.

10.7 Summary

Often it is the statistician who is at the interface of the trial design and the analysis plan. It is in the development of an analysis plan that the goals of the trial as well as the specific aims need to clarified. QOL and other patient reported outcomes can provide useful clinical information; their role needs to be carefully and explicitly defined. The goals, the role, and the actual domains that are to be measured specifically influence the procedures that will be used to minimize the multiple comparisons as well as the strategies for missing data.

Bibliography

[1] N. K. Aaronson, S. Ahmedzai, B. Bergman, M. Bullinger, A. Cull, N. J. Duez, A. Filiberti, H. Flechtner, S. B. Fleishman, J. C. de Haes, S. Kaasa, et al. The European Organization for Research and Treatment of Cancer QLQ-C30: a quality-of-life instrument for use in international clinical trials in oncology. *Journal of the National Cancer Institute*, 85(5):365–76, 1993.

[2] E. Basch, B. B. Reeve, S. A. Mitchell, S. B. Clauser, L. M. Minasian, A. C. Dueck, T. R. Mendoza, J. Hay, T. M. Atkinson, A. P. Abernethy, et al. Development of the National Cancer Institute's patient-reported outcomes version of the common terminology criteria for adverse events (PRO-CTCAE). *Journal of the National Cancer Institute*, 106(9), 2014.

[3] P. Bonomi, K. Kim, D. Fairclough, D. Cella, J. Kugler, E. Rowinsky, M. Jiroutek, and D. Johnson. Comparison of survival and quality of life in advanced non-small cell lung cancer patients treated with two dose levels of paclitaxel combined with cisplatin versus etoposide with cisplatin: results of an Eastern Cooperative Oncology Group trial. *Journal of Clinical Oncology*, 18(3):623–31, 2000.

[4] J. Carpenter and M. Kenward. Missing data in randomised controlled trials - a practical guide. Birmingham: National Institute for Health Research, Publication RM03/JH17/MK, 2008. http://www.missingdata.org.uk.

[5] D. F. Cella, D. S. Tulsky, G. Gray, B. Sarafian, E. Linn, A. Bonomi, M. Silberman, S. B. Yellen, P. Winicour, and J. Brannon. The Functional Assessment of Cancer Therapy scale: development and validation of the general measure. *Journal of Clinical Oncology*, 11(3):570–9, 1993.

[6] Y. Y. Chi and J. G. Ibrahim. Joint models for multivariate longitudinal and multivariate survival data. *Biometrics*, 62(2):432–45, 2006.

[7] J. D. Dawson. Stratification of summary statistic tests according to missing data patterns. *Statistics in Medicine*, 13(18):1853–63, 1994.

[8] A. Dempster, N. Laird, and D. Rubin. Maximum likelihood estimation from incomplete data via the EM algorithm (with discussion). *Journal of the Royal Statistical Society: Series B*, 39:1–38, 1977.

[9] P. Diehr, D. Patrick, S. Hedrick, M. Rothman, D. Grembowski, T. E. Raghunathan, and S. Beresford. Including deaths when measuring health status over time. *Medical Care*, 33(4 Suppl):As164–72, 1995.

[10] P. Diggle and M. Kenward. Informative dropout in longitudinal data analysis (with discussion). *Journal of the Royal Statistical Society: Series C*, 43:49–93, 1994.

[11] A. Dmitrienko, W. W. Offen, and P. H. Westfall. Gatekeeping strategies for clinical trials that do not require all primary effects to be significant. *Statistics in Medicine*, 22(15):2387–400, 2003.

[12] R. M. Elashoff, G. Li, and N. Li. An approach to joint analysis of longitudinal measurements and competing risks failure time data. *Statistics in Medicine*, 26(14):2813–35, 2007.

[13] D. L. Fairclough, J. H. Fetting, D. Cella, W. Wonson, and C. M. Moinpour. Quality of life and quality adjusted survival for breast cancer patients receiving adjuvant therapy. Eastern Cooperative Oncology Group (ECOG). *Quality of Life Research*, 8(8):723–31, 1999.

[14] D.L. Fairclough. *Design and Analysis of Quality of Life Studies in Clinical Trials.* CRC Press, Boca Raton, FL, 2nd edition, 2010.

[15] D. Feeny. Preference-based measures: utility and quality-adjusted life years. In P. Fayers and R. Hays, editors, *Assessing Quality of Life in Clinical Trials*. Oxford University Press, 2nd edition, 2006.

[16] P. Franks, E. I. Lubetkin, M. R. Gold, and D. J. Tancredi. Mapping the SF-12 to preference-based instruments: convergent validity in a low-income, minority population. *Medical Care*, 41(11):1277–83, 2003.

[17] N. Freemantle, M. Calvert, J. Wood, J. Eastangh, and C. Griffin. Composite outcomes in randomized trials: great precision but with greater uncertainty? *Journal of the American Medical Association*, 239:2554–2559, 2003.

[18] S. F. Garcia, D. Cella, S. B. Clauser, K. E. Flynn, T. Lad, J. S. Lai, B. B. Reeve, A. W. Smith, A. A. Stone, and K. Weinfurt. Standardizing patient-reported outcomes assessment in cancer clinical trials: a patient-reported outcomes measurement information system initiative. *Journal of Clinical Oncology*, 25(32):5106–12, 2007.

[19] P. P. Glasziou, R. J. Simes, and R. D. Gelber. Quality adjusted survival analysis. *Statistics in Medicine*, 9(11):1259–76, 1990.

[20] A. Goldhirsch, R. D. Gelber, R. J. Simes, P. Glasziou, and A. S. Coates. Costs and benefits of adjuvant therapy in breast cancer: a quality-adjusted survival analysis. *Journal of Clinical Oncology*, 7(1):36–44, 1989.

[21] J. Hicks, M. Lampert, L. Gerber, E. Glastein, and J. Danoff. Functional outcome update in patients with soft tissue sarcoma undergoing wide local excision and radiation (abstract). *Archives of Physical Medicine and Rehabilitation*, 66:542–543, 1985.

[22] Y. Hochberg. A sharper Bonferroni procedure for multiple tests of significance. *Biometrika*, 75(4):800–802, 1988.

[23] J. Hogan, J. Roy, and C. Korkontzelou. Tutorial in biostatistics: handling drop-out in longitudinal studies. *Statistics in Medicine*, 23:1455–1497, 2004.

[24] S. Holm. A simple sequentially rejective multiple test procedure. *Scandinavian Journal of Statistics*, 6:65–70, 1979.

[25] R. I. Jennrich and M. D. Schluchter. Unbalanced repeated-measures models with structured covariance matrices. *Biometrics*, 42(4):805–20, 1986.

[26] E. L. Korn and J. O'Fallon. Statistical considerations, statistics working group. Quality of life assessment in cancer clinical trials. In *Report on Workshop on Quality of Life Research in Cancer Clinical Trials, Division of Cancer Prevention and Control. Bethesda: National Cancer Institute*, 1990.

[27] N. J. Law, J. M. Taylor, and H. Sandler. The joint modeling of a longitudinal disease progression marker and the failure time process in the presence of cure. *Biostatistics*, 3(4):547–63, 2002.

[28] R. Little. A test of missing completely at random for multivariate data with missing values. *Journal of the American Statistical Association*, 83:1198–1202, 1988.

[29] R. Little. Pattern-mixture models for multivariate incomplete data. *Journal of the American Statistical Association*, 88:125–134, 1993.

[30] R. Little. Modeling the dropout mechanism in repeated-measures studies. *Journal of the American Statistical Association*, 90:1112–1121, 1995.

[31] R. J. A. Little. A class of pattern-mixture models for normal incomplete data. *Biometrika*, 81(3):471–483, 1994.

[32] R. Marcus, E. Peritz, and K. Gabriel. On closed testing procedures with special reference to ordered analysis of variance. *Biometrika*, 63:655–660, 1976.

[33] C. M. Moinpour, M. J. Savage, A. Troxel, L. C. Lovato, M. Eisenberger, R. W. Veith, B. Higgins, R. Skeel, M. Yee, B. A. Blumenstein, E. D. Crawford, and F. L. Meyskens, Jr. Quality of life in advanced prostate cancer: results of a randomized therapeutic trial. *Journal of the National Cancer Institute*, 90(20):1537–44, 1998.

[34] R. J. Motzer, B. A. Murphy, J. Bacik, L. H. Schwartz, D. M. Nanus, T. Mariani, P. Loehrer, G. Wilding, D. L. Fairclough, D. Cella, and M. Mazumdar. Phase III trial of interferon alfa-2a with or without 13-cis-retinoic acid for patients with advanced renal cell carcinoma. *Journal of Clinical Oncology*, 18(16):2972–80, 2000.

[35] D. K. Pauler, S. McCoy, and C. Moinpour. Pattern mixture models for longitudinal quality of life studies in advanced stage disease. *Statistics in Medicine*, 22(5):795–809, 2003.

[36] J. M. Raboud, J. Singer, A. Thorne, M. T. Schechter, and S. D. Shafran. Estimating the effect of treatment on quality of life in the presence of missing data due to drop-out and death. *Quality of Life Research*, 7(6):487–94, 1998.

[37] H. J. Ribaudo, S. G. Thompson, and T. G. Allen-Mersh. A joint analysis of quality of life and survival using a random effect selection model. *Statistics in Medicine*, 19(23):3237–50, 2000.

[38] J. L. Schafer and J. W. Graham. Missing data: our view of the state of the art. *Psychological Methods*, 7(2):147–77, 2002.

[39] M. D. Schluchter. Methods for the analysis of informatively censored longitudinal data. *Statistics in Medicine*, 11(14-15):1861–70, 1992.

[40] M. Schumacher, M. Olschewski, and G. Schulgen. Assessment of quality of life in clinical trials. *Statistics in Medicine*, 10(12):1915–30, 1991.

[41] M. Staquet, N. Aaronson, and S. Ahmedzai. Health-related quality of life research. *Quality of Life Research*, 1(1):3, 1992.

[42] P. H. Sugarbaker, I. Barofsky, S. A. Rosenberg, and F. J. Gianola. Quality of life assessment of patients in extremity sarcoma clinical trials. *Surgery*, 91(1):17–23, 1982.

[43] G. Touloumi, S. J. Pocock, A. G. Babiker, and J. H. Darbyshire. Estimation and comparison of rates of change in longitudinal studies with informative drop-outs. *Statistics in Medicine*, 18(10):1215–33, 1999.

[44] E. F. Vonesh, T. Greene, and M. D. Schluchter. Shared parameter models for the joint analysis of longitudinal data and event times. *Statistics in Medicine*, 25(1):143–63, 2006.

[45] J. Ware, K. Snow, M. Kosinski, and B. Gandek. *SF-36 Health Survey: Manual and Interpretation Guide.* CRC Press, Boca Raton, FL, 1993.

[46] K. Webster, D. Cella, and K. Yost. The Functional Assessment of Chronic Illness Therapy (FACIT) Measurement System: properties, applications, and interpretation. *Health and Quality of Life Outcomes*, 1:79, 2003.

[47] M. C. Wu and K. R. Bailey. Estimation and comparison of changes in the presence of informative right censoring: conditional linear model. *Biometrics*, 45(3):939–55, 1989.

[48] K. R. Yabroff, B. P. Linas, and K. Schulman. Evaluation of quality of life for diverse patient populations. *Breast Cancer Research and Treatment*, 40(1):87–104, 1996.

[49] K. J. Yost, D. T. Eton, S. F. Garcia, and D. Cella. Minimally important differences were estimated for six Patient-Reported Outcomes Measurement Information System-Cancer scales in advanced-stage cancer patients. *Journal of Clinical Epidemiology*, 64(5):507–16, 2011.

[50] M. Yu, N. Law, J. Taylor, and H. Sandler. Joint longitudinal-survival-cure models and their applications to prostate cancer. *Statistica Sinica*, 14:835–862, 2004.

Part IV

Personalized Medicine

11

Biomarker-based Clinical Trials

Edward L. Korn

Boris Freidlin

CONTENTS

11.1 Introduction

Biomarkers offer the potential to improve patient care by directing therapies to specific patients for whom they are most likely to work. This is especially true in the era of targeted therapies, for which it is thought that an understanding of the characteristics of a patient's tumor and how a targeted agent interacts with those characteristics should help personalize therapy for patients. How to incorporate biomarkers into the clinical trials used to develop and establish the benefit of a new agent (possibly in a subset of patients defined by their biomarker status) is not completely straightforward. The outline of this chapter is as follows. The chapter begins with a brief discussion of assessing the analytic performance of biomarker; before using a biomarker clinically, one would want to ensure that the biomarker is accurately measuring what it is supposed to be measuring. Next, we consider the distinction between prognostic versus predictive biomarkers. Prognostic and predictive biomarkers would be used in different ways in patient care, and so the careful assessment of the prognostic and predictive ability of a biomarker in clinical trials is important. We then discuss biomarkers and their potential roles in phase I, II, and III trials in successive sections. We end with a brief summary.

11.2 Analytic Performance of a Biomarker

Before definitively assessing a biomarker in clinical trials for its potential clinical utility, it is important to assure its analytic validity (accuracy and precision). That is, the biomarker assay should consistently capture the biological characteristic it is supposed to be measuring. Assessing analytic performance includes a number of considerations: The biomarker assay should yield reproducible results. If the same specimen is analyzed twice, then one should obtain very similar results each time; that is, the assay should have good precision. If different laboratories or different specimen-handling procedures (including timing between specimen collection and assay testing) are going to be used in practice, then reproducibility needs to be assessed across these different conditions. Although not part of the analytic performance of the biomarker assay, it can also be important in some applications to have the assay results be reproducible if multiple specimens are obtained from the same individual. The biomarker should be measuring what it is supposed to be measuring; that is, the assay should be accurate. This can be relatively easy to assess if the biomarker is measuring a chemical in the blood, but in general can be difficult if the biomarker is measuring something more nebulous. Sometimes there exist more costly or invasive techniques that can be used as a reference standard for comparison to help with this assessment. The biomarker assay should be "locked down" (i.e., prospectively specified). As well as the assay protocol not changing, the numerical methods used must be precisely defined: "Tuning parameters" (if any) need to stop being tuned, what assay results are considered valid versus "not determined" needs to be defined, and, in general, cut-points for continuous-valued assays that need to be dichotomized for binary biomarkers should be fixed. After being locked down, the analytic performance of the biomarker assay will need to be reassessed on a new set of specimens for independent validation. Because of the importance of quickly assessing new agents, the development of the biomarker assay may still be in progress during the early clinical testing of the agent. However, for use in definitive clinical testing, the biomarker assay will need to be fixed and its analytic performance will need to be confirmed as sufficient. The analytic performance required may depend on how the biomarker is going to be used in the clinical trial: determining eligibility, directing treatment, or being used for stratification. Detailed discussion of validating the analytic performance of biomarkers, including reference to regulatory documents, is given elsewhere [8, 26, 47].

11.3 Prognostic and Predictive Biomarkers

A prognostic biomarker distinguishes between patients who will have relatively good outcomes versus relatively bad outcomes when they are treated with no treatment, or, more generally, with a standard treatment or any treatment. It can be considered as a measure of the natural history of the disease [9]. A predictive biomarker separates patients into subgroups where the relative treatment benefit of one specific treatment over another specific treatment is different depending upon the biomarker value. With a single treatment, a prognostic biomarker separates patients who do relatively well versus relatively poorly. When there are multiple treatments being considered, for any given treatment, patients need to do better with a positive biomarker value than a negative biomarker. A prognostic biomarker can be a useful stratification variable in a randomized clinical trial (RCT). It can also sometimes be directly clinically useful if it identifies a subgroup of patients who will do so well that they do not need further treatment, or will do so poorly that they should be offered experimental treatments.

Figure 11.1 displays survival curves for a hypothetical predictive biomarker for an experimental and standard treatment, showing patients do better with the experimental treatment when they are biomarker positive and do better with the standard treatment when they are biomarker negative. This is not an unusual scenario when the standard treatment is a nonspecific treatment (e.g., chemotherapy) that works moderately well on everyone and the experimental treatment is a targeted therapy that works very well on biomarker-positive patients and not at all on biomarker-negative patients. The curves in Figure 11.1 display a qualitative interaction between the treatment and the biomarker status, i.e., the treatment effect goes in opposite direction depending on biomarker status. The curves in Figure 11.2, on the other hand, display a quantitative interaction — the treatment effect is different depending on biomarker status (being larger for the biomarker-positive patients), but in the same direction. The biomarker in Figure 11.2 is also predictive (i.e., the treatment-by-biomarker interaction is not zero). However, whether

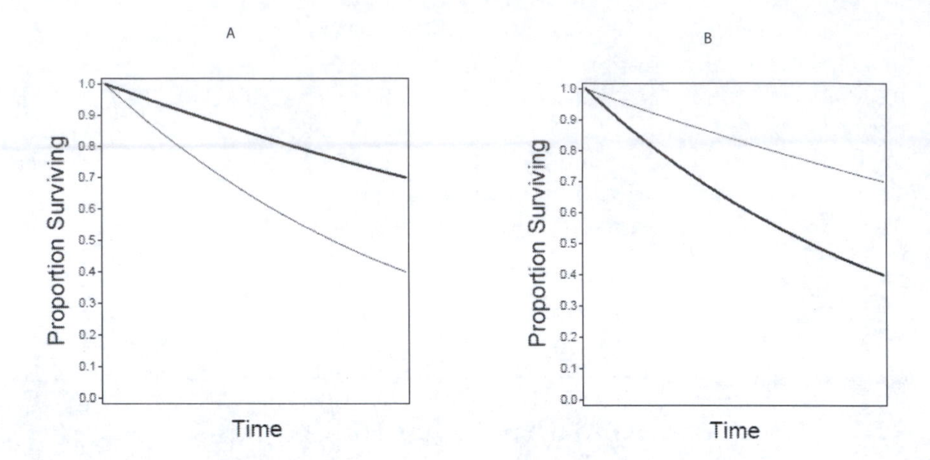

FIGURE 11.1: Survival curves for patients given a standard treatment (light lines) or an experimental treatment (dark lines) stratified by a hypothetical predictive biomarker showing a qualitative interaction. (A) Biomarker positive patients. (B) Biomarker negative patients.

this biomarker has clinical utility (i.e., could be useful in directing patient treatment) is questionable, and might depend on the relative benefit of one treatment over the other in the two biomarker subgroups, and the relative toxicity and costs of the two treatments.

Biomarkers can be both prognostic and predictive at the same time, and a biomarker can be predictive for a pair of treatments but not for another pair of treatments. Thus, it can sometimes be difficult to categorize a biomarker as prognostic and/or predictive. However, what is important is to examine the treatment-specific survival curves (or other appropriate clinical outcomes) stratified by biomarker status to assess whether the effects seen are sufficient that biomarker will be useful as a stratification variable in future trials and/or can be used to direct treatment for future patients. We now present some real examples of prognostic and predictive biomarkers.

Figure 11.3 displays the overall survival curves for a randomized trial of panitumumab versus best supportive care for metastatic colorectal cancer patients, stratified by KRAS status [2]. For these two treatments and with overall survival as the outcome variable, the biomarker (KRAS status) is not predictive (between treatment-arm hazard ratios = 1.02 and 0.99 for the mutant and wild-type KRAS groups), but is prognostic, with wild-type KRAS patients doing better than mutant KRAS patients (hazard ratio = 0.67) [2]. Figure 11.4 displays the progression-free survival curves for the predictive biomarker EGFR mutation status in the setting of gefitinib versus chemotherapy (carboplatin plus paclitaxel) for non-small cell lung cancer patients. In

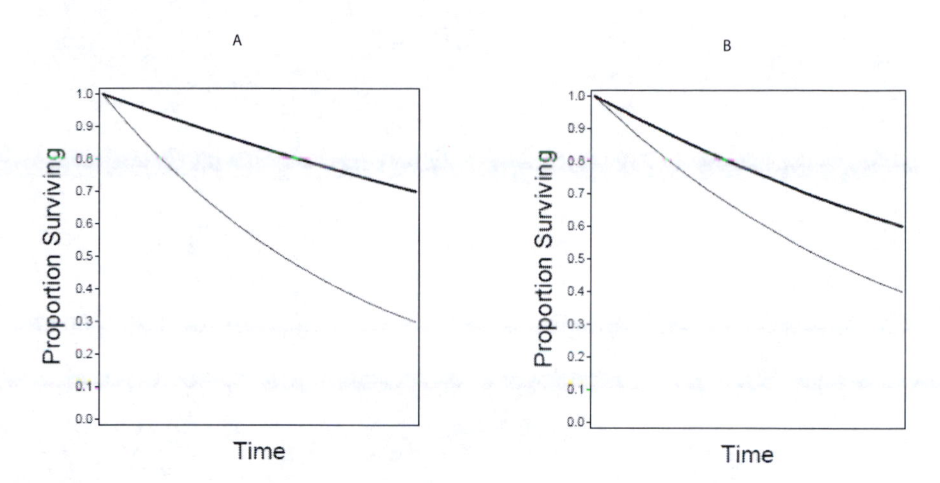

FIGURE 11.2: Survival curves for patients given a standard treatment (light lines) or an experimental treatment (dark lines) stratified by a hypothetical predictive biomarker showing a quantitative interaction. (A) Biomarker positive patients. (B) Biomarker negative patients.

fact, the interaction between biomarker and treatment arm is qualitative, with EGFR-mutation-positive patients doing better with the gefitinib (hazard ratio = 0.48) and EGFR-mutation-negative patients doing worse with the gefitinib (hazard ratio = 2.85) [44]. Clearly, this biomarker is quite useful in this setting to help decide which patients should get gefitinib versus standard chemotherapy. Our last example concerns a biomarker (IL-6) that is predictive but with only a quantitative interaction with treatment arm: Figure 11.5 displays the progression-free survival curves for pazopanib versus placebo for locally advanced/metastatic renal cell carcinoma patients stratified by IL-6 status. For patients with high IL-6, the treatment effect is larger (hazard ratio = 0.31) than for patients with low IL-6 (hazard ratio = 0.55) [62]. Since the pazopanib is better than the placebo regardless of the biomarker status, it is not clear whether this biomarker would be useful in this setting.

Note that the examples given for predictive biomarkers involve patients receiving a standard and new treatment. In special circumstances, it may be possible to assess whether a biomarker is predictive with an evaluation of only patients treated with a new treatment: If it is known that the outcomes are invariably bad when patients are treated with a standard treatment (e.g., no clinical tumor responses), and patients have a good (bad) outcome when treated with the new agent when their biomarker status is positive (negative), then the biomarker is predictive. Care is required in this type of analysis because of the usual caveats when making historical comparisons, and because a prognostic biomarker could easily be misidentified as a predictive biomarker

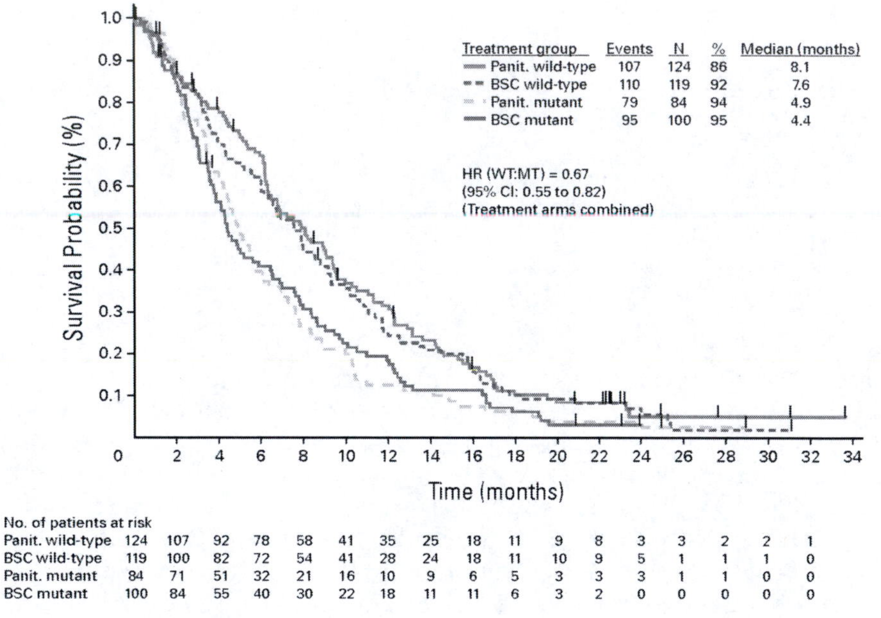

FIGURE 11.3: Overall survival curves by treatment arm (panitumumab versus best supportive care, BSC) and KRAS status (wild-type versus mutant) for metastatic colorectal cancer patients demonstrating that KRAS status is prognostic but not predictive in this setting. Figure is Figure 5 from Amado et al. [2] with permission.

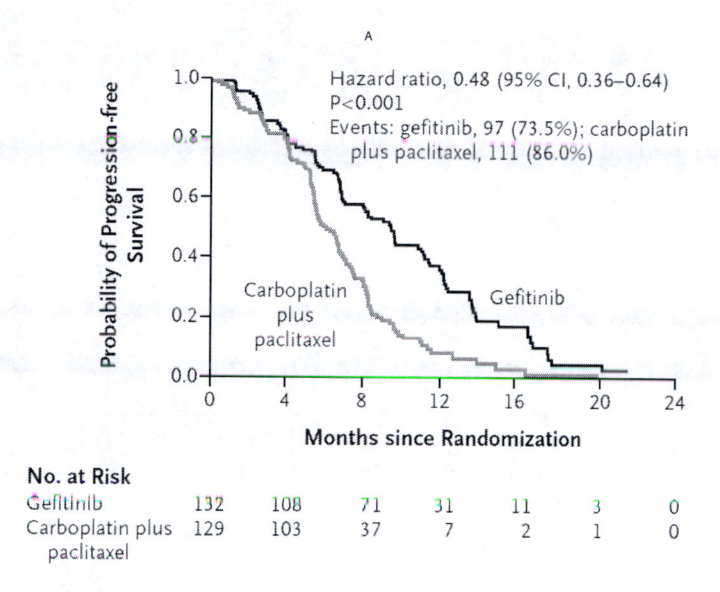

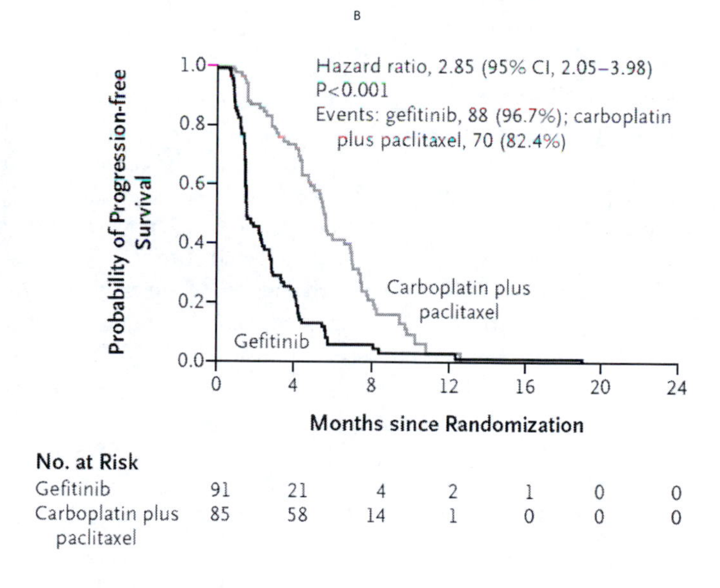

FIGURE 11.4: Progression-free survival curves by treatment arm (gefitinib versus carboplatin plus paclitaxel) for EGFR-mutation positive (A) and EGFR-mutation-negative (B) non-small cell lung cancer patients demonstrating the EGFR status is predictive and demonstrates a qualitative interaction with treatment arm in this setting. Figure is Figure 2B,C from Mok et al. [44] with permission.

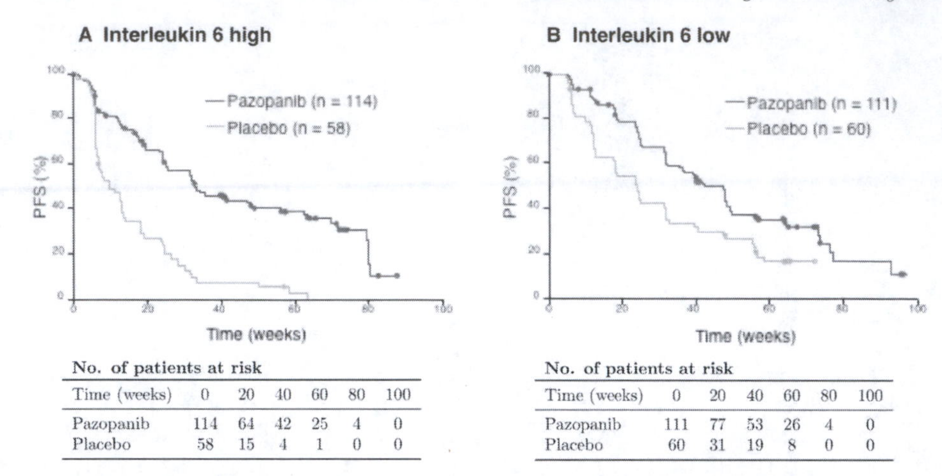

No. of patients at risk

Time (weeks)	0	20	40	60	80	100
Pazopanib	114	64	42	25	4	0
Placebo	58	15	4	1	0	0

No. of patients at risk

Time (weeks)	0	20	40	60	80	100
Pazopanib	111	77	53	26	4	0
Placebo	60	31	19	8	0	0

FIGURE 11.5: Progression-free survival (PFS) curves by treatment arm (pazopanib versus placebo) for interleukin-6 high (A) and interleukin-6 low (B) locally advanced/metastatic renal cell carcinoma patients demonstrating the interleukin-6 status is predictive and demonstrates a quantitative interaction with treatment arm in this setting. Figure is Figure 2A,B from Polley et al. [48] with permission, adapted from Figure 2A of Tran et al. [62].

unless the outcomes with standard treatments are known to be universally bad. This latter criterion may be hard to assess with survival-type (time-to-event) endpoints. For example, it would be tenuous to characterize a biomarker that categorizes five percent of the population as biomarker positive as predictive because these five percent of the patients treated with a new therapy have better survival than (i) patients previously treated with standard therapy and (ii) concurrent biomarker-negative patients treated with the new therapy. In some applications, the "biomarker" will offer predictions of responsiveness to a panel of potential treatments (chemoresponse assays). For example, Crystal et al. [11] developed cell lines from patient tumors that were resistant to first-line therapy and then tested these cell lines against a panel of 76 agents. Since the predictive ability of a biomarker is usually defined in terms of two treatments and a single prediction, there are some challenging conceptual issues as to what is meant by a predictive versus prognostic biomarker in this setting [34, 36, 61].

11.4 Biomarkers in Phase I Trials

Phase I trials are used to determine an appropriate dose level (and schedule) of a new agent (or a new combination of agents) to be used in further testing (Chapter 6). Historically, with cytotoxic chemotherapy, one assumes that (a) the clinical benefit of an agent increases with increasing dose, (b) the toxicity of an agent increases with increasing dose, and (c) there is a dose with acceptable toxicity that provides clinical benefit [31]. For targeted agents, there is the possibility of using biomarkers in a phase I trial to help find a dose level that has sufficient biologic activity below the maximum tolerated dose, and various trial designs have been suggested for this purpose [4, 21, 25, 40, 43, 50, 65]. Although trial designs using a biomarker to determine the recommended dose level sound appealing, they have been used little in practice [23, 46]. This could be because of concerns that the effects seen on a biomarker may not represent the target effect seen in the tumor, tumor target effects may not correlate with clinical benefit, and the agent may work by mechanisms other than the effect on the putative target because of an incomplete understanding of the tumor biology [51]. Even if a biomarker is not used to determine the recommended dose level, it makes sense to evaluate it in early trials to see if the target of the agent is being sufficiently affected [5]. Another design using a biomarker is the phase 0 design [55]. In this design the dose levels tested are assumed to be in a range that is pharmacodynamically active, but so low as not to have toxicity or clinical benefit. The aim of the design is to demonstrate dose levels where the agent has sufficient pharmacodynamic effects on the target as a method to eliminate inactive agents or potentially choose among competing analogues.

11.5 Biomarkers in Phase II Trials

Phase II trials assess preliminary efficacy of a new therapy to determine whether further development in definitive phase III trials is warranted (Chapter 7). Historically, single-arm trials using objective response rate as the endpoint have been widely used to show activity for cytotoxic agents. In these situations, it is expected that no responses would be seen without treatment. However, a single-arm trial design is generally not appropriate when it is expected that the agent may be effective but not yield responses, for example, when the agent is cytostatic [33]. The exception to this would be when one is expecting a very large treatment effect on a non-response endpoint, which could then be targeted for the outcome. For example, if one-year survival is less than 5% with standard agents, one might find an observed one-year survival of 30% with a new agent compelling enough to proceed with development of the agent. A single-arm trial is also generally not appropriate when the experimental agent is being combined with a standard agent that has activity. An exception to this would be there is an extensive meta-analysis available of trials with standard agents so that the trial-to-trial variability of the outcome results can be factored into whether the combination therapy is sufficiently active [35]. In cases where single-arm trials are inappropriate, randomized screening phase II trial designs have been proposed that randomize the therapy between the new agent and a control agent [54]. In a randomized phase II trial, a biomarker could potentially be used as an endpoint instead of a clinical endpoint. One would desire some evidence that the biomarker is a surrogate for clinical outcome, i.e., changes in the biomarker (e.g., relative to a control treatment) will lead to changes in clinical outcome. However, even if one has evidence that a biomarker is a reasonable surrogate for a set of treatments (perhaps from a meta-analysis [32]), there will be an extrapolation to assume that it will be a reasonable surrogate for a new agent, especially if the new agent has a different mechanism of action than previous treatments. With a one-armed trial, it can be difficult to define the change from baseline biomarker value that would be considered sufficient biologic activity to warrant proceeding to a phase III trial. The more promising application of biomarkers in phase II trials is to help define how, if at all, the biomarker should be used to define the population to be tested in a future phase III trial. We consider separately trial designs with and without control treatment arms.

11.5.1 Trials without a Control Arm

With a response rate endpoint and a single biomarker, one could perform a single-arm trial restricted to biomarker-positive patients and look for activity. Care is required here, as the biomarker could be prognostic, so that the biomarker-positive patients would do better no matter what therapy they received. This would be a problem if one were using a non-response endpoint or a combination therapy with a known active agent (the two exceptions mentioned above), as the new therapy could incorrectly appear better than the historical data which is not restricted to biomarker-positive patients [42].

A trial of a new agent could estimate response rates in the biomarker-positive and biomarker-negative subgroups. One might want to consider enrolling a sufficient number of biomarker-positive patients for evaluation in that subgroup. This could be done with two-stage design that enrolls differing numbers of patients in the subgroups in the second stage of accrual based on the number of responders in the two subgroups in the first stage [29, 49]. Sometimes an evaluation can be done retrospectively by evaluating the biomarker on stored specimens of patients treated with the agent. For example, the first demonstrations that EGFR mutation status was predictive of response to gefitinib (an EGFR inhibitor) were done retrospectively [39, 45]. With multiple biomarkers, there are two situations to consider. In the first, each biomarker has its own associated targeted agent. An example is the NCI MATCH trial, in which solid-tumor or lymphoma patients who have progressed on standard therapy are assigned to one of a set of 20–25 targeted agents based on having a relevant molecular abnormality [1]. The outcome is the response rate for each of the targeted agents. When the multiple biomarkers do not each have an associated targeted therapy, a retrospective approach is possible that examines in an exploratory fashion a number of biomarkers to see which, if any, are associated with good responses to a group of patients given the same (or a set of) treatments. A prospective approach randomizes patients to different treatments and evaluates a (small) set of biomarkers on the patients to look for associations. An example is the BATTLE trial, where chemorefractory non-small cell lung cancer patients were randomly assigned to four therapies and were simultaneously categorized into five biomarker subgroups [30]. These types of exploratory approaches would be appropriate when one has little idea about the relationships between the biomarkers and the therapies.

11.5.2 Randomized Screening Trials with a Control Arm

When a phase II randomized comparison with a control therapy is required, one can formally design a trial to examine the treatment effect (e.g., hazard ratio) in the biomarker-positive and biomarker-negative subgroups [18]. For example, Figure 11.6 shows a design that is targeting a hazard ratio of 2.0 in the biomarker-positive group: First the treatment is tested in the biomarker-positive subgroup (Step 1). If that test does not reject (the null hypothesis), the treatment is tested in the overall group (Step 2A). If that test does not reject, it is recommended that there be no phase III testing of the new therapy. If the test does reject in Step 2A, it is recommended that a phase III trial be done without using the biomarker. If the new therapy is statistically significantly better than the control therapy in the biomarker-positive subgroup (Step 1), then the 80% confidence interval for the hazard ratio in the biomarker-negative subgroup is examined (Step 2B) to decide whether to recommend a phase III enrichment design (described in Section 11.6.1) where the enrollment is restricted to biomarker-positive patients (when the new therapy does not appear to work in the biomarker-negative subgroup), a phase III trial without the biomarker (when the new therapy appears to work very well in the biomarker-negative subgroup), or a biomarker-stratified design (described in Section 11.6.2) in which the treatment effect is assessed in both the biomarker-positive and biomarker-negative subgroups. This randomized phase II design presumes that if the new therapy does not work in the biomarker-positive subgroup then it will now work in the biomarker-negative subgroup, and has good properties when this assumption is true [18].

When there are multiple biomarkers, one can randomize patients to an agent suggested by their biomarker versus a control treatment. For example, the NCI MPACT trial (NCT01827384) randomizes advanced cancer patients with tumor mutations in one of three genetic pathways to an agent targeting

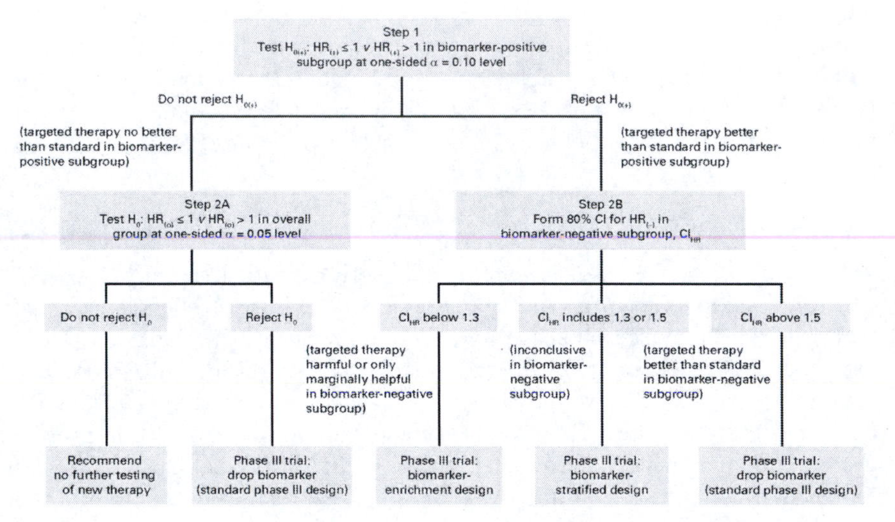

FIGURE 11.6: Decision algorithm for recommendation of phase III trial design based on the outcome of the phase II biomarker trial design. H_0 = null hypothesis in the overall group; $H_{0(+)}$ = null hypothesis in the biomarker-positive subgroup; $HR_{(+)}$ = hazard ratio of standard therapy relative to targeted therapy in biomarker-positive subgroup; $HR_{(-)}$ = hazard ratio of standard therapy relative to targeted therapy in biomarker-negative subgroup; $HR_{(o)}$ = hazard ratio of standard therapy relative to targeted therapy in overall group. Figure is Figure 1 from Freidlin et al. [18] with permission.

that pathway or to an agent not targeting that pathway. In a more exploratory vein, the I-SPY 2 trial randomly assigns locally advanced breast cancer patients to differing investigational neoadjuvant therapies and simultaneously assesses multiple biomarkers [3]. As with phase II trials without control arms, it is possible to analyze biomarkers retrospectively on a completed randomized phase II trial.

11.6 Biomarkers in Phase III Trials

The final stage of clinical development for a new therapy is a definitive phase III RCT. With a predictive biomarker, one can not only determine that the new treatment works better than a standard treatment, but also identify a subpopulation where it works [13]. At the time when a phase III RCT is being designed, the degree of confidence in the biomarker's ability to reliably separate a subpopulation that benefits versus a subpopulation that does not may vary considerably. The choice of an appropriate phase III design depends on the strength of the biomarker credentials [15]. In this section, we review how to select suitable phase III statistical trial designs based on the degree of confidence in the biomarker. In particular, we will consider situations where the credentials for the biomarker are compelling, strong, or weak.

11.6.1 Biomarkers with Compelling Credentials

If the biomarker credentials are compelling, that is, there is convincing evidence that the benefit of the new treatment, if any, is limited to the biomarker-positive subgroup, it is appropriate to restrict eligibility to that biomarker-defined subset of patients. This simple and efficient approach, displayed in Figure 11.7, is called an enrichment design. Because large treatment effects would be targeted in the sensitive subpopulation, enrichment trials typically require relatively small sample sizes. At the same time, a substantial number of patients may have to be screened to enroll the required number of biomarker-positive patients if the prevalence of biomarker positivity in the broad population is low. In general, sample size considerations and the analysis plans for enrichment designs are straightforward. The analysis is based on assessing overall treatment effect in the randomized study population (biomarker-positive patients) with the sample size determined to provide adequate power to detect the desired treatment effect (at a one-sided significance level appropriate for phase III studies, typically 0.025). Because the enrichment design is focused on the subpopulation where the new treatment works, it can require a considerably smaller sample size than a trial in the overall population [58].

The enrichment approach was used to design a phase III trial of the BRAF inhibitor vemurafenib in patients with metastatic melanoma [7]. The

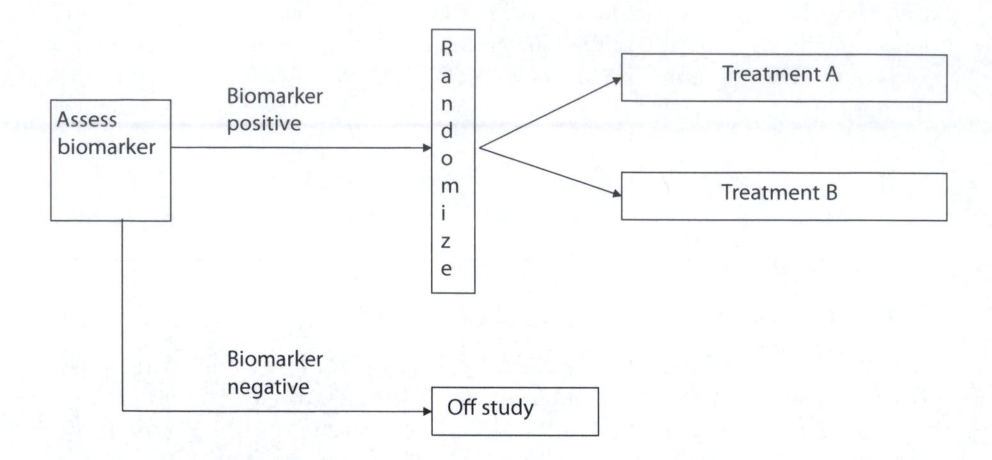

FIGURE 11.7: Enrichment design (Treatment A is thought to be potentially useful for biomarker-positive patients and Treatment B is standard therapy.) Figure is Figure 1B from Freidlin et al. [17] with permission.

biomarker was defined as presence of the BRAF V600E mutation. The trial screened 2107 melanoma patients to identify 675 patients who were biomarker positive and then were randomly assigned to treatment with either vemurafenib or standard chemotherapy. The results demonstrated improvements in both overall survival and progression-free survival (PFS) with the use of vemurafenib in BRAF mutation-positive patients. The enrichment trial-design approach is focused on the biomarker-positive population and provides no information on the treatment effect in the biomarker-negative population. Consequently, in the absence of compelling evidence that treatment benefit is limited to the biomarker-positive subgroup, a positive enrichment study fails to address the key issue of whether the biomarker has clinical utility. That is, the enrichment design does not provide evidence on whether the costs and inconvenience associated with using the biomarker to select patients for treatment in routine clinical practice are worthwhile, as the treatment may also work in the biomarker-negative subgroup. Furthermore, use of an enrichment trial design in the absence of compelling evidence of the lack of treatment benefit in biomarker-negative patients leads to uncertainty with regard to application of the new treatment in future clinical practice. For example, consider the adjuvant use of trastuzumab (a monoclonal HER2 receptor antibody) in breast cancer. Trastuzumab was assessed in two adjuvant RCTs that used enrichment designs, in which eligibility was restricted to the approximately 20% of patients whose tumours were considered HER2-positive [52]. Although these studies established a significant benefit for adjuvant trastuzumab therapy in this enriched HER2-positive population, questions about a possible trastuzumab benefit in the HER2-negative population remain open [37, 41]. When there are multiple biomarkers (with associated targeted agents) it can be efficient to have a "master protocol" in which patients are screened for the biomarkers and then offered participation in different randomized trials depending upon which they are eligible for. This can be especially useful when the biomarker-defined subgroups are small proportions of the population. For example, the ALCHEMIST trial considers the adjuvant treatment of non-small cell lung adenocarcinoma; approximately 8000 patients will be screened for the 15% with EGFR mutations and the 5% with ALK-fusion genes. These positive-screened patients will be offered participation in a trial of erlotinib (an EGFR inhibitor) versus placebo or crizotinib (an ALK inhibitor) versus placebo, respectively [1].

11.6.2 Biomarkers with Strong Credentials

Next we consider predictive biomarkers with strong but less than compelling credentials. That is, there is sufficiently convincing evidence to assume that the treatment is more likely to be effective in the biomarker-positive than in the biomarker-negative subgroup, but a clinically meaningful effect in biomarker-negative patients cannot be ruled out. In particular, if the biomarker is ineffective in the biomarker-positive subgroup then it will be ineffective in the biomarker-negative subgroup. In this scenario, a biomarker-stratified trial design is the preferred option [17]. Biomarker-stratified designs randomly assign both biomarker-positive and biomarker-negative patients to the treatments under investigation. There are two approaches to this. In one, all patients are randomized with their biomarker assessed concurrently to the treatment or later (Figure 11.8A). In the other, the biomarker status is determined before randomization (Figure 11.8B), and thus can be used to exclude patients from the study who do not have an evaluable biomarker status or to stratify the randomization by biomarker status. A potential advantage of the second approach is that it promotes sufficient specimen collection for biomarker evaluation, although this goal can be achieved by requiring specimen collection for a patient to be eligible for the trial. A disadvantage of the second approach is that it requires waiting for the biomarker evaluation in order for patients to start treatment. Some concerns have been raised related to estimation of the biomarker-subgroup treatment effect if the first approach is used, in particular, when only a small fraction of patients have biomarker status determined [64]. However, if the biomarker ascertainment is done independently of treatment assignment, the treatment comparisons should have internal validity [57].

The goal of the biomarker-stratified design is to provide a reliable assessment of the treatment effect in each biomarker subgroup to maximize the probability of recommending a new treatment to only those patients who ben-

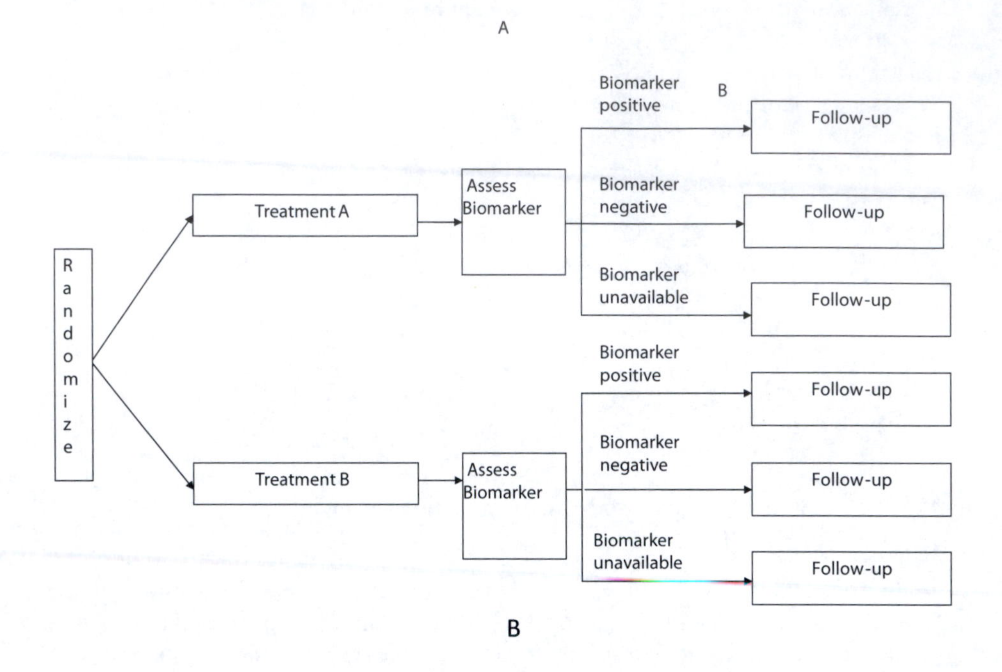

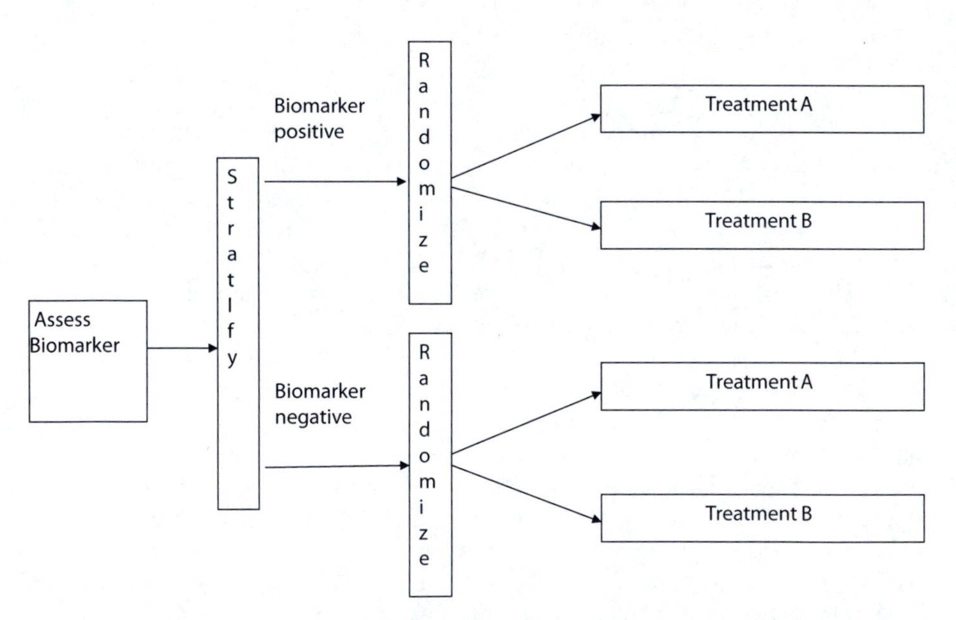

FIGURE 11.8: Biomarker-stratified designs. A. Biomarker assessed concurrently with treatment or later. B. Biomarker status determined before randomization. Figure 11.8B is Figure 1A from Freidlin et al. [17] with permission.

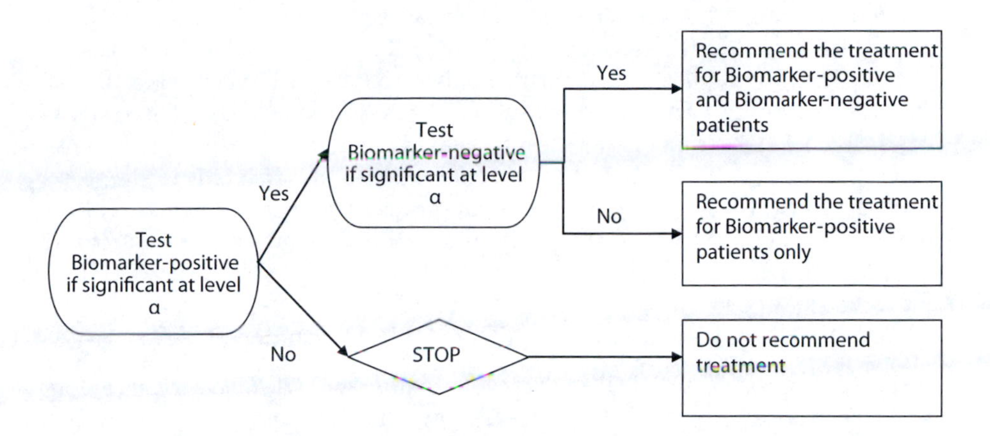

FIGURE 11.9: Sequential subgroup-specific strategy for analysis of biomarker-stratified design.

efit from it. There are several hypothesis testing strategies that can be used to analyze a biomarker-stratified trial, which will now be discussed.

11.6.2.1 Subgroup-specific Testing Strategies

A straightforward approach to analyze a biomarker-stratified trial is to use a parallel subgroup-specific strategy which tests the treatment effect separately in the biomarker-positive and the biomarker-negative populations. A common approach to controlling the type I error at level α is to use a Bonferroni correction: allocate the α between the tests of the null hypotheses of no treatment effect in each of the biomarker subgroups. For example, with α=0.025, one could use a 0.015 level for testing the biomarker-positive subgroup and a 0.010 level for testing the biomarker-negative subgroup. Because the underlying assumption for biomarkers with strong credentials is that the new treatment is unlikely to be effective in the biomarker-negative patients unless it is effective in the biomarker-positive ones, a sequential version of the subgroup-specific strategy is often used to improve design efficiency: First test for the treatment effect in the biomarker-positive patients using the significance level α; if this test is significant, then test the treatment effect in the biomarker-negative patients using the same α (Figure 11.9).

As an example of this strategy, consider the trial that evaluated the addition of panitumumab (an anti-EGFR monoclonal antibody) to standard chemotherapy in the first-line treatment of patients with metastatic colorectal cancer [12]. A retrospective analysis had previously suggested that having a tumor bearing KRAS mutations was predictive of a poor response to treatment with anti-EGFR monoclonal antibodies. The trial was designed to assess the effect of the addition of panitumumab in KRAS wild-type and mutated subgroups separately; the assessment in the mutated KRAS subgroup was conditional on observing a significant result in the KRAS wild-type patients. In this study the addition of panitumumab resulted in a significant improvement in PFS in the KRAS wild-type subgroup of patients, whereas a worse outcome was observed with the addition of panitumumab in the subgroup of patients with KRAS mutations [12].

11.6.2.2 Biomarker-positive and Overall Strategies

Another approach to the analysis of biomarker-stratified trials is the biomarker-positive/overall testing strategy. This commonly used, albeit flawed, approach formally tests the treatment effect in the overall population and in the biomarker-positive patients, but not in the biomarker-negative patients. In the parallel version of this strategy, the treatment effect is assessed separately in the overall population and the biomarker-positive patients, with type I error typically controlled by allocating α between the two tests of the null hypotheses. For example, the SATURN trial that evaluated erlotinib in patients with non-small cell lung cancer was designed to simultaneously test the EGFR-positive subgroup (at a one-sided significance level of 0.01) and the overall population (at a one-sided significance level of 0.015), to result in an overall type I error rate controlled at $\alpha = 0.025$ [6]. In the sequential version of the biomarker-positive/overall testing strategy, one first tests the biomarker-positive subgroup using significance level α; if the test is significant then the treatment effect in the overall population is tested using the same α (Figure 11.10). For example, a randomized study evaluating the addition of lapatinib (which inhibits HER2) to letrozole in patients with metastatic breast cancer was designed to first evaluate this treatment in the HER2-positive subgroup, using a test with a one-sided significance level α of 0.025; if the HER2-positive subgroup test results were significant, testing of the overall population (using the same α of 0.025) would follow [28].

A fundamental problem with the biomarker-positive/overall approach is that when the benefit of the new therapy is restricted to the biomarker-positive patients, the strategy may inappropriately recommend the treatment for the biomarker-negative subgroup [20, 53]. This is because even with no benefit in biomarker-negative patients, a statistically significant effect can still be observed in the overall population if the treatment effect in the biomarker-positive patients is large enough. (In theory, for treatments with a dramatic effect limited to the biomarker-positive patients, the probability of formally recommending ineffective therapy for the biomarker-negative patients approaches 100%.) In the context of the biomarkers with strong credentials, the scientific flaw in the biomarker-positive/overall approach becomes particularly appar-

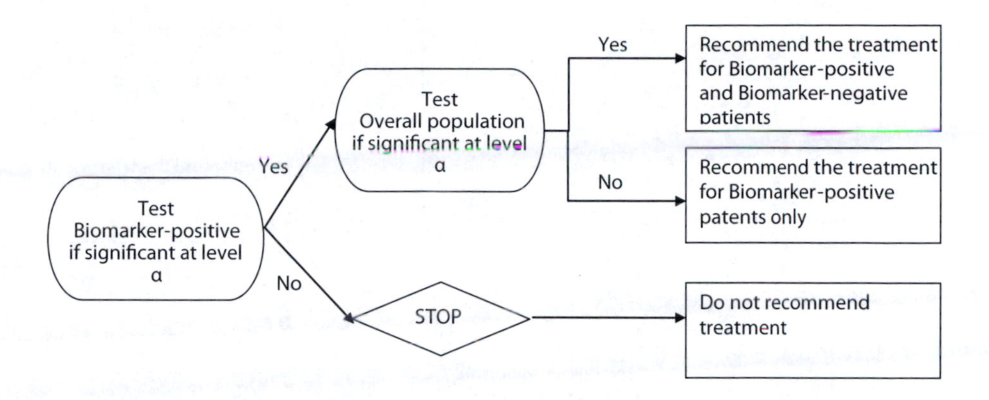

FIGURE 11.10: Sequential biomarker-positive/overall strategy for analysis of biomarker-stratified design.

ent in the sequential version of the design which proceeds to testing the overall effect after demonstration of treatment benefit in the biomarker-positive patients: After clinical benefit has been established in the biomarker-positive patients, the only clinically relevant issue is whether the treatment is beneficial in the biomarker-negative patients, not whether the average treatment effect in the overall population is significant. For example, in the lapatinib trial, the results of the protocol-specified biomarker-positive and overall population testing strategy indicated a statistically significant effect for lapatinib in the overall population [28]. Nevertheless, the investigators rightfully concluded that lapatinib should not be recommended for all patients because no evidence of a clinically meaningful benefit could be observed in the HER2-negative patients (even though the protocol-specified trial design did not involve a separate evaluation of the biomarker-negative subgroup).

11.6.2.3 Marker Sequential Test Design

An appealing feature of the biomarker-positive/overall strategy is that testing of the overall population allows borrowing of information from the biomarker-positive patients in providing a treatment recommendation for the biomarker-negative subgroup. This is an attractive approach when the treatment effect is homogeneous across the biomarker-defined subgroups, provided that the probability of recommending an ineffective treatment for the biomarker-negative patients is adequately controlled [20]. It is utilized in the Marker Sequential Test (MaST), which incorporates analyses of biomarker-positive and biomarker-negative subgroups, as well as the overall population while

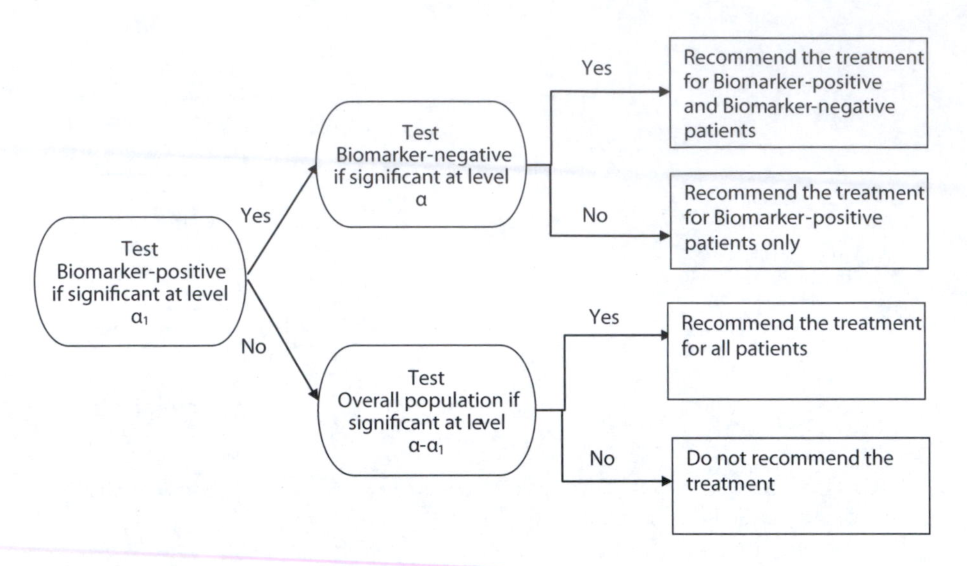

FIGURE 11.11: Marker sequential test (MaST) design. (α is the overall significance level.)

controlling the false-positive probability for the biomarker-negative subgroup [16]: First, the biomarker-positive subgroup is tested at a reduced significance level (α_1), which can be any value less than the desired overall significance level α of the trial (e.g., α_1=0.023 when α=0.025). If the results of this test are significant, then the biomarker-negative subgroup is tested at significance level α. If the results in the biomarker-positive subgroup are not significant, the overall population is tested at significance level $\alpha - \alpha_1$ (Figure 11.11).

An example of a trial using the MaST design is E1910, a phase III RCT investigating the addition of blinatumomab to chemotherapy in patients with acute lymphoblastic leukemia being conducted by the ECOG-ACRIN cancer research group. Minimal residual disease (MRD) is believed to be a predictor of blinatumomab benefit in this setting. Therefore, the study was designed using the MaST design with MRD as the biomarker. In this trial, $\alpha = 0.025$ and $\alpha_1 = 0.020$ [20]. The MaST design controls the overall type I error rate at significance level α when the treatment does not work in either subgroup. Furthermore, as this strategy only tests the overall population when no significant effect is detected in the biomarker-positive subgroup, it reduces the risk of erroneously concluding that the treatment is beneficial in the overall population when positive findings in the overall group are driven by a benefit limited to biomarker-positive patients.

11.6.2.4 Sample Size Considerations

Biomarker-stratified trials are used when there are strong credentials for the predictive value of the biomarker. Therefore, the sample size considerations for these trials are generally driven by the biomarker-positive subgroup. For example, for a trial using a sequential group-specific strategy, the study sample size is determined by the need to enroll sufficient number of biomarker-positive patients to have the required power for a desired treatment effect in this subgroup (with significance level α). (Note that this is the same sample size as needed to be screened for the enrichment design.) For the MaST design, one can calculate sample size of the biomarker-positive subgroup using significance level α_1 (instead of α). This results in only a minor increase in sample size compared to the corresponding sequential subgroup-specific design. For example, for α=.025, less than a 4% increase in sample size would be required to have the same power for an agent that is only effective in the biomarker-positive patients. Note that since the loss of power is negligible, in practice one can use the MaST design with the same sample size as the subgroup-specific strategy.

11.6.3 Biomarkers with Weak Credentials

At the time a phase III trial is designed, there sometimes is no clear evidence that the biomarker can separate sensitive versus non-sensitive subgroups. That is, there is a good possibility that the treatment is broadly effective. For these weak-biomarker-credential settings, a "fallback" design that sequentially tests the overall population and biomarker-positive subgroup can be used [59]: First, the treatment is tested in the overall population using a reduced significance level α_1 ($< \alpha$). If the results are significant, the treatment is considered effective in the overall population; if the results of the overall test are not significant, then the treatment effect is evaluated in the biomarker-positive subgroup, using significance level of $\alpha - \alpha_1$ (Figure 11.12). Note that one can utilize the correlation between the overall and biomarker-positive test statistics to modestly increase the significance level used for the biomarker-positive subgroup [22]. From a formal hypothesis-testing perspective this analysis strategy is similar to the biomarker-positive/overall strategy for analysis of biomarker-stratified designs. However, unlike the biomarker-stratified design that is used for biomarkers with strong predictive credentials, the fallback design is based on the assumption that the treatment is very likely to be beneficial for all (or almost all) patients. The 'fallback' component that tests the biomarker-positive subgroup provides for the unlikely contingency that the benefit is limited to a relatively small biomarker-positive subgroup. The main goal of a fallback design is to have sufficient number of patients to achieve good power for a meaningful effect in the overall population. In contrast, sample size considerations for the biomarker-stratified designs that

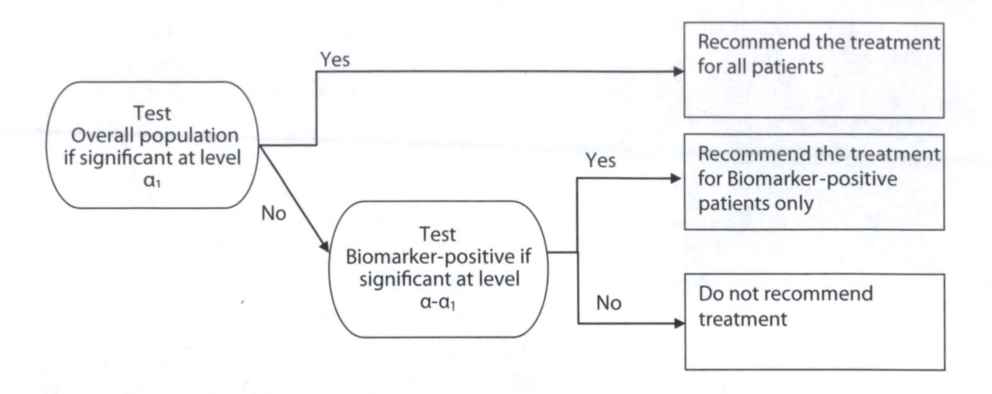

FIGURE 11.12: Fallback strategy for settings with weak biomarker credentials. (α is the overall significance level.)

focused on biomarkers with strong predictive credentials are typically driven by having sufficient power in the biomarker-positive subgroup.

The fallback strategy can also be used in settings where the biomarker has not been fully developed; since the treatment is expected to be effective in the overall population, the intent is to formally develop a biomarker only if the test in the overall population is negative. For example, in situations where a continuous or ordinal predictive score is available, but an optimal cutoff point for selecting the sensitive subgroup has not been established, a biomarker-adaptive threshold design can be used: First the treatment effect is tested in the overall population. If this overall test is statistically significant then the treatment is recommended for all patients. If results of the overall test are not significant, then the design provides a statistically rigorous assessment of whether there is a cutoff that defines a subgroup that benefits from the treatment [27]. When, no biomarker is available at the start of the phase III trial, the adaptive signature design [14, 19] utilizes the fallback strategy to carry out a prospectively defined development and validation of a biomarker based on high-dimensional data (e.g., multigene marker panels) if no treatment benefit is detected in the overall population.

11.6.4 Interim Monitoring

Most RCTs incorporate interim monitoring for ethical and efficiency reasons. It allows early stopping of a trial when accumulating outcome data demonstrate that (1) the new treatment is clearly superior to standard therapy (superiority), or (2) the new treatment will not be better than the standard therapy (inefficacy/futility) [24]. For enrichment trial designs, superiority and inefficacy monitoring can be performed in the usual manner on the randomized population. For biomarker-stratified trial designs (using sequential subgroup-specific or MaST analyses), it is important for the design to include interim monitoring for inefficacy in the biomarker-negative subgroup, as there is a good chance that the new therapy may be ineffective for these patients [17]. The trial could continue for the biomarker-positive subgroup even if it is stopped for inefficacy in the biomarker-negative subgroup. Additionally, superiority monitoring of the biomarker-positive subgroup can be conducted, and if that group crosses a superiority boundary at an interim analysis, one could stop the trial in the biomarker-positive subgroup and continue the trial with the biomarker-negative subgroup (and start superiority monitoring for this subgroup). A modification to studies with these designs is to first accrue only to the biomarker-positive group and, only if the results appear sufficiently promising, begin accruing to the whole population [38]. For the fallback design using a biomarker with weak credentials, interim monitoring is performed on the overall population. If the overall population crosses an inefficacy boundary, accrual stops for the biomarker-negative subgroup; the trial could continue in the biomarker-positive subgroup with interim monitoring for both inefficacy and superiority in that subgroup. Inefficacy monitoring would typically not be conducted in the biomarker-negative subgroup.

11.6.5 Retrospective Biomarker Analysis of Phase III Trial Data

Frequently, pre-randomization patient specimens are collected during a phase III trial that can be potentially used for a later biomarker evaluation. This can be done in an exploratory fashion, or it can be done rigorously in a "prospective-retrospective study" [60, 63]. To perform such a rigorous evaluation, the biomarker assay needs to be locked down, the procedures for the retrospective evaluation of the specimens must reproduce the results that would have been obtained if the specimens had been evaluated when first collected, the specimens need to be evaluated blinded with respect to treatment assignment and patient outcome, and the analysis plan needs to be prespecified in a protocol [48, 60].

11.6.6 Biomarker-strategy Designs

The biomarker-strategy design is sometimes used to compare a biomarker-guided treatment strategy to an alternative standard treatment. For a simplest case with two therapies A and B and a binary biomarker, the biomarker-strategy design proceeds as follows: Patients are randomly assigned to a control-arm standard treatment B or a biomarker-directed treatment arm where a patient receives treatment A if the biomarker is positive and treatment B if the biomarker is negative (Figure 11.13). Indeed, in this design the

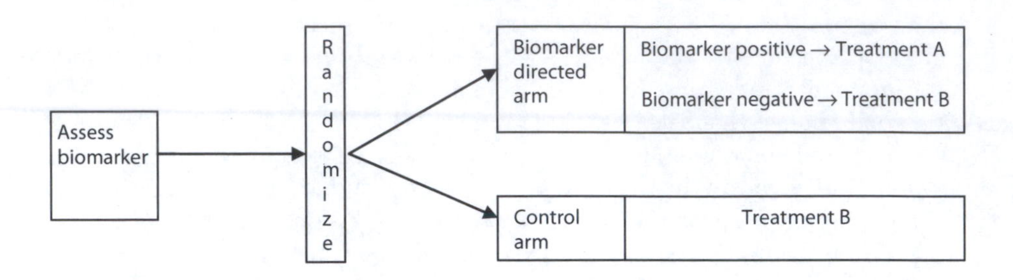

FIGURE 11.13: Biomarker-strategy design. (Treatment A is thought to be potentially useful for biomarker-positive patients and Treatment B is the standard therapy.) Figure is Figure 1C from Freidlin et al. [17] with permission.

experimental arm accurately reflects the therapeutic strategy under investigation. However, the design is not efficient because many patients on both arms will be treated with the same therapy, treatment B. Instead of using this inefficient design, one can use the arm-specific outcomes of a biomarker-stratified or enrichment design to estimate the same between-arm difference that would be seen in a biomarker-strategy design, but with a smaller required sample size. The loss of efficiency associated with biomarker-strategy design can be quantified in the context of hypothesis testing: For a setting with a biomarker population prevalence of p, approximately $1/p$ times more patients will have to be randomized in the biomarker-strategy design than randomized in the biomarker-stratified design (or screened in the enrichment design) to achieve the same power to detect the effect associated with the biomarker-guided treatment strategy [17]. For example, suppose the biomarker positivity rate was $1/3$ and one was considering performing a trial with 900 patients using a biomarker-strategy design. One could perform a biomarker-stratified design with 300 patients (or screen 300 patients and randomize 100 patients in an enrichment design) to achieve the same power.

Consequently, for simple settings involving few treatments there is no rationale for use of the biomarker-strategy design. In settings, where a biomarker is selecting among many alternative treatments (e.g., chemosensitivity assays) it may be impractical to perform a stratified design with a dozen strata or an enrichment design that has sufficient numbers of patients in each biomarker category. Under such circumstances the biomarker-strategy design may be considered if its limitations are understood and found acceptable: (1) The overall results of the trial can be negative even if the biomarker does identify a highly effective agent for a small subset of patients if the agents in the many of the other subsets are no better than the control treatment, (2) It is possible that the biomarker-strategy arm is deemed superior even if for a small biomarker-defined subgroup the biomarker-strategy assigns patients to an inferior treatment, and (3) The overall results of the trial can be positive even if the biomarker has no predictive ability if the agents being used in the biomarker-directed arm are better agents than those used in the control arm. To ameliorate this last limitation, one can randomly assign patients in the control arm to the standard and experimental treatments being used on the biomarker-directed arm [56]. An example of a trial using a biomarker-strategy design was a trial of docetaxel/cisplatin (standard arm) versus a biomarker-directed treatment arm for patients with metastatic non-small cell lung cancer [10]. In the biomarker-treatment directed arm, patients with low ERCC1 received docetaxel/cisplatin and patients with high ERCC1 received docetaxel/gemcitabine. Fifty-seven percent of the patients randomly assigned to the biomarker-directed arm received the same therapy (docetaxel/cisplatin) as the standard arm. Because there were only two treatment regimens involved, this was not a good use of the biomarker-strategy design.

11.7 Summary

The use of biomarkers to determine therapy on an individual basis is becoming more prevalent as improved understanding of cancer biology allows targeting of signaling pathways that are causing the cancer in specific individuals. The development of a targeted agent and its associated biomarker assay will frequently occur concurrently. Therefore, the biomarker will not be completely "locked down" when clinical trials that incorporate it are begun. However, the basic analytic validity of the biomarker should be assessed and verified on clinical specimens before it is used to direct therapy. Once a new targeted agent enters clinical trials, there are a number of choices needed to be made. In phase I, one could consider using effects on the target to choose a dose level rather than the conventionally used levels of acceptable toxicity. Even if this is not done, one can use the phase I data to ensure that target effects are sufficient at the recommended phase II dose, as well as to refine further the biomarker assay. In phase II, there is a choice between restricting accrual to patients who are positive for the biomarker, or having broad eligibility with a separate assessment of the activity in the biomarker-positive patients. When there are multiple biomarkers (that may define small subsets of patients) and multiple associated targeted agents, a master protocol that assigns patients to different agents is an efficient way to look for activity for the different agents. In phase III, depending upon the pre-trial level of evidence that the activity of the agent is restricted to biomarker-positive patients, one could consider an enrichment design (which restricts accrual to biomarker-positive patients) or a biomarker-stratified design (which accrues all comers). Although statistical methods have been developed that allow for some tuning of the biomarker assay quantification during a phase III trial, generally the biomarker assay should be completely defined at the start of a phase III trial. As more biomarkers and targeted agents are developed, the use of efficient phase III master protocols will become more prevalent.

Bibliography

[1] J. Abrams, B. Conley, M. Mooney, J. Zwiebel, A. Chen, J. J. Welch, N. Takebe, S. Malik, L. McShane, E. Korn, M. Williams, L. Staudt, and J. Doroshow. National Cancer Institute's precision medicine initiative for the new National Clinical Trials Network. *ASCO Educational Book 2014*, pages 71–76, 2014.

[2] R. G. Amado, M. Wolf, M. Peeters, E. Van Cutsem, S. Siena, D. J. Freeman, T. Juan, R. Sikorski, S. Suggs, R. Radinsky, S. D. Patterson, and D. D. Chang. Wild-type KRAS is required for panitumumab efficacy in patients with metastatic colorectal cancer. *Journal of Clinical Oncology*, 26(10):1626–34, 2008.

[3] A. D. Barker, C. C. Sigman, G. J. Kelloff, N. M. Hylton, D. A. Berry, and L. J. Esserman. I-SPY 2: an adaptive breast cancer trial design in the setting of neoadjuvant chemotherapy. *Clinical Pharmacology & Therapeutics*, 86(1):97–100, 2009.

[4] B. N. Bekele and Y. Shen. A Bayesian approach to jointly modeling toxicity and biomarker expression in a phase I/II dose-finding trial. *Biometrics*, 61(2):343–54, 2005.

[5] C. M. Booth, A. H. Calvert, G. Giaccone, M. W. Lobbezoo, L. K. Seymour, and E. A. Eisenhauer. Endpoints and other considerations in phase I studies of targeted anticancer therapy: recommendations from the task force on Methodology for the Development of Innovative Cancer Therapies (MDICT). *European Journal of Cancer*, 44(1):19–24, 2008.

[6] F. Cappuzzo, T. Ciuleanu, L. Stelmakh, S. Cicenas, A. Szczesna, E. Juhasz, E. Esteban, O. Molinier, W. Brugger, I. Melezinek, G. Klingelschmitt, B. Klughammer, and G. Giaccone. Erlotinib as maintenance treatment in advanced non-small cell lung cancer: a multicentre, randomised, placebo-controlled phase 3 study. *Lancet Oncology*, 11(6):521–9, 2010.

[7] P. B. Chapman, A. Hauschild, C. Robert, J. B. Haanen, P. Ascierto,

J. Larkin, R. Dummer, C. Garbe, A. Testori, M. Maio, D. Hogg, P. Lorigan, C. Lebbe, et al. Improved survival with vemurafenib in melanoma with BRAF V600E mutation. *New England Journal of Medicine*, 364(26):2507–16, 2011.

[8] G. M. Clark and L. M. McShane. Biostatistical considerations in development of biomarker-based tests to guide treatment decisions. *Statistics in Biopharmaceutical Research*, 3:549–560, 2011.

[9] G. M. Clark, D. M. Zborowski, J. L. Culbertson, M. Whitehead, M. Savoie, L. Seymour, and F. A. Shepherd. Clinical utility of epidermal growth factor receptor expression for selecting patients with advanced non-small cell lung cancer for treatment with erlotinib. *Journal of Thoracic Oncology*, 1(8):837–46, 2006.

[10] M. Cobo, D. Isla, B. Massuti, A. Montes, J. M. Sanchez, M. Provencio, N. Vinolas, L. Paz-Ares, G. Lopez-Vivanco, M. A. Munoz, E. Felip, et al. Customizing cisplatin based on quantitative excision repair cross-complementing 1 mRNA expression: a phase III trial in non-small cell lung cancer. *Journal of Clinical Oncology*, 25(19):2747–54, 2007.

[11] A. S. Crystal, A. T. Shaw, L. V. Sequist, L. Friboulet, M. J. Niederst, E. L. Lockerman, R. L. Frias, J. F. Gainor, A. Amzallag, P. Greninger, D. Lee, A. Kalsy, M. Gomez-Caraballo, L. Elamine, E. Howe, W. Hur, et al. Patient-derived models of acquired resistance can identify effective drug combinations for cancer. *Science*, 346(6216):1480–6, 2014.

[12] J. Y. Douillard, S. Siena, J. Cassidy, J. Tabernero, R. Burkes, M. Barugel, Y. Humblet, G. Bodoky, D. Cunningham, J. Jassem, F. Rivera, et al. Randomized, phase III trial of panitumumab with infusional fluorouracil, leucovorin, and oxaliplatin (FOLFOX4) versus FOLFOX4 alone as first-line treatment in patients with previously untreated metastatic colorectal cancer: the PRIME study. *Journal of Clinical Oncology*, 28(31):4697–705, 2010.

[13] U.S. Food and Drug Administration. Draft Guidance: Enrichment Strategies for Clinical Trials to Support Approval of Human Drugs and Biological Products, 2012.
http://www.fda.gov/downloads/Drugs/{\protect\newline}
GuidanceComplianceRegulatoryInformation/Guidances/UCM332181.
pdf.

[14] B. Freidlin, W. Jiang, and R. Simon. The cross-validated adaptive signature design. *Clinical Cancer Research*, 16(2):691–8, 2010.

[15] B. Freidlin and E. L. Korn. Biomarker enrichment strategies: matching trial design to biomarker credentials. *Nature Reviews Clinical Oncology*, 11(2):81–90, 2014.

[16] B. Freidlin, E. L. Korn, and R. Gray. Marker sequential test (mast) design. *Clinical Trials*, 11(1):19–27, 2014.

[17] B. Freidlin, L. M. McShane, and E. L. Korn. Randomized clinical trials with biomarkers: design issues. *Journal of the National Cancer Institute*, 102(3):152–60, 2010.

[18] B. Freidlin, L. M. McShane, M. Y. Polley, and E. L. Korn. Randomized phase II trial designs with biomarkers. *Journal of Clinical Oncology*, 30(26):3304–9, 2012.

[19] B. Freidlin and R. Simon. Adaptive signature design: an adaptive clinical trial design for generating and prospectively testing a gene expression signature for sensitive patients. *Clinical Cancer Research*, 11(21):7872–8, 2005.

[20] B. Freidlin, Z. Sun, R. Gray, and E. L. Korn. Phase III clinical trials that integrate treatment and biomarker evaluation. *Journal of Clinical Oncology*, 31(25):3158–61, 2013.

[21] H. S. Friedman, D. M. Kokkinakis, J. Pluda, A. H. Friedman, I. Cokgor, M. M. Haglund, D. M. Ashley, J. Rich, M. E. Dolan, A. E. Pegg, et al. Phase I trial of O6-benzylguanine for patients undergoing surgery for malignant glioma. *Journal of Clinical Oncology*, 16(11):3570–5, 1998.

[22] S. L. George. Statistical issues in translational cancer research. *Clinical Cancer Research*, 14(19):5954–8, 2008.

[23] B. H. Goulart, J. W. Clark, H. H. Pien, T. G. Roberts, S. N. Finkelstein, and B. A. Chabner. Trends in the use and role of biomarkers in phase I oncology trials. *Clinical Cancer Research*, 13(22 Pt 1):6719–26, 2007.

[24] S. Green, J. Benedetti, and J. Crowley. *Clinical Trials in Oncology, Second Edition.* Chapman & Hall. Boca Raton, USA, 2003.

[25] S. Hunsberger, L. V. Rubinstein, J. Dancey, and E. L. Korn. Dose escalation trial designs based on a molecularly targeted endpoint. *Statistics in Medicine*, 24(14):2171–81, 2005.

[26] L. Jennings, V. M. Van Deerlin, and M. L. Gulley. Recommended principles and practices for validating clinical molecular pathology tests. *Archives of Pathology & Laboratory Medicine*, 133(5):743–55, 2009.

[27] W. Jiang, B. Freidlin, and R. Simon. Biomarker-adaptive threshold design: a procedure for evaluating treatment with possible biomarker-defined subset effect. *Journal of the National Cancer Institute*, 99(13):1036–43, 2007.

[28] S. Johnston, J. Pippen, Jr., X. Pivot, M. Lichinitser, S. Sadeghi, V. Dieras, H. L. Gomez, G. Romieu, A. Manikhas, M. J. Kennedy, et al. Lapatinib combined with letrozole versus letrozole and placebo as first-line therapy for postmenopausal hormone receptor-positive metastatic breast cancer. *Journal of Clinical Oncology*, 27(33):5538–46, 2009.

[29] C. L. Jones and E. Holmgren. An adaptive Simon two-stage design for phase 2 studies of targeted therapies. *Contemporary Clinical Trials*, 28(5):654–61, 2007.

[30] E. S. Kim, R. S. Herbst, I. I. Wistuba, J. J. Lee, G. R. Blumenschein, Jr., A. Tsao, D. J. Stewart, M. E. Hicks, J. Erasmus, Jr., S. Gupta, et al. The BATTLE trial: personalizing therapy for lung cancer. *Cancer Discovery*, 1(1):44–53, 2011.

[31] E. L. Korn. Nontoxicity endpoints in phase I trial designs for targeted, non-cytotoxic agents. *Journal of the National Cancer Institute*, 96(13):977–8, 2004.

[32] E. L. Korn, P. S. Albert, and L. M. McShane. Assessing surrogates as trial endpoints using mixed models. *Statistics in Medicine*, 24(2):163–82, 2005.

[33] E. L. Korn, S. G. Arbuck, J. M. Pluda, R. Simon, R. S. Kaplan, and M. C. Christian. Clinical trial designs for cytostatic agents: are new approaches needed? *Journal of Clinical Oncology*, 19(1):265–72, 2001.

[34] E. L. Korn and B. Freidlin. Evaluation of chemoresponse assays as predictive markers. *British Journal of Cancer*, 112(4):621–3, 2015.

[35] E. L. Korn, P. Y. Liu, S. J. Lee, J. A. Chapman, D. Niedzwiecki, V. J. Suman, J. Moon, V. K. Sondak, M. B. Atkins, et al. Meta-analysis of phase II cooperative group trials in metastatic stage IV melanoma to determine progression-free and overall survival benchmarks for future phase II trials. *Journal of Clinical Oncology*, 26(4):527–34, 2008.

[36] E. L. Korn, V. K. Sondak, C. A. Bertelsen, and D. H. Kern. Analysis of the clinical utility of a predictive chemosensitivity assay. *Statistics in Medicine*, 4(4):527–34, 1985.

[37] I. E. Krop and H. J. Burstein. Trastuzumab: qui bono? *Journal of the National Cancer Institute*, 105(23):1772–5, 2013.

[38] A. Liu, C. Liu, Q. Li, K. F. Yu, and V. W. Yuan. A threshold sample-enrichment approach in a clinical trial with heterogeneous subpopulations. *Clinical Trials*, 7(5):537–45, 2010.

[39] T. J. Lynch, D. W. Bell, R. Sordella, S. Gurubhagavatula, R. A. Okimoto, B. W. Brannigan, P. L. Harris, S. M. Haserlat, J. G. Supko, et al.

Activating mutations in the epidermal growth factor receptor underlying responsiveness of non-small cell lung cancer to gefitinib. *New England Journal of Medicine*, 350(21):2129–39, 2004.

[40] S. J. Mandrekar, Y. Cui, and D. J. Sargent. An adaptive phase I design for identifying a biologically optimal dose for dual agent drug combinations. *Statistics in Medicine*, 26(11):2317–30, 2007.

[41] S. J. Mandrekar and D. J. Sargent. Clinical trial designs for predictive biomarker validation: theoretical considerations and practical challenges. *Journal of Clinical Oncology*, 27(24):4027–34, 2009.

[42] L. M. McShane, S. Hunsberger, and A. A. Adjei. Effective incorporation of biomarkers into phase II trials. *Clinical Cancer Research*, 15(6):1898–905, 2009.

[43] H. Meany, F. M. Balis, A. Aikin, P. Whitcomb, R. F. Murphy, S. M. Steinberg, B. C. Widemann, and E. Fox. Pediatric phase I trial design using maximum target inhibition as the primary endpoint. *Journal of the National Cancer Institute*, 102(12):909–12, 2010.

[44] T. S. Mok, Y-L. Wu, S. Thongprasert, C-H. Yang, D-T. Chu, N. Saijo, P. Sunpaweravong, B. Han, B. Margono, Y. Ichinose, Y. Nishiwaki, et al. Gefitinib or carboplatin-paclitaxel in pulmonary adenocarcinoma. *New England Journal of Medicine*, 361:947–957, 2009.

[45] J. G. Paez, P. A. Janne, J. C. Lee, S. Tracy, H. Greulich, S. Gabriel, P. Herman, F. J. Kaye, N. Lindeman, T. J. Boggon, K. Naoki, H. Sasaki, et al. EGFR mutations in lung cancer: correlation with clinical response to gefitinib therapy. *Science*, 304(5676):1497–500, 2004.

[46] W. R. Parulekar and E. A. Eisenhauer. Phase I trial design for solid tumor studies of targeted, non-cytotoxic agents: theory and practice. *Journal of the National Cancer Institute*, 96(13):990–7, 2004.

[47] G. A. Pennello. Analytical and clinical evaluation of biomarkers assays: when are biomarkers ready for prime time? *Clinical Trials*, 10(5):666–76, 2013.

[48] M. Y. Polley, B. Freidlin, E. L. Korn, B. A. Conley, J. S. Abrams, and L. M. McShane. Statistical and practical considerations for clinical evaluation of predictive biomarkers. *Journal of the National Cancer Institute*, 105(22):1677–83, 2013.

[49] L. Pusztai, K. Anderson, and K. R. Hess. Pharmacogenomic predictor discovery in phase II clinical trials for breast cancer. *Clinical Cancer Research*, 13(20):6080–6, 2007.

[50] O. E. Rahma, E. Gammoh, R. M. Simon, and S. N. Khleif. Is the "3+3" dose-escalation phase I clinical trial design suitable for therapeutic cancer vaccine development? A recommendation for alternative design. *Clinical Cancer Research*, 20(18):4758–67, 2014.

[51] M. J. Ratain and R. H. Glassman. Biomarkers in phase I oncology trials: signal, noise, or expensive distraction? *Clinical Cancer Research*, 13(22 Pt 1):6545–8, 2007.

[52] E. H. Romond, E. A. Perez, J. Bryant, V. J. Suman, C. E. Geyer, Jr., N. E. Davidson, E. Tan-Chiu, S. Martino, S. Paik, P. A. Kaufman, et al. Trastuzumab plus adjuvant chemotherapy for operable HER2-positive breast cancer. *New England Journal of Medicine*, 353(16):1673–84, 2005.

[53] M. D. Rothmann, J. J. Zhang, L. Lu, and T. R. Fleming. Testing in a pre-specified subgroup and the intent-to-treat population. *Drug Information Journal*, 46(2):175–179, 2012.

[54] L. V. Rubinstein, E. L. Korn, B. Freidlin, S. Hunsberger, S. P. Ivy, and M. A. Smith. Design issues of randomized phase II trials and a proposal for phase II screening trials. *Journal of Clinical Oncology*, 23(28):7199–206, 2005.

[55] L. V. Rubinstein, S. M. Steinberg, S. Kummar, R. Kinders, R. E. Parchment, A. J. Murgo, J. E. Tomaszewski, and J. H. Doroshow. The statistics of phase 0 trials. *Statistics in Medicine*, 29:1072–1076, 2010.

[56] D. Sargent and C. Allegra. Issues in clinical trial design for tumor marker studies. *Seminars in Oncology*, 29(3):222–30, 2002.

[57] R. Simon. Stratification and partial ascertainment of biomarker value in biomarker-driven clinical trials. *Journal of Biopharmaceutical Statistics*, 24(5):1011–21, 2014.

[58] R. Simon and A. Maitournam. Evaluating the efficiency of targeted designs for randomized clinical trials. *Clinical Cancer Research*, 10(20):6759–63, 2004.

[59] R. Simon and S. J. Wang. Use of genomic signatures in therapeutics development in oncology and other diseases. *Pharmacogenomics Journal*, 6(3):166–73, 2006.

[60] R. M. Simon, S. Paik, and D. F. Hayes. Use of archived specimens in evaluation of prognostic and predictive biomarkers. *Journal of the National Cancer Institute*, 101(21):1446–52, 2009.

[61] C. Tian, D. J. Sargent, T. C. Krivak, M. A. Powell, M. J. Gabrin, S. L. Brower, and R. L. Coleman. Evaluation of a chemoresponse assay as a predictive marker in the treatment of recurrent ovarian cancer: further

analysis of a prospective study. *British Journal of Cancer*, 111(5):843–50, 2014.

[62] H. T. Tran, Y. Liu, A. J. Zurita, Y. Lin, K. L. Baker-Neblett, A. M. Martin, R. A. Figlin, T. E. Hutson, C. N. Sternberg, R. G. Amado, L. N. Pandite, and J. V. Heymach. Prognostic or predictive plasma cytokines and angiogenic factors for patients treated with pazopanib for metastatic renal-cell cancer: a retrospective analysis of phase 2 and phase 3 trials. *Lancet Oncology*, 13(8):827–37, 2012.

[63] S. J. Wang, N. Cohen, D. A. Katz, G. Ruano, P. M. Shaw, and B. Spear. Retrospective validation of genomic biomarkers- what are the questions, challenges and strategies for developing useful relationships to clinical outcomes- workshop summary. *Pharmacogenomics Journal*, 6(2):82–8, 2006.

[64] S. J. Wang, R. T. O'Neill, and H. J. Hung. Statistical considerations in evaluating pharmacogenomics-based clinical effect for confirmatory trials. *Clinical Trials*, 7(5):525–36, 2010.

[65] Y. Zang, J. J. Lee, and Y. Yuan. Adaptive designs for identifying optimal biological dose for molecularly targeted agents. *Clinical Trials*, 11(3):319–327, 2014.

12

Adaptive Clinical Trial Designs in Oncology

J. Jack Lee

Lorenzo Trippa

CONTENTS

12.1 Introduction

In this chapter, we focus on adaptive clinical trial designs that aim to improve the efficiency of research by more quickly answering the important questions posed in the research protocol, identifying effective treatments and dropping ineffective treatments early, and providing the best treatments to the individual patients enrolled in clinical trials.

Clinical trials are costly endeavors. When added to the expense of the laboratory research that precedes a trial and all the costs during clinical development, drug development costs are rapidly increasing. However, the notable investments in R&D costs have not resulted in commensurate increases in the number of new drugs approved for medical use, nor in the success rates in such clinical trials. For example, as recorded by BioMedTracker, for 4275 clinical trials for which results were released from 2003 to 2010, the overall success rate for final approval of the trial drug or intervention was only 9% [16]. In oncology, only 13% of the experimental drugs evaluated in phase I trials between 1993 and 2004 were eventually approved by the United States Food and Drug Administration (FDA) [29], and significant results were obtained from only 34% of confirmatory phase III trials conducted between 2003 and 2010 [118]. In a review of new drug candidates evaluated in 2011 and 2012, Arrowsmith and Miller [3] reported that a lack of efficacy was found in 59% of unsuccessful phase II studies of new drugs and in 52% of unsuccessful studies in phase III or thereafter. In addition, patient safety concerns were the cause of 22% of the unsuccessful phase II studies of new drugs and in 35% of the unsuccessful studies in phase III or thereafter.

One potential solution to this low success rate is to reconfigure the framework under which we design and conduct clinical trials. The FDA released a critical path opportunities list in 2006 for the purpose of stimulating the development and implementation of innovative clinical trial designs [34]. The list specifically cited statistical designs that use the information accruing in the trial to guide the further conduct of the trial, i.e., adaptive designs.

The definition of an adaptive trial design is one that directs planned, well-defined modifications of the primary clinical trial design parameters during the conduct of the trial on the basis of data from that trial to achieve goals of scientific validity, efficiency, and safety. This is different from the conduct of a standard clinical trial design that allows for little or no adaption in the trial conduct. The adaptive trial captures interim data and considers the meaning of that data in regard to the overall objectives of the trial. This consideration may then result in alterations of the trial conduct according to predetermined guidelines [38]. Adaptations can be configured in many aspects of a trial, such as to guide adaptive dose escalation or de-escalation; to modify a randomization scheme on the basis of patient covariates and/or outcomes; to re-estimate the sample size; to use biomarkers to guide treatment allocation; to drop a treatment arm for inferiority or add a new treatment arm; to employ a seamless transition between the phases of a study; and to stop the trial early because of ample evidence of toxicity or highly probable efficacy or futility [9, 26]. Bayesian methods work well with adaptive trial designs because such methods are inherently adaptive. Frequentist methods can also be used in adaptive trial designs; some frequentist approaches will be covered in this chapter. The primary focus of this chapter, however, will be the Bayesian framework and its application to adaptive clinical trials. The objectives of an adaptive design are (i) to provide the best answers to the scientific questions of interest in the trial; (ii) to operate efficiently, allowing a trial to terminate when the answer becomes apparent; and (iii) to increase the individual ethics of the trial by determining the best dose/schedule of a treatment or, in a multi-arm trial, the superior treatment as the trial progresses and then modifying the randomization scheme so that new patients have greater likelihood of being assigned to the superior treatment, all while maintaining the scientific validity and integrity of the trial as planned in the clinical protocol.

In oncology trials that evaluate new drugs, clinicians do not know the efficacy or toxicity of the investigational drug at the beginning of the trial. Thus, it is reasonable to use the information collected in the trial, then adapt the trial conduct and assess the subsequent information collected in the trial. This is considered the "learn as we go" approach. As a patient cohort is enrolled in the trial, is treated, and data are gathered, an adaptive design will determine the efficacy and toxicity profiles of the treatment and use that accumulating data to direct the trial conduct as it proceeds. Used this way, an adaptive design can provide the advantages of reducing the overall sample size and associated cost of the study, shortening the length of the study and the drug development time, increasing the statistical power of the study, treating more patients with more effective treatments, and correctly identifying the most efficacious drugs for specific subgroups of patients on the basis of biomarker profiles.

Multi-arm, multi-stage trial designs have been developed to improve the efficiency and cost-effectiveness of the drug development process. More radical innovations have been proposed, such as the nationwide master protocol, which has been initiated for lung cancer research. New concepts in trial design have been proposed: "umbrella trials," which enroll patients with one disease and multiple molecular aberrations, and "basket trials," which enroll patients with different diseases but align each molecular aberration with the corresponding treatment. In addition, platform-based designs allow for combining multiple studies under a common valuation platform to increase efficiency. These will be further discussed in subsequent sections.

The goal of this chapter is to review the methodology, development, and implementation of adaptive designs in clinical research. This chapter is organized as follows. In Sections 12.2 through 12.9, we introduce adaptive design methods commonly employed in clinical trials, which include adaptive dose-finding methods; adaptive randomization; interim analysis; early stopping rules; sample size re-estimation; biomarker-guided randomization; group sequential designs; and seamless phase I/II and II/III designs. In Section 12.10, we discuss multi-arm, multi-stage designs, and in Section 12.11, we describe master protocols, umbrella trials, basket trials, and platform-based designs. In Section 12.12, we introduce two clinical trials that were recently conducted using adaptive designs and discuss practical issues encountered in the implementation of such designs. In Section 12.13, we briefly review statistical software and tools to assist in the planning and conduct of adaptive trials. We provide concluding remarks in Section 12.14.

12.2 History of Adaptive Designs

Adaptive clinical trial designs are increasingly being used in many areas of research [8, 11, 15, 26, 47, 138]. Indeed, academic journals have published special sections or issues on the topic of adaptive designs (e.g., Biometrics, Statistics in Medicine, the Journal of Biopharmaceutical Statistics, Statistics in Bioscience, and others) [38]. The pharmaceutical industry and regulatory agencies have found adaptive designs attractive because of their potential advantages and because they reflect medical practice in the real world. For example, several organizations have established adaptive design working groups, which have proposed strategies, methodologies, and implementation policies for consideration by regulatory agencies. These include the Pharmaceutical Research and Manufacturers of America, Biotechnology Industry Organization, the Biopharmaceutical section of the American Statistical Association, and the Drug Information Association (DIA).

The first time a new treatment was approved in the United States on the basis of an adaptive analysis of treatment efficacy was in 2003, when the Center for Drug Evaluation and Research (CDER) of the FDA approved a new combination form of pravastatin for the treatment of high cholesterol in individuals with coronary artery disease, with the goal of decreasing the risk of heart attack, stroke, or other cardiovascular complication [9]. That trial implemented a Bayesian adaptive design. In 2004, the FDA sponsored a workshop with the Johns Hopkins University on the topic of improving regulatory decision making through the use of Bayesian methods in drug development [137]. Five years later, the Medicare Evidence Development and Coverage Advisory Committee convened to publicly share information on the use of Bayesian inference to make decisions regarding medical insurance coverage [22]. The "Guidance for the use of Bayesian statistics in medical device clinical trials" was first published by the Center for Devices and Radiological Health (CDRH) branch of the FDA in 2006. The final guidance was published in 2010 [89]. Thereafter, the Center for Biologics Evaluation and Research and the CDER at the FDA jointly issued a guidance document for planning and implementing adaptive designs in clinical trials [88]. In 2011, the DIA formed a Bayesian Scientific Working Group with the aim of disseminating educational opportunities in the use of Bayesian methods for the development of medical products and to better inform decision making in the research and development environments, regulatory environment, and among economic policy makers. In February 2015, the DIA Global Center held a 2-day educational conference:

the Joint Adaptive Design and Bayesian Statistics Conference: Drivers of Efficiency in Modern Medical Product Development, which featured experts from industry, regulatory agencies, and academia [43].

12.3 Bayesian Framework and Its Use in Clinical Trials

Bayesian inference is based on the observed data related to and gathered in a trial and not conditioned on the postulated unobserved data or sampling method; therefore, it is particularly applicable when researchers choose to incorporate informed flexibility into trial conduct. Such flexibility is provided by an adaptive trial design. This framework provides three steps for modeling the parameters of interest: (i) determine the prior distribution, then (ii) gather the data and perform likelihood calculations, and (iii) update the information by using Bayes' theorem to compute the posterior distribution. Bayesian inference requires proper determination of the prior distribution and the probability model. The Bayesian method is adaptive by definition, which makes it a natural framework for adaptive trial designs [70].

Merits of the Bayesian framework include the ability to (i) use valuable information collected before, during and external to the trial, and apply that knowledge for real-time decision making; (ii) incorporate varying levels of uncertainty for unknown parameters through the use of probability distributions; (iii) enact frequent monitoring of the data and make interim decisions; (iv) formally incorporate gain/loss functions to aid in medical decision making; and (v) maintain scientific validity as the trial adapts. For more details, see [70].

The Bayesian framework offers four approaches. The two most commonly applied to clinical trial design are the "proper Bayes" approach and the "reference Bayes" approach. The reference Bayes approach uses an objective prior to make the inference more objective. The proper Bayes approach uses the available evidence to achieve informative prior distributions and uses posterior distributions to reach conclusions, but does not definitively incorporate a utility (gain/loss) function.

In contrast, the "decision-theoretic Bayes" approach employs definitive gain/loss functions to guide decisions, thereby augmenting the expected gain or diminishing the expected loss [130]. This approach can best answer research questions in the context of complex issues and opposing objectives; however, it requires sophisticated programming, demanding computations, and includes the challenge of determining an appropriate gain/loss function. For these reasons, clinical trial designs do not commonly employ the decision-theoretic Bayes approach. As the first step of the traditional Bayesian framework enumerated in the first paragraph of this section, the prior distribution is determined before any data are observed. In contrast, the fourth approach, the "empirical Bayes approach," uses observed data to derive the prior distribution. This approach employs the most probable values of the hyperparameters in a hierarchical model.

The feasibility of designing experiments under the Bayesian framework has been tremendously assisted by the development of modern algorithms, namely the Markov chain Monte Carlo (MCMC) algorithm [41, 42], and several extensions of general computing tools, which started with Bayesian inference using Gibbs sampling (BUGS) [78]. In addition to the many computing tools that are now available, the conduct of a trial under the Bayesian framework will often require customized computer programs and web-based applications. Expediency is particularly important when new observations and ongoing data analyses inform the next decisions made within the trial.

Currently, only a small proportion of clinical trials are conducted under a Bayesian framework. One common application is in the phase I trial designs to determine the optimal dose of a new drug or evaluate its pharmacokinetics or pharmacodynamics. In addition, numerous Bayesian methods are currently applied within more traditional trial designs to evaluate the efficacy or toxicity of a new treatment or to guide diagnostic and treatment decisions.

12.4 Adaptive Dose-finding Designs for Identifying Optimal Biologic Dose

In the development of new drugs, a phase I clinical trial examines the potential of the new drug to be toxic in humans to find safe doses. For additional background information and details, we refer the reader to Chapter 6: Phase I Trials and Dose-finding.

The statistical designs that direct phase I dose-finding trials fall into one of two general types: an up-and-down design based on an algorithm, and an adaptive design based on a statistical model. The first type, the up-and-down design, generally follows rigid rules that are determined in advance of the trial. The "3+3" design (for review, see, e.g., [117]) and the accelerated titration design [112] are examples of this type of dose-finding design. The second type, the adaptive dose-finding design, applies the data accumulating in the phase I trial to compute the curve that relates the dose level to the toxicity level, and then uses that information to prompt either dose escalation or de-escalation within the trial. The model-based design is more adept and yielding than the algorithm-based design.

Three examples of the model-based dose-finding design are the continual reassessment method (CRM) [33, 44, 91], the escalation with overdose control design [5], and the Bayesian model averaging continual reassessment method (BMA-CRM) [142]. Statisticians have also developed dose-finding designs for when the toxic effects of a new drug are not expected to be observable soon after the dose is administered, but only after a delay. These designs include the time-to-event CRM [23], the expectation-maximization CRM [147], and the data augmentation CRM [75]. Other model-based designs have been developed for trials of drugs used in combination [81, 120, 141, 143, 144], and for phase I/II trials [97, 121, 145, 148, 150]. Braun [19] wrote a comprehensive review of adaptive designs for phase I dose-finding trials.

Compared to traditional anti-cancer drugs, which are highly toxic, biologics are expected to have low toxicity within therapeutic dose ranges. Thus, the goal of determining the maximum tolerated dose (MTD) in an early dose-finding trial is replaced by the goal of determining an optimal biological dose (OBD), which is generally defined as the lowest safe dose of the targeted agent with the highest rate of efficacy. Statisticians have developed methods to determine the OBD in clinical trials using nonparametric and semiparametric designs which yield consistently good operating characteristics suitable for practical use [50, 57, 81, 148].

12.5 Multi-stage Designs, Group Sequential Designs, Interim Analysis, Early Stopping for Toxicity, Efficacy, or Futility

The safe dose recommended in the phase I trial of a new drug is subsequently evaluated for its beneficial effects in a phase II trial. Sequential designs for phase II trials have been developed to evaluate the efficacy of a new treatment. Commonly used single-arm designs are two-stage designs [40, 109], which control the type I and type II error rates in order to reach a predetermined target rate of efficacy. Thall and Simon [124] used a binary outcome measure and simulations to adjust the bounds that direct the stopping rules of a phase II Bayesian adaptive trial design. That work was expanded by Thall, Simon and Estey [125] through modeling the outcomes of both efficacy and toxicity, and by Thall, Wooten and Tannir [127], through modeling the trial duration until the occurrence of a specific event of interest. Lee and Liu [73] developed an adaptive Bayesian design that continuously monitors the trial and guides the termination decisions at each interim analysis through the use of a predictive probability, which is the probability of a successful trial conclusion based on the interim data should the current trend within the trial continue. Compared to frequentist designs, Bayesian adaptive designs are more flexible in trial conduct but can still preserve the type I and type II error rates with higher early stopping probability when the treatment is inefficacious.

Upon establishing the initial evaluation of treatment efficacy, further testing is followed by randomized phase II studies or phase III studies. Group sequential designs provide interim monitoring for studies with two or more treatment arms. By using interim analyses to direct the future course of the trial, group sequential designs are efficient because they can stop the trial early if the interim data analysis indicates that the new treatment is significantly associated with severe adverse effects (stopping for toxicity), that there is no significant benefit from the new treatment compared to the standard treatment (stopping for futility [no difference] or inferiority), or that there is a clear significant benefit from the new treatment (stopping for efficacy). The group sequential design of Pocock [95] applied bounds for the stopping rule that carried equal probability throughout the trial. The design of O'Brien and Fleming [86] started the trial with stricter probability bounds for the stopping rule, and then loosened the bounds near the end of the trial. These designs were combined and generalized by Wang and Tsiatis [132]. DeMets and Lan [28] gave the group sequential design greater flexibility via the alpha spending function approach. Further discussion of group sequential designs can be found in the work of Jennison and Turnbull [60].

Despite the statistical advances in group sequential designs, which address multiplicity by controlling the overall type I error rate, frequentist adaptive designs face many challenges. For example, the proposed treatment effect can be overestimated or underestimated, which will have an impact on the sample size (see Section 12.6). The fixed number and timing of the interim analyses under the typical group sequential designs are rigid; whereas in practice, many factors can influence the actual timing of the interim analysis. The alpha spending function approach provides some flexibility; however, the choice of the spending function is somewhat subjective. [131] provided regulatory perspectives on multiplicity in adaptive designs throughout a drug development process. For explorative adaptive trials, the goal is to maximize the probability of correctly selecting the design features such as dose, effect size, and probability of the correct "go" or "no go" decisions. For the confirmatory adaptive trials, controlling the type I and type II error rates in the study is of paramount importance.

Bayesian adaptive designs offer greater flexibility because inference under the Bayesian framework is not affected when the interim analysis is performed, nor when a trial is terminated early; rather, the posterior distribution is repeatedly updated as new data accumulate in the trial. A consistent inference framework based on the posterior probability of the parameter of interest or the predictive probability can be formulated. Interim analyses are a natural part of Bayesian analysis. The cutoff values for declaring significance can be calibrated to control the type I and type II error rates.

12.6 Sample Size Re-estimation

Adaptive designs have been developed to correct an improper sample size that may arise when the historical data used to determine the effect size (the standardized treatment difference) are not accurate, perhaps because of sampling bias or dissimilar study conditions. An overestimated or underestimated sample size is possible in a group sequential design that uses a predetermined and fixed sample size that is based on historical data. These adaptive designs use the data accumulating in the trial to re-estimate the sample size [108].

Proschan and Hunsberger [98] incorporated sample size re-estimation after the first stage of a two-stage design. They use the data from the first stage to estimate the effect size, which then forms the basis of the re-estimation of the sample size for the second stage. Cui, Hung, and Wang [27] provided a sample size re-estimation procedure in group sequential clinical trials based on the observed data. By modifying the weights used in the traditional repeated significance test, the test provides a substantial gain in power with an increase in sample size while controlling the type I error probability at the target level. Shen and Fisher [106] developed the self-designing strategy, which does not require a prespecified maximum sample size, but uses the accruing data in the trial to guide the decision to stop for futility or continue the trial to obtain the intended statistical power. Statisticians should apply caution, however, when designing studies that use sample size re-estimation. Tsiatis and Mehta [129] showed that a typical group sequential design guided by the sequentially computed likelihood ratio test can be more efficient than the adaptive design that uses sample size re-estimation. However, it does not preclude the use of sample size re-estimation or early stopping based on the posterior probability or predictive probability calculations.

Brutti, De Santis, and Gubbiotti [20] developed a flexible sample size calculation and re-estimation method that uses a predictive Bayesian approach. Rather than depending on a specific choice of the prior distribution, this method is based on mixtures of prior distributions that characterize the multiple sources of prior information or data for estimating the unknown parameters. Choosing proper weights for the mixture distribution gives this approach the advantage of helping to avoid sample size underestimation and low predictive probability of trial success.

12.7 Adaptive Randomization, Individual Ethics versus Group Ethics

Randomized assignment of trial participants to any one of two or more treatment arms prevents treatment assignment bias by balancing the determinant factors between the various treatment groups. The randomization strategies most often used in clinical trials are equal randomization to each treatment arm, or a fixed ratio randomization, such as a 2:1 rate. In contrast, adaptive randomization allows the probability of assigning patients to specific treatments to vary as the trial progresses and data accumulate. There are two main types of adaptive randomization, namely, covariate-adjusted adaptive randomization and outcome-adaptive randomization. These two adaptive randomization schemes can be combined to form a covariate-adjusted outcome-adaptive randomization scheme.

Covariate-adjusted adaptive randomization designs may use baseline measurements of particular characteristics that are associated with the prognosis (prognostic markers) for each participant to direct the treatment assignment, which will balance the determinant factors among the treatment groups [31, 96]. In contrast, outcome-adaptive randomization uses the treatment responses accumulating in the trial to direct the treatment assignment, which will tend to assign more participants to the treatment arms that are resulting in better outcomes [135, 149]. The strategy of equal randomization maximizes the statistical power of the study, which generally increases the efficiency of the trial. Equal randomization is considered to benefit the overall population that is relevant to the study, which strengthens the "group ethics" of the trial [92]. Outcome-adaptive randomization, however, allows for a change in the randomization probability as the trial proceeds. It directs the assignment of newly enrolling trial participants on the basis of the data accumulating in the trial, creating a greater probability that more participants will be assigned to the more efficacious treatment. This strategy benefits the trial participants, which strengthens the "individual ethics" of the trial [92].

Outcome-adaptive randomization can be constructed under both the frequentist and Bayesian frameworks. Taking the frequentist approach, Hu and Rosenberger [52, 53] derived the optimal randomization probability under various criteria. For example, in a two-arm trial with a binary endpoint, assuming the response rates of the two treatment arms, 1 and 2, are, respectively, p_1 and p_2, the optimal randomization probability of assigning patients to arm 1 (ϕ_1) to maximize the power of the test for comparing two response rates (also called Neyman allocation) is $\phi_1 = \dfrac{\sqrt{p_1 q_1}}{(\sqrt{p_1 q_1} + \sqrt{p_2 q_2})}$, where $q_i = 1 - p_i$ for $i = 1, 2$. Alternatively, the optimal ϕ_1 to minimize the expected number of non-responders is $\sqrt{p_1}/(\sqrt{p_1} + \sqrt{p_2})$.

Since we do not know the true response rates, they can be replaced by the estimated response rates based on the interim data available at the time of randomization as the trial progresses [100]. This strategy can be improved by accounting for the proportion of participants assigned to each treatment and the current estimate of the desired allocation proportion to compute the randomization probability to achieve optimal design properties with less variability, such as in the "doubly adaptive biased coin" design [32, 54].

Under the Bayesian framework, several adaptive randomization strategies have been proposed. The most intuitive approach is simple Bayesian adaptive randomization, which assigns patients to arm 1 with $\phi_1 = Prob(\theta_1 > \theta_2)$, where θ_i is the posterior probability of p_i for $i = 1, 2$ at the time of randomization. Thall and Wathen [126] extended simple Bayesian adaptive randomization by applying a power transformation:

$$\phi_1 = \frac{Prob(\theta_1 > \theta_2)^c}{Prob(\theta_1 > \theta_2)^c + Prob(\theta_1 < \theta_2)^c}.$$

To lessen the variability of the randomization probability, they proposed using $c = n/(2N)$, where n is the number of currently enrolled patients and N is the maximum number of patients in the trial. As a result, the randomization probability is close to 0.5 at the beginning of the trial. As more data accumulate, the randomization probability can move away from 0.5, depending on how much difference there is between the response rates for the two treatments. One can similarly use equal randomization in the first part of a clinical trial, and then switch to adaptive randomization or restricting the randomization probability within, say, 0.2 to 0.8, to lessen its variability. The randomization probability can also be constructed from the posterior mean (or median) of the treatment effect, $\phi_1 = \widehat{\theta_1}/(\widehat{\theta_1} + \widehat{\theta_2})$, where $\widehat{\theta_i}$ is the posterior mean (or median) of θ_i for $i = 1, 2$ [30, 72]. As shown in Figure 12.1, an adaptive randomization strategy can be coupled with early stopping rules for futility and/or efficacy, which are frequent components of a Bayesian adaptive clinical trial design [139].

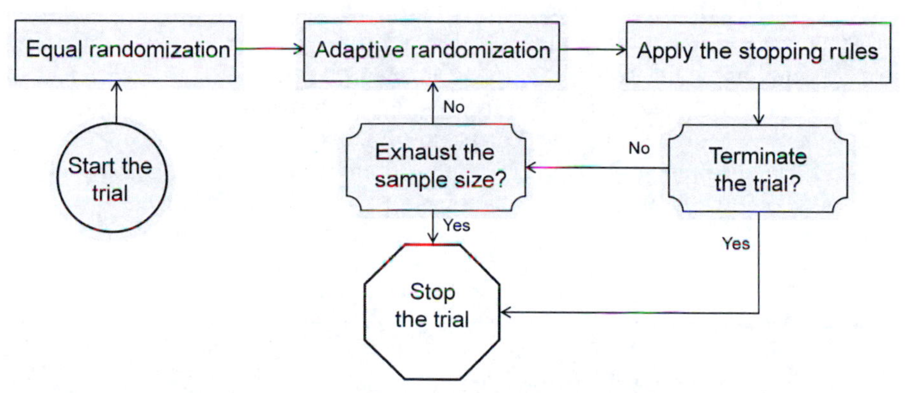

FIGURE 12.1: Diagram of a phase II trial design that begins with equal randomization, followed by Bayesian adaptive randomization. Early stopping rules for toxicity, futility, and/or efficacy can be applied to terminate the trial early when the prespecified conditions are met.

Is outcome-adaptive randomization useful? The answer is still under debate in the clinical trial communities from statistical, trial conduct, and ethical perspectives. Advantages in different scenarios are provided by equal and adaptive randomization methods. For a two-arm trial with a binary endpoint, Korn and Freidlin [65] claimed that equal randomization is preferable because it results in smaller sample sizes and fewer non-responders. These authors also argue that the increased complexity of implementing the adaptive strategy does not justify the resulting benefit. Hey and Kimmelman [48] examined outcome-adaptive randomization from the perspective of drug development, informed consent, and validity, and concluded that outcome-adaptive allocation is not ethical for two-arm trials. That article was accompanied by six commentaries and a rejoinder. When there is a large difference between the effects of the treatments examined in a trial, the adaptive randomization strategy provides a much higher overall rate of favorable response to treatment (superior individual ethics) and can also result in better statistical power [69]. However, this difference wanes when an early stopping rule is added to the trial design. Adaptive randomization may be advantageous when studying a rare disease and is preferable when the trial design involves multiple treatment arms and multiple stages of study. It is particularly advantageous when one treatment is much more beneficial than the others [14, 133].

For trials that use adaptive randomization to evaluate multiple treatments, one must be careful to monitor the different treatment groups throughout the trial to check for population drift, which may lead to biased comparisons of the various treatments. Population drift is a more severe problem under an adaptive randomization strategy that favors the more beneficial treatments because the strategy may result in an imbalance in participant characteristics across the treatment groups [65]. A severe population drift can result in a high degree of confounding between the patient characteristics and the adaptive treatment assignment, which can invalidate proper inference. Several methods can be applied to address this issue. For example, regression analysis can be used to account for an imbalance in prognostic covariates among treatments. The problem can be partially corrected by incorporating a reference or a control arm and placing bounds on the randomization probability to ensure a non-negligible randomization probability for each treatment arm.

12.8 Seamless Designs

Upon determining the recommended safe dose of a new drug in a phase I trial, a second phase of study is entered to assess the intended beneficial effects of the drug. If the phase II trial finds the drug to have sufficient beneficial effects, then a longer, phase III trial is generally entered to validate those findings by comparing the effects of the new drug to those achieved by the standard treatment. Each phase of a trial (phases I–III) is traditionally run separately and sequentially to reach a defined but partial conclusion of whether a new drug is safe and efficacious. This overall trial scheme is simple to design and conduct; however, it is costly, inefficient, and is not flexible; therefore, statisticians have developed trial designs that will seamlessly direct these three phases of study.

Several seamless trial designs have been developed and evaluated (e.g., [45, 90, 123, 140]). Some designs consolidate dose finding (toxicity assessment) with treatment efficacy [55, 121, 145], which includes a design for trials evaluating drug combinations [146], and a design for evaluating targeted agents [50]. Other pertinent adaptive designs are the trinomial CRM design [150] and the two-stage design [97].

Seamless designs that combine phase II and phase III have also been developed (e.g., [17, 56, 64, 116]). The overall goal is to shorten the lengthy drug development process, while also improving the success rate of clinical trials, wherein success is achieved when a beneficial new treatment is identified and then enters the market after receiving FDA approval. To attain this goal, these designs often use multiple treatments (drugs) and multiple dose levels of the new drug [15]. In a study that compared the seamless trial design and others that have the same operating characteristics, Inoue, Thall, and Berry [58] demonstrated sample size reductions of 30% to 50% on average and shorter overall trials when the seamless design was used. In an inferentially seamless design, some data from the dose selection stage can be added to the final data analysis, provided that the participants in both stages are given the same treatments and have the same primary endpoints [11]. The final data analysis under the inferentially seamless design must include calibration simulations to control the potential increase in the overall type I error rate caused by using data to conduct and analyze the confirmatory phase of a trial.

In oncology, the beneficial effect of a new treatment often may be assessed through the measure of tumor response at a certain point after treatment for a solid tumor, generally whether the tumor has shrunk or grown larger. If a phase II study indicates that the new treatment causes diminution of the tumor, then the treatment moves to phase III, where its long-term effect is evaluated. A long-term endpoint for a phase III oncology trial is often the overall survival time of the participants in the trial. The seamless phase II/III oncology trial can use the short-term endpoint to inform the long-term endpoint when selecting the dose of the new drug that is associated with the highest efficacy or selecting the most efficacious yet safe drug and dropping the less beneficial one among multiple drugs. Then, the selected best dose or best new drug can be entered directly into a smaller confirmatory study in which the new drug is evaluated in comparison to the standard treatment. Of note, it has been reported that, in lung cancer and on a trial level, there is a strong association between the overall response rate (ORR) and progression-free survival (PFS). However, an association between ORR and the overall survival time (OS) and between PFS and OS has not been established. This could arise from the crossover and longer survival time realized after treatment with targeted therapy. The corresponding patient-level analysis showed that responders have better PFS and OS compared with non-responders [18]. There are mixed reports regarding whether PFS is a good surrogate for OS in different diseases and different settings [1, 66, 93, 107]. The proper choice of endpoints is essential to the success of seamless phase II/III trials.

12.9 Biomarker-guided Adaptive Designs

The transition in oncology from using chemotherapy and radiotherapy to using therapies that target specific molecules or functional molecular pathways in a cell has resulted in greater treatment efficacy with reduced toxicities in selected settings [105, 115]. Our ability to take full advantage of targeted therapies depends upon our ability to identify within trial participants the predictive biomarkers that directly correlate with the favorable outcomes achieved by the targeted therapies [36, 82, 83, 104].

Several adaptive trial designs have been developed for the purpose of identifying and confirming biomarkers that correlate with specific treatment outcomes, as well as trial designs that then apply those predictive biomarkers to direct treatment assignment [37, 72, 74, 80, 87, 102, 103, 110, 113, 114, 136]. Figure 12.2 provides flowcharts of the equally randomized marker-stratified design [110] and the Bayesian adaptively randomized mark-stratified design [72]. Simon [111] provides a comprehensive review of biomarker-guided designs.

12.10 Multi-arm Adaptive Designs

Controlled multi-arm studies, which test multiple experimental treatments, are substantially more efficient than two-arm balanced studies with patients equally randomized to a control arm and a single experimental treatment arm. There are multiple explanations for the efficiency gain attributed to multi-arm trials (e.g., [10, 35]). First, multi-arm studies test several experimental treatments while sharing the control arm, which, in contrast, is replicated in each separate study if drugs are evaluated using two-arm studies. Second, the use of response-adaptive assignment algorithms and sequential designs can further increase the efficiency gap between multi-arm and two-arm studies [128].

During the trial, adaptive algorithms for multi-arm studies (e.g., [126, 139]) typically increase the randomization probabilities toward the most promising treatments. This often translates into higher sample sizes for the treatment arms that are associated with beneficial treatment effects and, in turn, into higher power of detecting the best treatments at the completion of the study. Response-adaptive randomization can be combined with decision rules to drop arms for futility or toxicity and to allow for variations during the trial of the eligibility criteria specific to a given treatment arm. Moreover, individual randomization probabilities can be tailored to the patient's profile, defined by biomarkers, thus reflecting the possibility of treatment-biomarker interactions suggested by the outcome data (e.g., [2, 151]).

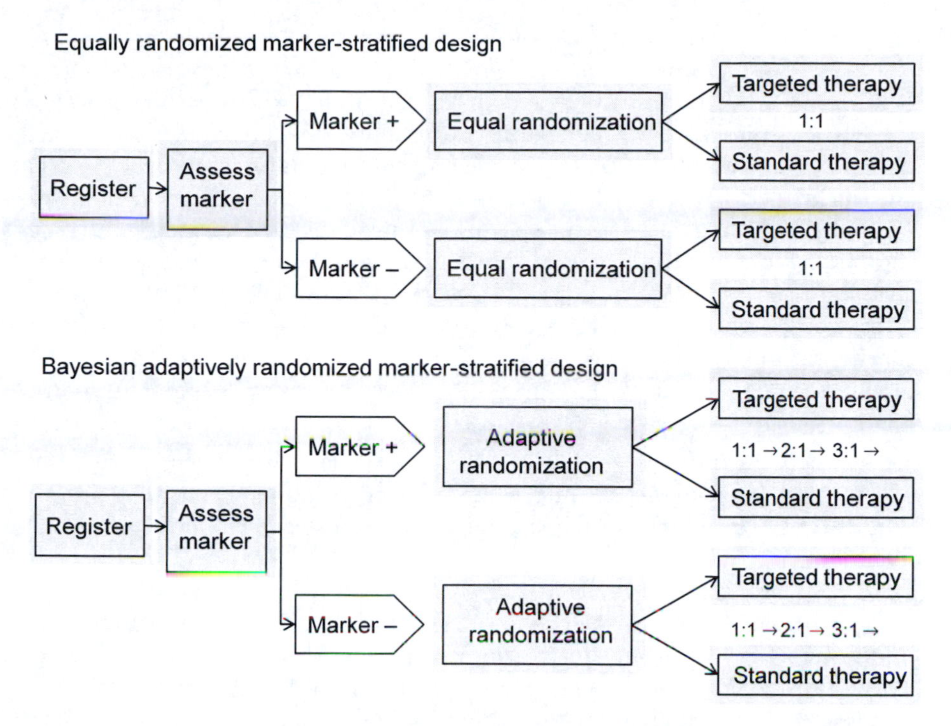

FIGURE 12.2: Diagrams of the marker-stratified design. A fixed 1:1 randomization ratio is used in the equally randomized marker-stratified design. Examples of possible variations in the randomization ratio for the Bayesian adaptively randomized marker-stratified design: the marker-positive group starts at 1:1, then changes to 2:1 in favor of the targeted therapy, then 4:1; whereas the marker-negative group starts at 1:1, then changes to 1:2 in favor of the standard therapy, then 1:3, assuming that the targeted therapy is more effective for the marker-positive form of the disease and the standard therapy is more effective for the marker-negative form.

Despite these advantages, multi-arm study designs are not frequently used in early-stage clinical studies, both in cancer and in several other diseases. The main goal of this section is to review statistical methods, evaluation criteria, and simulation approaches to use in planning and designing adaptive multi-arm clinical trials. We start from a simple example that points to the efficiency gain of multi-arm controlled clinical trials compared to standard two-arm balanced designs. For simplification, we consider only balanced randomized designs that do not include early stopping rules for futility, toxicity or early evidence of efficacy. The plan consists of comparing three experimental treatments to the current standard of care. We focus on only two alternative approaches. The first consists of three separate two-arm controlled studies, one for each experimental treatment; whereas the second consists of a single multi-arm study, with four arms, three experimental treatment options, and one control. If a desired level of power for detecting a clinically relevant effect, say 80%, requires a sample size of 200 patients for each of the two-arms studies, then the first strategy requires a total of $3 \times 200 = 600$ patients. In contrast, the balanced multi-arm trial requires a sample size of only 400 patients. The multi-arm strategy achieves the same uncertainty level for the treatment effects, with a 1/3 reduction in the number of enrolled patients. This 1/3 reduction is unrelated to the specific setting and type of primary outcome, such as the response to the treatment. It is also unrelated to the desired power level and the specific plan of the statistical analyses. The 1/3 reduction is a direct consequence of simultaneously testing multiple experimental drugs by sharing the same control arm instead of replicating the control arm three times in three separate studies. More generally, if we contrast K separate two-arm studies that test K treatments with a trial that has $(K+1)$ treatment arms, we find that identical power levels can be achieved with a $\frac{(K-1)}{(2K)}$ reduction in the total number of patients. This first simple observation points to an important efficiency gain. Adaptive allocation rules can further increase this difference.

A response-adaptive multi-arm design is defined by an algorithm that is used at regular time intervals or at the enrollment of each new patient. The inputs into the algorithm are the data that the clinical trial has generated at the time of the possible adaptation, which typically includes patient characteristics, such as individual biomarker profiles, enrollment dates, treatment assignments, treatment dates, treatment doses and schedules, follow-up dates, measurements of response to treatment, and other outcome measures. In other words, the input is an exhaustive representation of what happened during the study up to a specific time point. The output of the algorithm guides the enrollment of new patients and the randomization of subsequent cohorts of patients; it provides updated randomization probabilities and indicates whether some of the treatment arms should be dropped and whether the study should be terminated.

It is useful to represent an adaptive design as the application of an algorithm, a set of rules that are included in the study protocol, which has a clearly defined input and output and which constitutes the backbone of the adaptive design. How do we distinguish between a good and a bad adaptive design? In most cases, the major criteria for comparing candidate designs include the overall costs, the total number of patients who will be randomized, the number of patients who will benefit from the experimental treatments during the study, projected estimates of the final treatment effects, and recommendations for all the treatments to be evaluated. Simulations are perhaps the most powerful tool for comparing and optimizing candidate designs. After iteratively simulating an adaptive clinical trial, the major criteria and the cost-benefit balance of the simulated experiment can be directly quantified and graphed.

A good adaptive algorithm optimizes the trade-off between the costs and benefits of the clinical trial. Simulations, conducted under realistic scenarios, provide the investigator with estimates and variability summaries of the operating characteristics of the trial. The variability summaries capture the possible variability due to randomness in the accrual time, patient characteristics, outcomes, etc. This information allows the investigator to contrast candidate adaptive designs (and non-adaptive designs as well) by comparing the resulting operating characteristics, which represent the efficiency of the study in detecting treatment effects, appropriate patient allocation, and other evaluation criteria.

Bayesian adaptive randomization for multi-arm designs can be viewed as a map that is used each time a patient is enrolled in the trial and which transforms the available data into suitable randomization probabilities. The algorithm translates the estimates and predictions into randomization probabilities. Bayesian modeling allows for meaningful prediction during the trial and can be used to answer key questions during an ongoing trial. These key questions include:

> What is the probability that a specific experimental treatment has higher efficacy than the control?
>
> Conditional on the specific design, treatment protocol, and available data, what is the probability that, upon completion of the trial, there will be significant evidence of a positive effect for a specific treatment arm?
>
> What is the predicted proportion of enrolled patients who will receive the best treatment option?

These questions can be answered by sequentially updating a Bayesian model that describes the uncertainty of the relevant unknown quantities such as the response rates or median survival times for each arm. Bayesian adaptive strategies sequentially map probabilistic statements obtained from the Bayesian model into randomization probabilities, or they select other decisions, such as the exclusion of an experimental treatment arm.

Most Bayesian adaptive algorithms transform the updated posterior probabilities of the treatment effects into the randomization probabilities $\pi_k^i, k = 0, \cdots, K$, for the next patient, at the i-th enrollment, to $(K+1)$ treatment arms. Note that π_k^i varies during the trial. The algorithm can also take into account other components, such as the number of individuals already enrolled and the planned overall sample size. The choice of the Bayesian model is fundamental; key guidelines for selecting a model include (i) simplicity and interpretability of the model, (ii) low sensitivity of posterior estimates to the prior parameterization, and (iii) robustness of posterior inference under reasonable deviations from the model assumptions. Also fundamental is the choice of the map that transforms the probabilistic statements into randomization probabilities.

We provide a possible definition of $\pi_k^i, k = 0, \cdots, K$, with $k = 0$ denoting the control and $k = 1, \cdots, K$, denoting the experimental treatment arms. We specify $\pi_i^k = pr$(i-th enrolled patient is randomized to arm k conditional on the data), $k = 0, 1, \cdots, K$, in two steps. First, the randomization probability π_i^0 for assigning a patient cohort to the control arm is set to be equal to

$$\frac{1}{K} exp\left(\max_{k=1,\cdots,K}[no.\,pts.\,assigned\,to\,arm\,k] - [no.\,pts.\,assigned\,to\,control]\right).$$

This randomization probability increases with the difference between the current sample size of the experimental treatment arm that has been assigned more frequently and the number of patients who have been randomized to the control arm.

Second, if the i-th patient is assigned to an experimental arm $k = 1, \cdots, K$, then the conditional probability $\pi_i^k/(1 - \pi_i^0)$ is set to be equal to

$$\frac{pr\,(\text{Arm } k \text{ has positive treatment effect conditional on the data})^{\gamma(i)}}{\sum_{j=1}^{K} pr\,(\text{Arm } j \text{ has positive treatment effect conditional on the data })^{\gamma(i)}}$$

for $k = 1, \cdots, K$ and is a function of the evidence of positive treatment effects in each of the experimental arms. The above expressions provide interpretable randomization probabilities π_k^i. At the completion of the trial, the first expression nearly matches the number of patients randomly assigned to the control arm to that of the patients randomly assigned to the experimental arm with the highest sample size. The goal is to sustain the number of allocations to the control arm, which in turn is necessary to show evidence of positive treatment effects. The second expression shows that when $\gamma(i)$ is positive, the probability of assigning the i-th patient to arm k increases with the evidence in favor of a positive treatment effect. The parameter $\gamma(i)$ modulates the trade-off between exploration versus exploitation. Typically, it is approximately close to or equal to zero for an initial cohort of patients, so that the members of this cohort are randomly assigned with approximately identical probabilities to each of the treatment arms, which may be desirable in the initial explorative stage of the trial. Then, the algorithm, with increasing values of $\gamma(i)$ for the patients who are subsequently randomized, exploits the available information and generates higher randomization probabilities for the most promising treatment arm(s).

Sensitivity analyses are important to evaluate the adaptive design's robustness to departures from the assumptions used to tune the assignment algorithm. In our example of sensitivity evaluations (Figure 12.3), we focus on the average number of patients assigned to each treatment arm. We use a proportional hazards model to define randomization probabilities, and compute the estimated operating characteristics, assuming stationary accrual rates that are invariant during the course of the trial. Figure 12.3 illustrates a relevant difference in the arm-specific average sample sizes. For each panel, we consider the same median survival times under each arm. Under a scenario without departures from the modeling assumptions (panel a), 44 patients are assigned to the control arm and 44 patients to the only experimental treatment arm that achieves a positive treatment effect (hazard ratio: 0.65); whereas 26 patients are assigned to the other two experimental arms that do not achieve positive treatment effects. We also show robustness to departures from the design assumptions. Panels (b) and (c) correspond to violations of the proportional hazards assumption, which is replaced by an accelerated failure time model (panel b), and by a proportional odds model (panel c). We also consider robustness when the accrual rate is higher than the initial estimate (panel d), and when there is a two-month delay in the data management process in providing the accumulating data for posterior calculations and adaptation (panel e).

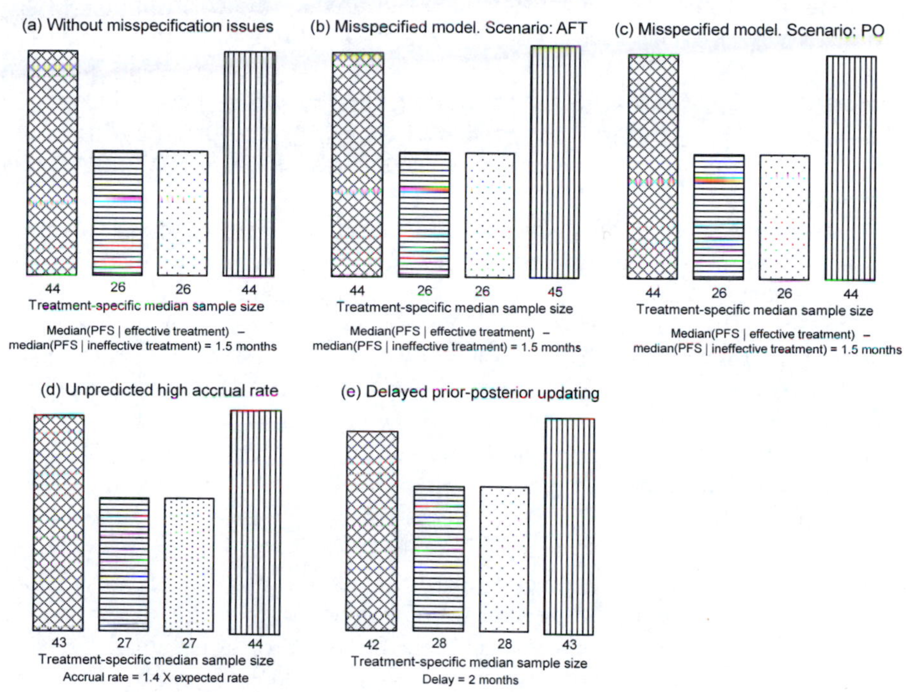

FIGURE 12.3: Sensitivity analyses of the ability of the adaptive trial design to adjust to unexpected developments during trial conduct. The four columns in each panel show the average number of patients assigned to each treatment arm; the control arm (cross-hatch), experimental arm with positive treatment effect (vertical stripes), and two experimental arms without positive treatment effects (horizontal stripes and dots). (a) The expected scenario when no misspecifications occur. (b) Accelerated failure time model (AFT) replaces proportional hazards model because of violations of the design assumptions. (c) Proportional odds model (PO) replaces proportional hazards model because of violations of the design assumptions. (d) Accrual rate is 1.4 times faster than expected. (e) Assessment of accumulating data is delayed by 2 months. PFS is progression-free survival time.

Variations of the adaptive algorithm, with the additional complexity of biomarkers and Bayesian modeling of treatment-biomarker interaction, have been applied in clinical trials, for example in the BATTLE trial [63] and the I-SPY 2 trial [6] (which are described in Section 12.12). Extending methods for simultaneously evaluating more than two agents (e.g., [79, 101]) resulted in the multi-arm multi-stage (MAMS) adaptive trial design (e.g., [133, 134]). The MAMS design uses interim data to identify treatment arms associated with positive treatment effects. This design differs from adaptive randomization designs in that the usual MAMS design does not change the allocation proportions, but sets the stopping thresholds on the basis of test statistics, and excludes a treatment from further allocation when the outcomes associated with that treatment are shown to violate the predetermined stopping boundaries. In MAMS trials, the number of patients randomized to each treatment arm during a single stage of the study is fixed. The MAMS design has been successfully implemented in trials, including the "Systemic therapy in advancing or metastatic prostate cancer: Evaluation of drug efficacy" (STAMPEDE) trial [4, 119] and the "Telmisartan and insulin resistance in HIV" (TAILoR) trial [134].

Using an extensive set of simulation scenarios, we compared the Bayesian adaptive design to the MAMS design, and also to balanced designs [133]. We used the same number of interim analyses, which, in the Bayesian adaptive design, were predetermined and used to compute the posterior probabilities. We also used nearly identical complexity levels for the MAMS and Bayesian adaptive designs. Our comparison demonstrated that the Bayesian adaptive design was more efficient in detecting treatment effects. This conclusion was driven mainly by comparing the required sample sizes under hypothetical scenarios to achieve desired power levels and comparing the precision of the treatment effect estimates for the best treatment options.

Upon completion of a Bayesian adaptive trial, the investigator can decide whether to use Bayesian or frequentist terms for reporting inference, including rigorous hypothesis testing and the confidence interval for the treatment effects. Typically, the control of the type I error rate is obtained by computing the summary statistics for each experimental arm and rejecting the corresponding null hypotheses for those arms for which the test statistics exceed a suitably chosen threshold. In our experience, we found two effective alternative computational approaches for controlling the type I error probability: bootstrap procedures and importance sampling. The first approach uses resampling to estimate the distribution of the summary statistics under the corresponding null hypotheses. Similarly, importance sampling can be used to approximate the distributions of the summary statistics under a continuum of possible scenarios that are simulated. The structure of the Bayesian adaptive algorithm offers a solution to the problem of using the available information during the course of the clinical trial to increase the efficiency in the discovery and estimation of positive treatment effects. Although this algorithm has practical advantages, including the fact that it is defined by interpretable transformations of posterior probabilities, the use of alternative strategies can be valuable.

For example, one can attempt to replace the posterior probabilities of positive effects in the adaptive algorithm with different characteristics of the posterior distributions, such as point estimates of the treatment effects. The anticipated construction of yet more computationally practical algorithms on the basis of Bayesian inference and prediction has the potential to further strengthen the advantages of Bayesian adaptive designs.

12.11 Master Protocols, Umbrella Trials, Basket Trials, and Platform-based Designs

A design in which individuals with specific pathologic diagnoses and disease characteristics are matched with clinical trials of investigational drugs that target their specific disease profiles is facilitated by the use of a "master protocol." The use of such a protocol requires the combined efforts of the clinical investigators, biopharmaceutical companies, individuals with cancer, patient advocates, FDA, and national cooperative groups. The lung cancer master protocol (LUNG-MAP), the first implementation of this framework (http://lung-map.org/), was conceived at the Conference on Clinical Cancer Research in 2012. Five pharmaceutical companies and a large number of research centers, community hospitals, and physician cooperatives throughout the United States are participating in the LUNG-MAP, which is managed by SWOG Cancer Research, a cooperative research group supported by the National Cancer Institute through the National Clinical Trials Network. More than 200 genes associated with cancer are screened for mutations in each potential participant in LUNG-MAP. The individual's resulting genomic profile is then used to match him or her with one of five trials that are evaluating various experimental treatments. The trials are adaptive, allowing for the addition of new therapies as they become available. The master protocol design is considered to be an "umbrella" trial as all patients with one disease are enrolled under one protocol then assigned to multiple arms with multiple drugs to address different molecular aberrations. Applications of the master protocol framework have already accelerated the FDA's approval of 14 new drugs and the initiation of the phase II/III cooperative trial for squamous cell lung cancer in more than 400 locations around the country [51]. Thus, the framework of the master protocol holds great promise for improving the efficiency and effectiveness of the drug development process.

In contrast to the umbrella trial, which deals with one disease and multiple molecular aberrations, the proposed "basket trial" enrolls many patients with different types of cancer (such as lung, colon, and breast cancers) that involve the same molecular aberrations. The basket trial then tests a drug or drug combination thought to be effective against that particular genomic abnormality. Hence, a basket trial deals with one molecular aberration in multiple diseases or histologic subtypes. In this design, all patients can be enrolled and screened for molecular aberrations. Depending on the specific molecular pathways involved, patients are treated with different drugs regardless of their varying histology or disease diagnosis. For example, the CUSTOM trial enrolled patients with lung cancer characterized by different histologic features. The patients were treated with standard-of-care therapies or with one of the following five biomarker-matched treatments: erlotinib for EGFR mutations; selumetinib for KRAS, NRAS, HRAS, or BRAF mutations; MK2206 for PIK3CA, AKT, or PTEN mutations; lapatinib for ERBB2 mutations or amplifications; and sunitinib for KIT or PDGFRA mutations or amplifications [77]. The basket trial accommodates efficient genomic screening to identify rare aberrations and to guide patients to the appropriate treatments.

One notable example is the NCI-Molecular Analysis for Therapy Choice (NCI-MATCH) trial [59], which is a clinical trial to analyze patients' tumors to determine whether they contain genetic abnormalities for which a targeted drug exists and assign treatment based on the abnormality. NCI-MATCH seeks to determine whether treating cancers according to their molecular abnormalities will show evidence of effectiveness. NCI-MATCH can add new treatments or drop treatments over time. Each treatment will be used in a unique arm, or substudy, of the trial. The trial opened for enrollment in July 2015, with 10 arms for patients with advanced, recurrent solid tumors, and lymphomas. The initial plan is to obtain tumor biopsy specimens from as many as 3000 patients. The specimens will undergo DNA sequencing to identify those that have genetic abnormalities that may respond to the targeted drugs selected for the trial. It is anticipated that 20 to 25 drugs will ultimately be tested, each in a different arm of the trial.

Another innovative proposal is the use of "platform-based designs" for clinical trials [49, 71]. A platform is an operational and statistical framework under which new agents or therapies for a particular pathological diagnosis can be screened simultaneously as they are developed. Each platform is specific to a given diagnosis rather than to a specific treatment protocol. The platform-based design uses Bayesian modeling and randomization to carry out the equivalent of several phase II trials of multiple treatment arms. This design is adaptive in that a new agent may be added after an appropriate dose has been selected in a phase I trial, and data accumulating in the screening process can guide the decision to drop an agent that is not achieving the desired results. The agent that is dropped may be returned to a phase I study to take a closer look at the optimal treatment dose or schedule of doses. And it may once again be screened if evidence indicates that an alternative dose or schedule of doses may prove beneficial.

Among the important statistical challenges of the platform-based design is the proper use of sequential adaptive strategies for monitoring the futility of the experimental agents while controlling the predetermined type I error rate in the face of a stochastic number of comparisons. With the addition of any new agent into an ongoing platform-based trial, a comparison between the effect of the new agent and that of another agent in the trial involves imbalances in the sample sizes. To account for this potentially ongoing imbalance, the proposed design defines the futility stopping rule on the basis of the posterior predictive probability of a successful trial. A Bayesian model is employed to accommodate the uncertainty that arises from interim estimations of the model parameters and the variability that arises from the treatment responses of future patients in the trial. Acceptable frequentist properties are obtained for the platform-based design through the use of simulations to calibrate the design parameters. Although the calculation of Bayesian posterior distributions and predictive probabilities are computationally intensive, once determined, the platform-based designs that use the predictive probability can operate continuously and perform ongoing screenings of new drugs or therapies without the need to conduct these Bayesian computations on an interim basis.

An informative discussion of the adaptive biomarker-driven trials spanning the master protocol, umbrella trial, basket trial, and platform design can be found in Berry [12]. Much of the work on multi-arm and/or multi-stage designs has proposed similar approaches to streamline and improve the process of drug development (e.g., [7, 35, 94, 133, 134]). The potential advantages of the platform-based design include decreasing the down time between phases I and II or phase II and III, decreasing the overall time needed to screen new drugs or therapies, greatly decreasing the number of times the standard treatment must be given to patients to serve as a control arm, increasing the number of available new treatment options for patients, decreasing the bias associated with inter-trial heterogeneity, improving the control of inherent multiplicities, and providing better information for decisions about future confirmatory trials.

12.12 Examples of Trials with Adaptive Designs — Lessons for Design and Conduct

An investigative team should consider using an adaptive trial design only if it will enhance the overall success of evaluating drugs or treatments, which includes the efficient operation of the trial. The planning process for such a trial can be considerably longer than that of the standard design when the trial is complex. In addition to measuring the statistical performance of a new drug or treatment based on the operating characteristics, the team should also consider how it will measure the success of the adaptive trial on the operational level.

Three essential parts of planning to conduct an adaptive trial are (i) simulations of the performance of the statistical design under the possible scenarios, (ii) simulations of the overall operations of the various components of the trial, and (iii) integration of the systems involved in the trial. The third step requires fully integrating the team, uniting researchers from clinical medicine, biostatistics, and pharmacy with members of clinical operations and regulatory operations. It also involves integrating the automated computational systems that will guide the conduct of the trial with the web-based applications for data input, monitoring, and reporting throughout the trial.

Simulation models are useful during the planning stage of the trial, as well as during trial conduct, when real data accumulating in the trial can be added to the model to study the trial's operating characteristics. The assumptions used to conduct the initial simulations and to guide the start of a trial can be based on historical data from related trials, data obtained from a full feasibility analysis, or estimations obtained from data mining. Simulations of the future trial are used to conceptualize the relation between the various data inputs, including the total patient enrollment, the enrollment and randomization rates, the treatment arms and doses to be evaluated, the endpoint measures, the timing of interim analyses, the occurrence of adverse events, the supply and administration of the experimental drug, the costs associated with the trial, and other relevant data. The simulation results are used to evaluate the statistical assumptions of the trial design under the different possible scenarios and outcomes. For multicenter trials, simulations will evaluate the use of different numbers of sites, various initiation and start-up dates, and variations in the supply of the experimental drug.

Planning also includes determining precisely what data will be collected during the trial, how and when the data will be collected, and how and when the data will be input into a central operational database, which will allow it to be used to inform the adaptivity of the trial. This will involve a clinical trial data management center, which will operate the central, integrated database for data collection, randomized treatment assignment, regulatory reporting, and data quality assessment. The database will provide a single source for data entry, storage, and dissemination and for the overall quality management of the clinical trial. Although strict data management procedures are required in the conduct of all clinical trials, the timeliness of the data collection and availability is crucial to the conduct of an adaptive trial. Timely data are essential to inform the ongoing randomization strategy and stopping rules. The particular endpoints used to assess a patient's treatment response and the timing of making that data available to inform the ongoing trial will directly affect the randomization rate for the trial. Adaptive randomization cannot be useful if the outcome data from previously enrolled patients are not available to inform the randomization strategy used for the patients who enroll thereafter. Thus, endpoints that can be measured over a shorter period of time (including appropriate surrogate endpoints) can be compatible with adaptive trial designs.

The ability to use an electronic data collection system, to remotely monitor the data, to transfer data efficiently, to automate the generation of reports and reminders for patient follow-up, and to work with integrated statistical analysis tools and trial conduct software will greatly enhance the implementation of an adaptive trial design. In addition to having the data management center oversee a trial, adaptive trials require the use of centralized remote monitoring as well as on-site monitoring of key data, such as data related to patient safety and treatment efficacy. These data inputs may trigger the statistical model guiding the trial, such as high toxicity triggering dose de-escalation for the next patient cohort, serious adverse events or evidence of futility triggering a stopping rule, or automated notification of missing patient data or protocol violations. To monitor the interim trial conduct, the role of the Data Safety and Monitoring Board (DSMB) is critical as the trial is adaptive in nature and the DSMB can view the unblinded data to assess whether the trial conduct is consistent with the trial design. If there are deviations, the DSMB can help to identify the issues and make appropriate course corrections to ensure the trial validity is not compromised. For detailed guidance on the various components of adaptive trial monitoring, see Marchenko et al. [84].

As examples of the application of adaptive designs, we describe two large, randomized, phase II clinical trials that use interim analyses to inform their randomization strategies. On the basis of the trial participant's biomarker profile, these trials use adaptive randomization to increase the probability of assigning that participant to the treatment that will be most effective for him or her. These two trials are the "Biomarker-integrated approaches of targeted therapy of lung cancer elimination" (BATTLE) trial and the "Investigation of serial studies to predict your therapeutic response with imaging and molecular analysis" (I-SPY 2) trial. The BATTLE trial [63, 151] uses response-adaptive randomization and imposes a stopping rule for futility. This stopping rule could exclude from the randomization choices the treatments that would not benefit a participant based on his or her biomarker profile. The I-SPY 2 trial [6] uses adaptive randomization within each biomarker subgroup and imposes a stopping rule for futility or efficacy.

The study population in the BATTLE trial consisted of patients with stage IV recurrent non-small cell lung cancer. The primary endpoint, a binary outcome, was the 8-week disease control rate. The trial evaluated four targeted therapies, each of which was matched with one of the four biomarker profiles evaluated (expressions of genes, gene mutations, copy numbers, and proteins measured by immunohistochemistry). The trial design used Bayesian methods to model the treatment-response interaction and borrowed strength across biomarker subgroups through the use of a hierarchical probit model. The overall goals of the trial were to test the treatment efficacy and biomarker effect and to determine the capacity to predict treatment outcomes on the basis of biomarker profiles. A total of 341 patients were enrolled in the BATTLE trial, and 255 were randomized equally at first (the first 97 patients) and then adaptively under the biomarker-guided strategy. The end results supported the prespecified scientific hypotheses of the study and discovered new predictive markers to be validated in future studies [63]. Using the results from the first trial, the BATTLE-2 trial was then initiated [13]. It uses adaptive randomization in a two-stage design to evaluate four treatments. That trial screens 10 to 15 candidate biomarkers by employing training, test, and validation processes to select the most appropriate biomarkers to use in the trial. Group lasso and adaptive lasso methods are applied for variable selection to identify both prognostic and predictive markers [46].

The I-SPY 2 trial is a multicenter trial involving neoadjuvant treatment (standard chemotherapy or radiation therapy before tumor removal surgery) plus the use of up to 12 experimental drugs in patients with breast cancer. The FDA approved the use of adaptive guidance for the I-SPY 2 trial, allowing the trial to move a successful drug directly into the confirmatory phase, to exclude an unsuccessful drug from further use in the trial, and to add a new drug during the trial rather than starting with a new protocol [21]. The trial evaluates 10 subgroups of patients according to their biomarker profiles (hormone-receptor status of the breast tumor and the MammaPrint signature, which is the expression level of specific genes associated with early breast cancer development [85]). The goal is to determine which biomarker profile correlates with a beneficial treatment outcome that is attributable to any of the experimental drugs. The tumor burden as assessed by magnetic resonance imaging is used to measure the treatment outcome. The phase II portion of this trial is used to screen the experimental drugs, and then the drugs that are predicted to be successful in a future phase III trial of 300 patients are moved forward into the confirmatory phase. The I-SPY 2 trial has randomized more than 700 patients, moved two experimental treatments to confirmatory studies, and successfully demonstrated that this adaptive trial design can reduce the cost of drug development and improve the efficiency of screening new drugs [6, 67].

12.13 Software for Adaptive Designs

Statisticians have many choices of software programs to use when designing, conducting, and analyzing clinical studies. Among the commonly used programs are SAS® (SAS Institute Inc., Cary, NC), S-Plus® (TIBCO Software Inc., Palo Alto, CA), SPSS® (IBM Software, Armonk, NY), and Stata® (Stata Corp, LP, College Station, TX). The R software environment is also commonly used for statistical analysis and computing. Specialty applications and tools have been designed and many are freely available online.

Three software programs are freely available online for planning and implementing a phase I dose-finding trial that uses the continual reassessment method [91]: the CRM simulator, the BMA-CRM, and the TITE-CRM. The CRM simulator uses one set of the prior means of toxicity to select the optimal dose level and allows the user to adjust the parameters until the desired output is achieved. The Bayesian model averaging continual reassessment method (BMA-CRM) [142] selects the optimal dose on the basis of multiple sets of probabilities of the prior means for toxicity. The time-to-event continual reassessment method (TITE-CRM) software [23] has a similar use when determining the optimal dose of a drug that is expected to show delayed toxicity.

For a dose-finding cancer trial, software known as dose escalation with overdose control (EWOC) [5], when compared to CRM, assigned fewer patients to subtherapeutic or severely toxic doses, treated more patients at doses near the maximum tolerated dose, and resulted in lower average bias and mean squared error when estimating the MTD. EWOC incorporates adaptive learning in its application. Another option for cancer trials is dose finding based on modified toxicity posterior intervals (mTPI) [61]. This software is available as R functions or as an Excel macro with an add-in file. The decision rules are based on a unit probability mass, using a Bayesian decision-theoretic framework.

A recently published design, the Bayesian optimal interval (BOIN) design for phase I clinical trials, identifies the MTD based on computing the optimal probability interval. It optimizes the dose assignment for each patient enrolled in the trial. The software (an R function called BOIN.r) implements the BOIN design of Liu and Yuan [76], which effectively treats patients and minimizes the chance of exposing them to subtherapeutic or overly toxic doses. Upon specifying the design parameters, the BOIN design is algorithm-based and can be implemented in a simple way, similar to the traditional 3+3 design. The performance of the BOIN design is comparable on average to that of the CRM in terms of selecting the MTD, but the BOIN has a substantially lower risk of assigning patients to subtherapeutic or overly toxic doses.

In drug development, it is useful for phase I/II cancer trials to evaluate both toxicity and efficacy simultaneously and incorporate a trade-off between the two for a given drug. The adaptive phase I/II design allows for adaptive learning during a trial by assigning patients to the most efficacious yet safe dose. This software is known as Eff-Tox [121, 122].

Software that is useful for designing a phase II clinical trial to evaluate a single treatment includes Multc99, the predictive probability design, and the BFDesigner. Multc99 [125] can be used to calculate the operating characteristics and stopping boundaries for different settings of a study that evaluates both efficacy and toxicity. A simplified version "Multclean" is also useful and is more user friendly in the design setup. The predictive probability design [73] can be used in trial design to determine the cutoff values of the predictive probability and the calculation of the associated stopping boundary for continuous trial monitoring on the basis of the input of the type I and type II error rates. The BFDesigner [62] is useful for obtaining efficient stopping rules.

Several software options are available for use in sequential trial designs. For group sequential designs, gsDesign, developed by Keavon Anderson of Merck Research Laboratories, is available through the Comprehensive R Archive Network repository. S + SeqTrial is an S-Plus software library integrated within the S-Plus software that can be used to plan, monitor, and analyze group sequential trials. Additional software for the planning and evaluation of sequential trials (PEST), developed by the MPS Research Unit at Lancaster University in Lancashire, U.K., is available for use with a SAS session; however, PEST is no longer maintained. Commercial software for sequential trial design and conduct includes the many tools available as East® (Cytel, Inc., Cambridge, MA).

Another commercial software program is Adaptive Designs-Plans and Analyses (ADDPLAN®, Aptiv Solutions, Inc., Reston, VA), which is specifically formulated to plan and conduct adaptive clinical trials. Additional useful computational tools include adaptive randomization software, available commercially and through free online repositories. Two other helpful computational tools that are freely available (https://biostatistics.mdanderson.org/SoftwareDownload/) are "parameter solver," which calculates the distribution parameters of a random variable given either two quantiles or the mean and variance, and "predictive probabilities," which, for a trial with two treatment arms and a binary endpoint, calculates the posterior predictive probabilities of concluding that one treatment arm or the other is superior or of stopping the trial due to futility [15].

12.14 Discussion

The need for improvements in the overall clinical trial process is well recognized by experts in all areas of this process, including drug developers and manufacturers, regulatory officials, clinicians, and biostatisticians. Whether the use of master protocols and other innovative approaches will provide an adequate level of improvement remains to be seen. Nevertheless, adaptive clinical trial designs are already playing important roles in the current clinical trial process. These designs have the potential to enhance the flexibility and efficiency of the conduct of clinical trials and reduce the overall sample size, while also tending to preserve the individual ethics of the trial and treat the participants in the trial with the best available treatment. An adaptive design that guides a multi-arm trial can identify the drugs or therapies that show the greatest benefit, exclude from further consideration the least beneficial drugs early, screen and confirm biomarkers, match the most beneficial treatments with specific subgroups of participants on the basis of their biomarker profiles, and shorten the drug development process.

There are several challenges to using adaptive designs in clinical trials. The overall logistics are much more complicated for adaptive designs compared to traditional trial designs [39]. This greater complexity requires more effort throughout the process of planning, designing and conducting the trial.

Close collaboration between the statisticians, clinicians, drug developer and pharmacists, operational agents, programmers, and data managers is vital to a successful adaptive trial. A central database for data storage should be integrated with the software that directs the interim analyses, randomization strategy, and stopping rules, as well as the software that directs the operational requirements such as follow-up reminders, data audits, and regulatory reporting. The timely collection of accurate data is crucial to an adaptive clinical trial. As with all randomized trials, maintaining the confidentiality of specific treatment assignments is necessary to prevent investigator bias. The modifications that may occur during an adaptive trial can lead investigators to make conclusions about the outcomes while the trial is underway; therefore, data collection and storage must be secure to protect the integrity of the trial, particularly for an unblinded, randomized trial [25]. The establishment of an independent DSMB is critical for monitoring the trial conduct to ensure the integrity of the study implementation, interim data analysis, and reporting.

Compared to a conventional clinical trial, an adaptive trial requires much more work from the statisticians who collaborate in its design and planning. They must carefully examine the operating characteristics of the statistical design under a range of possible conditions. This requires them to conduct extensive simulations of the trial performance to ensure that the type I error rate, power, and accuracy in estimating the treatment effect, rates of adverse events, or dose finding are well defined and acceptable across a wide range of possible true treatment effect sizes, dose-response relationships, and population characteristics. Timely data analyses and continuous monitoring of the trial require the use of specialized software and computational tools [68]. The ongoing monitoring of the trial by the statistician will include checking for population drift when adaptive randomization is used to assign patients among multiple treatment options. Despite the aforementioned challenges and slow adoption of adaptive designs in practice, much interest in this area has propelled more education, more methodologic research, and more software development in recent years, which in turn increasingly enable the implementation of adaptive designs [24, 99]. We need to continue innovation in both trial design and implementation to learn and improve beyond the status quo. With more applications of adaptive designs and adaptive learning, clinical trials can be integrated with clinical practice, using up-to-date knowledge to benefit more patients [12].

The decision to use an adaptive design should be an informed decision, made on the basis of simulated comparisons between conventional and adaptive methods. Statistical modeling should be used during the planning stages to examine the objectives of the study and to thoroughly evaluate the risk of using an adaptive design compared with the potential rewards. Such requirements should not discourage the use of these methods, however, but should enable the practitioner to determine and understand both the limitations of adaptive designs and their potential rewards. Adaptive designs can refine their performance as the trial proceeds; thereby increasing the knowledge we gain from the data. Careful planning and implementation of an adaptive design in a clinical trial can improve the drug development process, administer better therapy to the participants in the trial, and more effectively answer the scientific questions of interest.

Glossary

Basket trial: A set of trials that enroll patients with varying diseases, but with the same molecular aberration
Covariate-adjusted adaptive randomization: A randomization scheme that, at the time of a patient's enrollment, uses measurements of particular characteristics associated with prognosis to direct the treatment assignment; this scheme balances the determinant factors among the treatment groups
Decision-theoretic Bayes approach: A Bayesian statistical approach that uses definitive gain/loss functions to guide decisions, thereby augmenting the expected gain or diminishing the expected loss
Empirical Bayes approach: A Bayesian statistical approach that uses observed data to derive the prior distribution, employing the most probable values of the hyperparameters in a hierarchical model
Group ethics: A trial design that has the purpose of scientific learning so as to benefit future patients and the greater scientific community
Individual ethics: A trial design that has the purpose of scientific learning, while also tending to provide better treatment to the patients currently enrolled in the trial
Outcome-adaptive randomization: A randomization scheme that uses the treatment responses accumulating in the trial to direct the treatment assignment for subsequent patients; this scheme will tend to assign more patients to the treatment arms that are associated with better outcomes
Population drift: An imbalance in patient covariates across treatment groups that may lead to improper inference
Prognostic marker: A biological measurement that is determined to be associated with a patient's prognosis
Proper Bayes approach: A Bayesian statistical approach that uses the available evidence to achieve informative prior distributions and uses posterior distributions to reach conclusions, but does not definitively incorporate a utility (gain/loss) function
Reference Bayes approach: A Bayesian statistical approach that uses an objective prior to make the inference more objective
Umbrella trial: A set of trials that enroll patients with the same disease, but varying molecular aberrations

Acknowledgments

This work was supported in part by grant CA016672 from the United States National Cancer Institute. Lorenzo Trippa has been supported by the Burroughs Wellcome Fund and the Claudia Adams Barr Program in Cancer Research. The authors thank LeeAnn Chastain for her editorial assistance.

Bibliography

[1] B. M. Alexander and L. Trippa. Progression-free survival: too much risk, not enough reward? *Neuro-Oncology*, 16:615–616, 2014.

[2] B. M. Alexander, P. Y. Wen, L. Trippa, D. A. Reardon, W. K. Yung, G. Parmigiani, and D. A. Berry. Biomarker-based adaptive trials for patients with glioblastoma-lessons from I-SPY 2. *Neuro-Oncology*, 15:972–978, 2013.

[3] J. Arrowsmith and P. Miller. Trial watch: phase I and phase III attrition rates 2011-2012. *Nature Reviews Drug Discovery*, 12:569, 2013.

[4] G. Attard, M. R. Sydes, M. D. Mason, N. W. Clarke, D. Aebersold, J. S. de Bono, D. P. Dearnaley, C. C. Parker, A. W. S. Ritchie, J. M. Russell, et al. Combining enzalutamide with abiraterone, prednisone, and androgen deprivation therapy in the stampede trial. *European Urology*, 66:799–782, 2014.

[5] J. Babb, A. Rogatko, and S. Zacks. Cancer phase I clinical trials: efficient dose escalation with overdose control. *Statistics in Medicine*, 17:1103–1120, 1998.

[6] A. D. Barker, C. C. Sigman, G. J. Kelloff, N. M. Hylton, D. A. Berry, and L. J. Esserman. I-SPY 2: an adaptive breast cancer trial design in the setting of neoadjuvant chemotherapy. *Clinical Pharmacology Therapy*, 86:97–100, 2009.

[7] F. M. S. Barthel, M. K. B. Parmar, and P. Royston. How do multi-stage, multi-arm trials compare to the traditional two-arm parallel group design - a reanalysis of 4 trials. *Trials*, 10:21, 2009.

[8] P. Bauer and W. Brannath. The advantages and disadvantages of adaptive designs for clinical trials. *Drug Discovery Today*, 9:351–357, 2004.

[9] D. A. Berry. Bayesian clinical trials. *Nature Reviews Drug Discovery*, 5:27–36, 2006.

[10] D. A. Berry. Adaptive clinical trials: the promise and the caution. *Journal of Clinical Oncology*, 29:606–609, 2011.

[11] D. A. Berry. Adaptive clinical trials in oncology. *Nature Reviews Clinical Oncology*, 10:199–207, 2012.

[12] D. A. Berry. The brave new world of clinical cancer research: adaptive biomarker-driven trials integrating clinical practice with clinical research. *Molecular Oncology*, 9:951–959, 2015.

[13] D. A. Berry, R. S. Herbst, and E. H. Rubin. Reports from the 2010 Clinical and Translational Cancer Research Think Tank meeting: design strategies for personalized therapy trials. *Clinical Cancer Research*, 18:638–644, 2012.

[14] D. A. Berry, P. Muller, A. P. Grieve, M. Smith, T. Parke, T. Blazek, N. Mitchard, and M. Krams. Adaptive Bayesian designs for dose-ranging drug trials. In C. Gatsonis, R. E. Kass, B. Carlin, A. Carriquiry, A. Gelman, I. Verdinelii, and W. West, editors, *Case Studies in Bayesian Statistics, Volume V*, pages 99–181. Springer-Verlag, New York, NY, USA, 2001.

[15] S. M. Berry, B. P. Carlin, J. J. Lee, and P. Muller. *Bayesian Adaptive Methods for Clinical Trials.* Chapman and Hall/CRC Press, Boca Raton, FL, USA, 2010.

[16] Biotechnology Industry Organization. BioMedTracker: Clinical trial success rates study.
http://insidebioia.files.wordpress.com/2011/02/bio-ceo-biomedtracker-bio-study-handout-final-2-15-2011.pdf.

[17] W. Bischoff and F. Miller. A seamless phase II/III design with sample-size re-estimation. *Journal of Biopharmaceutical Statistics*, 19:595–609, 2009.

[18] G. M. Blumenthal, S. W. Karuri, H. Zhang, L. Zhang, S. Khozin, D. Kazandjian, S. Tang, R. Sridhara, P. Keegan, and R. Pazdur. Overall response rate, progression-free survival, and overall survival with targeted and standard therapies in advanced non-small cell lung cancer: U.S. Food and Drug Administration trial-level and patient-level analyses. *Journal of Clinical Oncology*, 33:1008–1014, 2015.

[19] T. M. Braun. The current design of oncology phase I clinical trials: progressing from algorithms to statistical models. *Chinese Clinical Oncology*, 3:1, 2014.

[20] P. Brutti, F. De Santis, and S. Gubbiotti. Mixtures of prior distributions for predictive Bayesian sample size calculations in clinical trials. *Statistics in Medicine*, 28:2185–2201, 2009.

[21] P. Carrie. I-SPY 2 breast cancer clinical trial launches nationwide. *Cancer*, 116:3308, 2010.

[22] Centers for Medicare and Medicaid Services. MEDCAC Meeting 6/17/2009 - Bayesian statistical methods and Medicare evidence. http://www.cms.gov/medicare-coverage-database/details/medcac-meeting-details.aspx?MEDCACId=49\&TAId=65\&bc=BAAgAAAAAIAAAA%3D%3D&.

[23] Y. K. Cheung and R. Chappell. Sequential designs for phase I clinical trials with late-onset toxicities. *Biometrics*, 56:1177–1182, 2000.

[24] S. Chevret. Bayesian adaptive clinical trials: a dream for statisticians only? *Statistics in Medicine*, 31:1002–1013, 2012.

[25] S. C. Chow and M. Chang. Adaptive design methods in clinical trials - a review. *Orphanet Journal of Rare Diseases*, 3:11, 2008.

[26] S. C. Chow and M. Chang. *Adaptive Design Methods in Clinical Trials. 2nd Edition.* Chapman and Hall/CRC Press, Boca Raton, FL, USA, 2011.

[27] L. Cui, H. M. J. Hung, and S. J. Wang. Modification of sample size in group sequential clinical trials. *Biometrics*, 55:853–857, 1999.

[28] D. L. DeMets and K. K. Lan. Interim analyses: the alpha spending function approach. *Statistics in Medicine*, 13:1341–1352, 1994.

[29] J. A. DiMasi, J. M. Reichert, L. Feldman, and A. Malins. Clinical approval success rates for investigational cancer drugs. *Clinical Pharmacology and Therapeutics*, 94:329–335, 2013.

[30] Y. Du, X. Wang, and J. J. Lee. Simulation study for evaluating the performance of response-adaptive randomization. *Contemporary Clinical Trials*, 40:15–25, 2015.

[31] B. Efron. Forcing sequential experiments to be balanced. *Biometrika*, 58:403–417, 1971.

[32] J. R. Eisele. The doubly adaptive biased coin design for sequential clinical trials. *Journal of Statistical Planning and Inference*, 38:249–262, 1994.

[33] D. Faries. Practical modification of the continual reassessment methods for phase I clinical trials. *Journal of Biopharmaceutical Statistics*, 4:147–164, 1994.

[34] U.S. Food and Drug Administration. Critical path opportunities list, 2006.
http://www.fda.gov/downloads/scienceresearch/specialtopics/

criticalpathinitiative/criticalpathopportunitiesreports/UCM077258.pdf.

[35] B. Freidlin, E. Korn, R. Gray, and A. Martin. Multi-arm clinical trials of new agents: some design considerations. *Clinical Cancer Research*, 14:4368–4371, 2008.

[36] B. Freidlin, L. M. McShane, and E. L. Korn. Randomized clinical trials with biomarkers: design issues. *Journal of the National Cancer Institute*, 102:152–160, 2010.

[37] B. Freidlin and R. Simon. Evaluation of randomized discontinuation design. *Journal of Clinical Oncology*, 23:5094–5098, 2004.

[38] P. Gallo, S. Chuang, V. Dragalin, B. Gaydos, M. Krams, and J. Pinheiro. Executive summary of the phrma working group on adaptive designs in clinical drug development. *Journal of Biopharmaceutical Statistics*, 16:275–283, 2006.

[39] B. Gaydos, K. M. Anderson, D. Berry, N. Burnham, C. Chuang-Stein, J. Dudinak, P. Fardipour, P. Gallo, S. Givens, R. Lewis, J. Maca, J. Pinheiro, Y. Pritchett, and M. Krams. Good practices for adaptive clinical trials in pharmaceutical product development. *Therapeutic Innovation and Regulatory Science*, 43:539–556, 2009.

[40] E. A. Gehan. The determination of the number of patients required in a follow-up trial of a new chemotherapeutic agent. *Journal of Chronic Diseases*, 13:346–353, 1961.

[41] A. E. Gelfand and A. F. M. Smith. Sampling-based approaches to calculating marginal densities. *Journal of the American Statistical Association*, 85:398–409, 1990.

[42] S. Geman and D. Geman. Stochastic relaxation, Gibbs distributions, and the Bayesian restoration of images. *IEEE Transactions on Pattern Analysis and Machine Intelligence*, 6:721–741, 1984.

[43] DIA Global. Joint Adaptive Design and Bayesian Statistics Conference: Drivers of Efficiency in Modern Medical Product Development, 2015. http://www.diahome.org/en-US/Meetings-and-Training/Find-Meetings-and-Training/Meeting-Details.aspx?ProductID=3556268\&EventType=Meeting.

[44] S. N. Goodman, M. L. Zahurak, and S. Piantadosi. Some practical improvements in the continual reassessment methods to phase I studies. *Statistics in Medicine*, 14:1149–1161, 1995.

[45] T. A. Gooley, P. J. Martin, L. D. Fisher, and M. Pettinger. Simulation as a design tool for phase I/II clinical trials: an example from bone marrow transplantation. *Controlled Clinical Trials*, 15:450–462, 1994.

[46] X. Gu, N. Chen, C. Wei, S. Liu, V.A. Papadimitrakopoulou, R. S. Herbst, and J. J. Lee. Bayesian two-stage biomarker-based adaptive design for targeted therapy development. *Statistics in Biosciences*, 2015.

[47] W. He, J. Pinheiro, and O. M. Kuznetsova. *Practical Considerations for Adaptive Trial Design and Implementation*. Springer, New York, NY, USA, 2014.

[48] S. P. Hey and J. Kimmelman. Are outcome-adaptive allocation trials ethical? *Clinical Trials*, 12:102–106, 2015.

[49] B. P. Hobbs, N. Chen, and J. J. Lee. Controlled multi-arm platform design using predictive probability. 2015 (under revision).

[50] A. Hoering, M. LeBlanc, and J. Crowley. Seamless phase I-II trial design for assessing toxicity and efficacy for targeted agents. *Clinical Cancer Research*, 17:640–646, 2011.

[51] R. Hohman. Lung-MAP demonstrates real change in cancer research and care possible through collaboration, 2014. http://catalyst.phrma.org/lung-map-demonstrates-real-change-in-cancer-research-and-care-possible-through-collaboration.

[52] F. Hu and W. Rosenberger. Optimality, variability, power: evaluating response-adaptive randomization procedures for treatment comparisons. *Journal of the American Statistical Association*, 98:671–678, 2003.

[53] F. Hu and W. F. Rosenberger. *The Theory of Response-adaptive Randomization in Clinical Trials*. John Wiley and Sons, New York, NY, USA, 2006.

[54] F. Hu and L. X. Zhang. Asymptotic properties of doubly adaptive biased coin designs for multitreatment clinical trials. *Annals of Statistics*, 32:268–301, 2004.

[55] X. Huang, S. Biswas, Y. Oki, J. P. Issa, and D. A. Berry. A parallel phase I/II clinical trial design for combination therapies. *Biometrics*, 63:429–436, 2007.

[56] X. Huang, J. Ning, Y. Li, E. Estey, J. P. Issa, and D. A. Berry. Using short-term response information to facilitate adaptive randomization for survival clinical trials. *Statistics in Medicine*, 28:1680–1689, 2009.

[57] S. Hunsberger, L. V. Rubinstein, J. Dancey, and E. L. Korn. Dose escalation trial designs based on a molecularly targeted endpoint. *Statistics in Medicine*, 24:2171–2181, 2005.

[58] L. Y. T. Inoue, P. Thall, and D. A. Berry. Seamlessly expanding a randomized phase II trial to phase III. *Biometrics*, 58:823–831, 2002.

[59] National Cancer Institute. NCI-Molecular Analysis for Therapy Choice Program (NCI-MATCH). http://www.cancer.gov/about-cancer/treatment/clinical-trials/nci-supported/nci-match.

[60] C. Jennison and B. W. Turnbull. *Group Sequential Tests with Application to Clinical Trials.* Chapman and Hall/CRC Press, Boca Raton, FL, USA, 2000.

[61] Y. Ji, P. Liu, Y. Li, and B. N. Bekele. A modified toxicity probability interval method for dose-finding trials. *Clinical Trials*, 7:653–663, 2010.

[62] V. E. Johnson and J. D. Cook. Bayesian design of single-arm phase II clinical trials with continuous monitoring. *Biometrics*, 6:217–226, 2009.

[63] E. S. Kim, R. S. Herbst, I. I. Wistuba, J. J. Lee, G. R. Blumenschein, Jr., A. Tsao, D. J. Stewart, M. E. Hicks, J. Erasmus, Jr., S. Gupta, et al. The BATTLE trial: personalizing therapy for lung cancer. *Cancer Discovery*, 1:44–53, 2000.

[64] P. K. Kimani, N. Stallard, and J. L. Hutton. Dose selection in seamless phase II/III clinical trials based on efficacy and safety. *Statistics in Medicine*, 28:917–936, 2009.

[65] E. L. Korn and B. Freidlin. Outcome-adaptive randomization: Is it useful? *Journal of Clinical Oncology*, 29:771–776, 2011.

[66] S. Laporte, P. Squifflet, N. Baroux, F. Fossella, V. Georgoulias, J. L. Pujol, J. Y. Douillard, S. Kudoh, J. P. Pignon, E. Quinaux, and M. Buyse. Prediction of survival benefits from progression-free survival benefits in advanced non-small cell lung cancer: Evidence from a meta-analysis of 2334 patients from 5 randomised trials. *BMJ Open*, 3:e001802, 2013.

[67] Quantum Leap. I-SPY 2 breast cancer clinical trial graduates two promising drugs. http://www.quantumleaphealth.org/spy-2-trial-graduates-2-new-drugs-press-release.

[68] J. J. Lee and N. Chen. Software for design of clinical trials. In J. Crowley and A. Hoering, editors, *Handbook of Statistics in Clinical Oncology, 3rd ed.*, pages 305–324. Chapman and Hall/CRC Press, Boca Raton, FL, USA, 2011.

[69] J. J. Lee, N. Chen, and G Yin. Worth adapting? revisiting the usefulness of outcome-adaptive randomization. *Clinical Cancer Research*, 18:4498–4507, 2012.

[70] J. J. Lee and C. T. Chu. Bayesian clinical trials in action. *Statistics in Medicine*, 31:2955–2972, 2012.

[71] J. J. Lee and C. T. Chu. Novel statistical models for NSCLC clinical trials. In J. A. Roth, W. K. Hong, and R. U. Komaki, editors, *Lung Cancer*, pages 488–503. John Wiley and Sons, New York, NY, USA, 2014.

[72] J. J. Lee, X. Gu, and S. Liu. Bayesian adaptive randomization designs for targeted agent development. *Clinical Trials*, 7:584–597, 2010.

[73] J. J. Lee and D. D. Liu. A predictive probability design for phase II cancer clinical trials. *Clinical Trials*, 5:93–106, 2008.

[74] E. O. Lillie, B. Patay, J. Diamant, B. Issell, E. J. Topol, and N. J. Schork. The n-of-1 clinical trial: the ultimate strategy for individualizing medicine? *Personalized Medicine*, 8:161–173, 2011.

[75] S. Liu, G. Yin, and Y. Yuan. Bayesian data augmentation dose finding with continual reassessment method and delayed toxicity. *Annals of Applied Statistics*, 7:2138–2156, 2013.

[76] S. Liu and Y. Yuan. Bayesian optimal interval designs for phase I clinical trials. *Journal of the Royal Statistical Society: Series C*, 64:507–523, 2015.

[77] A. Lopez-Chavez, A. Thomas, A. Rajan, M. Raffeld, B. Morrow, R. Kelly, C. A. Carter, U. Guha, K. Killian, C. C. Lau, et al. Molecular profiling and targeted therapy for advanced thoracic malignancies: a biomarker-derived, multiarm, multihistology phase II basket trial. *Journal of Clinical Oncology*, 33:1000–1007, 2015.

[78] D. Lunn, D. Spiegelhalter, A. Thomas, and N. Best. The BUGS project: evolution, critique and future directions. *Statistics in Medicine*, 28:3049–3067, 2009.

[79] D. Magirr, T. Jaki, and J. Whitehead. A generalized Dunnett test for multiarm-multistage clinical studies with treatment selection. *Biometrika*, 99:494–501, 2012.

[80] A. Maitournam and R. Simon. On the efficiency of targeted clinical trials. *Statistics in Medicine*, 24:329–339, 2005.

[81] S. J. Mandrekar, Y. Cui, and D. J. Sargent. An adaptive phase I design for identifying a biologically optimal dose for dual agent drug combinations. *Statistics in Medicine*, 26:2317–2330, 2007.

[82] S. J. Mandrekar and D. J. Sargent. Clinical trial designs for predictive biomarker validation: theoretical considerations and practical challenges. *Journal of Clinical Oncology*, 27:4027–4034, 2009.

[83] S. J. Mandrekar and D. J. Sargent. A review of phase II trial designs for initial marker validation. *Contemporary Clinical Trials.*, 36:597–604, 2013.

[84] O. Marchenko, V. Fedorov, J.J. Lee, C. Nolan, and J. Pinheiro. Adaptive clinical trials: overview of early-phase designs and challenges. *Therapeutic Innovation and Regulatory Science*, 48:20–30, 2014.

[85] S. Mook, M. K. Schmidt, G. Viale, G. Pruneri, I. Eekhout, A. Floore, A. M. Glas, J. Bogaerts, F. Cardoso, M. J. Piccart-Gebhart, E. T. Rutgers, and L. J. Van't Veer. The 70-gene prognosis-signature predicts disease outcome in breast cancer patients with 1-3 positive lymph nodes in an independent validation study. *Breast Cancer Research and Treatment*, 116:295–302, 2009.

[86] P. C. O'Brien and T. R. Fleming. A multiple testing procedure for clinical trials. *Biometrics*, 35:549–556, 1979.

[87] Friends of Cancer Research. Design of a lung cancer master protocol, 2013.
http://www.focr.org/events/design-lung-cancer-master-protocol.

[88] U.S. Department of Health, Food Human Services, and Drug Administration (CDER/CBER). Guidance for industry: adaptive design clinical trials for drugs and biologics.
http://www.fda.gov/downloads/{\protect\newline}
DrugsGuidanceComplianceRegulatoryInformation/Guidances/
UCM201790.pdf.

[89] U.S. Department of Health, Food Human Services, and Drug Administration (CDRH). Guidance for the use of Bayesian statistics in medical device clinical trials, Draft May 2006, February 2010.
http://www.fda.gov/RegulatoryInformation/Guidances/ucm071072.
htm.

[90] J. O'Quigley, M. D. Hughes, and T. Fenton. Dose-finding designs for HIV studies. *Biometrics*, 57:1018–1029, 2001.

[91] J. O'Quigley, M. Pepe, and L. D. Fisher. Continual reassessment method: a practical design for phase I clinical trials in cancer. *Biometrics*, 46:33–48, 1990.

[92] C. R. Palmer and W. F. Rosenberger. Ethics and practice: alternative designs for phase III randomized clinical trials. *Controlled Clinical Trials*, 20:172–186, 1999.

[93] X. Paoletti, K. Oba, Y. J. Bang, H. Bleiberg, N. Boku, O. Bouché, P. Catalano, N. Fuse, S. Michiels, M. Moehler, S. Morita, Y. Ohashi, et al. Progression-free survival as a surrogate for overall survival in

advanced/recurrent gastric cancer trials: a meta-analysis. *Journal of the National Cancer Institute*, 105:1667–1670, 2013.

[94] M. K. B. Parmar, J. Carpenter, and M. R. Sydes. More multiarm randomised trials of superiority are needed. *Lancet*, 384:283–284, 2014.

[95] S. J. Pocock. Group sequential method in the design and analysis of clinical trials. *Biometrika*, 64:191–199, 1977.

[96] S. J. Pocock and R. Simon. Sequential treatment assignment with balancing for prognostic factors in the controlled clinical trials. *Biometrics*, 31:103–115, 1975.

[97] M. Y. Polley and Y. K. Cheung. Two-stage designs for dose-finding trials with a biologic endpoint using stepwise tests. *Biometrics*, 64:232–241, 2008.

[98] M. A. Proschan and S. A. Hunsberger. Designed extension of studies based on conditional power. *Biometrics*, 51:1315–1324, 1995.

[99] A. Rogatko, D. Schoeneck, W. Jonas, M. Tighiouart, F. R. Khuri, and A. Porter. Translation of innovative designs into phase I trials. *Journal of Clinical Oncology*, 25:4982–4986, 2007.

[100] W. F. Rosenberger, N. Stallard, A. Ivanova, C. Harper, and M. Ricks. Optimal adaptive designs for binary response trials. *Biometrics*, 57:909–913, 2001.

[101] P. Royston, M. Parmar, and W. Qian. Novel designs for multi-arm clinical trials with survival outcomes with an application in ovarian cancer. *Statistics in Medicine*, 22:2239–2256, 2003.

[102] D. J. Sargent and C. Allegra. Issues in clinical trial design for tumor marker studies. *Seminars in Oncology*, 29:222–230, 2002.

[103] D. J. Sargent, B. A. Conley, C. Allegra, and L. Collette. Clinical trial designs for predictive marker validation in cancer treatment trials. *Journal of Clinical Oncology*, 23:2020–2027, 2005.

[104] D. J. Sargent and S. J. Mandrekar. Statistical issues in the validation of prognostic, predictive, and surrogate biomarkers. *Clinical Trials*, 10:647–652, 2013.

[105] C. Sawyers. Targeted cancer therapy. *Nature*, 432:294–297, 2004.

[106] Y. Shen and L. Fisher. Statistical inference for self-designing clinical trials with a one-sided hypothesis. *Biometrics*, 55:190–197, 1999.

[107] Q. Shi, A. De Gramont, A. Grothey, J. Zalcberg, B. Chibaudel, H. J. Schmoll, M. T. Seymour, R. Adams, L. Saltz, R. M. Goldberg, et al. Individual patient data analysis of progression-free survival versus overall survival as a first-line end point for metastatic colorectal cancer in modern randomized trials: Findings from the analysis and research in cancers of the digestive system database. *Journal of Clinical Oncology*, 33:22–28, 2015.

[108] W. J. Shih. Sample size re-estimation - journey for a decade. *Statistics in Medicine*, 20:515–518, 2001.

[109] R. Simon. Optimal two-stage designs for phase II clinical trials. *Controlled Clinical Trials*, 10:1–10, 1989.

[110] R. Simon. The use of genomics in clinical trial design. *Clinical Cancer Research*, 14:5984–5993, 2008.

[111] R. Simon. Biomarker based clinical trial design. *Chinese Clinical Oncology*, 3:39, 2014.

[112] R. Simon, B. Freidlin, L. Rubinstein, S. G. Arbuck, J. Collins, and M. C. Christian. Accelerated titration designs for phase I clinical trials in oncology. *Journal of the National Cancer Institute*, 89:1138–1147, 1997.

[113] R. Simon and A. Maitournam. Perspective evaluating the efficiency of targeted designs for randomized clinical trials. *Clinical Cancer Research*, 10:6759–6763, 2004.

[114] F. A. Sinicrope and D. J. Sargent. Molecular pathways: microsatellite instability in colorectal cancer: prognostic, predictive, and therapeutic implications. *Clinical Cancer Research*, 18:1506–1512, 2012.

[115] G. W. Sledge. What is targeted therapy? *Journal of Clinical Oncology*, 23:1614–1615, 2005.

[116] N. Stallard. A confirmatory seamless phase II/III clinical trial design incorporating short-term endpoint information. *Statistics in Medicine*, 29:959–971, 2010.

[117] B. E. Storer. Design and analysis of phase I clinical trials. *Biometrics*, 45:925–937, 1989.

[118] S. Sutter and L. Lamotta. Internal Medicine News Digital Network: cancer drugs have worst phase III track record. http://www.internalmedicinenews.com.

[119] M. R. Sydes, M. K. Parmar, N. D. James, N. W. Clarke, D. P. Dearnaley, M. D. Mason, R. C. Morgan, K. Sanders, and P. Royston. Issues in applying multi-arm multi-stage methodology to a clinical trial in prostate cancer: the MRC STAMPEDE trial. *Trials*, 10:39, 2009.

[120] P. Thall, R. Millikan, P. Muller, and S. J. Lee. Dose-finding with two agents in phase I oncology trials. *Biometrics*, 59:487–496, 2003.

[121] P. F. Thall and J. D. Cook. Dose-finding based on efficacy-toxicity trade-offs. *Biometrics*, 60:684–693, 2004.

[122] P. F. Thall and J. D. Cook. Adaptive dose-finding based on efficacy-toxicity trade-offs. In S.C. Chow, editor, *Encyclopedia of Biopharmaceutical Statistics*, pages 1–5. Marcel Dekker, New York, NY, USA, 2nd edition, 2006.

[123] P. F. Thall and K. E. Russell. A strategy for dose-finding and safety monitoring based on efficacy and adverse outcomes in phase I/II clinical trials. *Biometrics*, 54:251–264, 1998.

[124] P. F. Thall and R. Simon. Practical Bayesian guidelines for phase IIB clinical trials. *Biometrics*, 50:337–349, 1994.

[125] P. F. Thall, R. Simon, and E. H. Estey. Bayesian sequential monitoring designs for single-arm clinical trials with multiple outcomes. *Statistics in Medicine*, 14:357–379, 1995.

[126] P. F. Thall and K. J. Wathen. Practical Bayesian adaptive randomisation in clinical trials. *European Journal of Cancer*, 43:859–866, 2007.

[127] P. F. Thall, L. Wooten, and N. Tannir. Monitoring event times in early phase clinical trials: some practical issues. *Clinical Trials*, 2:467–478, 2005.

[128] L. Trippa, E. Q. Lee, P. Y. Wen, T. T. Batchelor, T. Cloughesy, G. Parmigiani, and B. M. Alexander. Bayesian adaptive randomized trial design for patients with recurrent glioblastoma. *Journal of Clinical Oncology*, 30:3258–3263, 2012.

[129] A. A. Tsiatis and C. Mehta. On the inefficiency of the adaptive design for monitoring clinical trials. *Biometrika*, 90:367–378, 2003.

[130] S. Ventz and L. Trippa. Bayesian designs and the control of frequentist characteristics: a practical solution. *Biometrics*, 71:218–226, 2015.

[131] S. J. Wang, H. M. Hung, and R. O'Neill. Regulatory perspectives on multiplicity in adaptive design clinical trials throughout a drug development program. *Journal of Biopharmaceutical Statistics*, 21:846–859, 2011.

[132] S. K. Wang and A. A. Tsiatis. Approximately optimal one-parameter boundaries for group sequential trials. *Biometrics*, 43:193–199, 1987.

[133] J. M. Wason and L. Trippa. A comparison of Bayesian adaptive randomization and multi-stage designs for multi-arm clinical trials. *Statistics in Medicine*, 33:2206–2221, 2014.

[134] J. M. S. Wason and T. Jaki. Optimal design of multi-arm multi-stage trials. *Statistics in Medicine*, 31:4269–4279, 2012.

[135] L. J. Wei and S. Durham. The randomized play-the-winner rule in medical trials. *Journal of the American Statistical Association*, 73:840–843, 1978.

[136] C. Willyard. Basket studies will hold intricate data for cancer drug approvals. *Nature Medicine*, 19:655, 2013.

[137] J. Woodcock. FDA introduction comments: clinical studies design and evaluation issues. *Clinical Trials*, 2:273–275, 2005.

[138] G. Yin. *Clinical Trial Design: Bayesian and Frequentist Adaptive Methods*. John Wiley and Sons, New York, NY, USA, 2012.

[139] G. Yin, N. Chen, and J. J. Lee. Phase II trial design with Bayesian adaptive randomization and predictive probability. *Journal of the Royal Statistical Society: Series C*, 61:219–235, 2012.

[140] G. Yin, Y. Li, and Y. Ji. Bayesian dose-finding in phase I/II trials using toxicity and efficacy odds ratio. *Biometrics*, 62:777–784, 2006.

[141] G. Yin and Y. Yuan. Bayesian dose-finding in oncology for drug combination by copula regression. *Journal of the Royal Statistical Society: Series C*, 58:211–224, 2009.

[142] G. Yin and Y. Yuan. Bayesian model averaging continual reassessment method in phase I clinical trials. *Journal of the American Statistical Association*, 104:954–968, 2009.

[143] G. Yin and Y. Yuan. A latent contingency table approach to dose-finding for combinations of two agents. *Biometrics*, 65:866–875, 2009.

[144] Y. Yuan and G. Yin. Sequential continual reassessment method for two-dimensional dose findings. *Statistics in Medicine*, 27:5664–5678, 2008.

[145] Y. Yuan and G. Yin. Bayesian dose finding by jointly modeling toxicity and efficacy as time-to-event outcomes. *Journal of the Royal Statistical Society: Series C*, 58:719–736, 2009.

[146] Y. Yuan and G. Yin. Bayesian phase I/II drug-combination trial design in oncology. *Annals of Applied Statistics*, 5:924–942, 2011.

[147] Y. Yuan and G. Yin. Robust EM continual reassessment method in oncology dose finding. *Journal of the American Statistical Association*, 106:818–831, 2011.

[148] Y. Zang, J. J. Lee, and Y. Yuan. Adaptive designs for identifying optimal biological dose for molecularly targeted agents. *Clinical Trials*, 11:319–327, 2014.

[149] M. Zelen. Play the winner rule and the controlled clinical trial. *Journal of the American Statistical Association*, 64:131–146, 1969.

[150] W. Zhang, D. J. Sargent, and S. J. Mandrekar. An adaptive dose-finding design incorporating both toxicity and efficacy. *Statistics in Medicine*, 25:2365–2383, 2006.

[151] X. Zhou, S. Liu, E. S. Kim, R. R. Herbst, and J. J. Lee. Bayesian adaptive design for targeted therapy development in lung cancer - a step toward personalized medicine. *Clinical Trials*, 5:181–193, 2008.

13

Dynamic Treatment Regimes

Marie Davidian

Anastasios (Butch) Tsiatis

Eric Laber

CONTENTS

13.1 Introduction

Cancer treatment ordinarily involves a series of treatment decisions made over the course of a patient's disease. Key decision points may correspond to milestones in the disease process, such as remission, progression, or recurrence; or decisions may be necessitated by, for example, occurrence of an adverse event. In practice, at each decision point, a clinician will synthesize the accrued information on the patient, which might include demographic and genetic/genomic information as well as evolving physiologic and other clinical variables, to select a treatment from among the available options, with the goal of "personalizing" the decision to the patient to achieve the "best" clinical outcome.

There has been considerable interest in approaches to making such clinical decision making evidence-based. A *dynamic treatment regime* can be viewed as formalizing this objective. A dynamic treatment regime is a set of sequential *decision rules*, each corresponding to a key point in the disease at which a treatment decision is required. Each rule dictates the treatment to be given from among the available options based on the accrued information on the patient to that point. Taken together, the rules define an algorithm for making treatment decisions. Such treatment regimes are referred to as *dynamic* because the treatment actions they dictate may vary depending on the accrued information; dynamic treatment regimes thus *personalize* the decisions to the patient. Also possible are treatment regimes that do not use accrued information to determine treatment but instead specify the treatments to be given in advance; these have been called *static* [8] or *non-dynamic* (in the early literature). In the next section, we present examples of both, and we use *treatment regime* to refer to any approach to selecting treatment over a single or multiple decision points. Some authors prefer the term *treatment regimen* [24] on the basis of interpretability by clinicians.

An extensive literature has emerged on methods for learning about and developing dynamic treatment regimes from data from clinical and observational studies and on the conception and design of so-called *sequential, multiple assignment, randomized trials* (SMARTs), which are clinical trials suited to these goals [24, 40]. Data-based study of dynamic treatment regimes is thus a major step toward providing clinicians with evidence-based decision support.

In this chapter, we introduce the notion of a dynamic treatment regime and discuss an appropriate statistical framework in which treatment regimes of any type may be studied. In the context of a running example, presented in the next section, we discuss regimes of varying complexity and the idea that common questions can be represented as finding the optimal regime within a particular class of regimes of interest, where "optimal" is defined precisely within the statistical framework. We then discuss SMARTs as an ideal trial design for collecting data that may be used for studying dynamic treatment regimes and present statistical methods for studying the optimal regime within a specified class of interest. We further demonstrate that many common treatment challenges can be shown to involve dynamic treatment regimes and that this can lead to novel approaches to addressing them. In principle, an infinitude of possible sets of rules, and thus treatment regimes, can be conceived. We review methods for estimating an optimal treatment regime within a rich class of possible treatment regimes, where the notion of optimal is precisely defined, and which provide formal approaches to evidence-based personalized medicine. We conclude with a discussion of extensions and further challenges relevant in the study of cancer treatment.

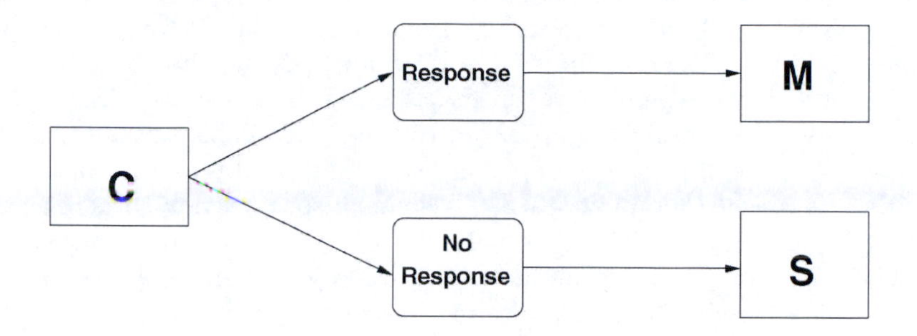

FIGURE 13.1: Schematic of two sequential decision points in cancer treatment. Decision 1: Induction chemotherapy (two options C_1 and C_2). Decision 2: For responders to induction therapy, maintenance therapy (two options M_1 and M_2); for non-responders to induction therapy, salvage therapy (two options S_1 and S_2).

Throughout, we assume that there is a health outcome by which treatment benefit can be assessed, which we take to be coded so that larger values reflect greater benefit; e.g., a survival time or a binary indicator of response to treatment. We focus on the situation where, at each decision point, the set of possible treatment options is finite, so we do not consider the case where, for example, the options span a continuous range of doses.

13.2 Characterization of Treatment Regimes

13.2.1 Decision Rules and Regimes

As a running example, we focus on the setting depicted in Figure 13.1, which is representative of that in acute leukemias. The considerations discussed in this context regarding sequential treatment decisions are relevant more generally in other cancer settings. For a patient presenting with disease of a particular type and stage, an initial decision must be made on induction chemotherapy, C, which is intended to induce a suitable response, e.g., complete or partial response or remission. Assume that there are two available induction chemotherapy options, which we denote by C_1 and C_2, from which the clinician can choose at this first decision point (Decision 1). After some specified number of cycles of induction therapy or other time frame, response status is evaluated. If the patient is deemed to have achieved response, a second decision is made on maintenance therapy, M, which is administered to sustain the response; otherwise, if the patient has not achieved satisfactory response, the second decision involves choosing a second line or salvage therapy, S. Assume that at this second decision point (Decision 2) there are two maintenance options, M_1 and M_2, from which the clinician can choose for patients who respond, and two salvage options, S_1 and S_2, for patients who do not respond.

The objective of the clinician in practice is to make these decisions, and thus choose an induction therapy from the set of available options $\{\mathsf{C}_1, \mathsf{C}_2\}$ followed by a maintenance therapy chosen from $\{\mathsf{M}_1, \mathsf{M}_2\}$ if the patient responds or a salvage therapy from $\{\mathsf{S}_1, \mathsf{S}_2\}$ if he or she does not, so as to achieve maximal expected benefit for the patient with respect to some outcome, as disease-free or overall survival time. In our presentation here, we focus on maximizing expected outcome; however, the development is applicable more broadly. For example, for a binary outcome such as response to treatment, maximizing expected outcome corresponds to maximizing the probability of response. Likewise, for a continuous measure such as survival time, the probability of exceeding the threshold is maximized.

In this example, then, we focus on two key decision points at which decisions on treatment are to be made; in general, depending on the context, there may be $K \geq 1$ decision points of interest. In practice, a clinician makes these decisions based on the information available on the patient up to the time of the decision. A dynamic treatment regime corresponding to our situation thus consists of $K = 2$ decision rules, each taking as input the accrued information on the patient and returning the treatment to be given from among the set of available options. In our example, we consider two options for each of induction, maintenance, and salvage therapy, but the principles we now discuss generalize to any numbers of options.

To define decision rules, we adopt the following standard notation. Let x_1 be patient information that may be available on a patient at Decision 1; this might include genetic and genomic information, demographic variables, clinical and physiological variables, variables describing prior medical history and concomitant conditions, and so on. Let a_1 denote a treatment option in the set of available options at Decision 1, $\mathcal{A}_1$, say; in our example, $\mathcal{A}_1 = \{\mathsf{C}_1, \mathsf{C}_2\}$. Let x_2 be additional patient information that may accrue between Decisions 1 and 2; that is, in the period immediately following initiation of the selected treatment option at Decision 1 up until the time of the second decision. This could include evolving levels of markers such as carcinoembryonic antigen (CEA) or prostate-specific antigen (PSA); physiological variables; occurrence and timing of adverse events; and so on. Let a_2 denote a treatment option in the set of available options $\mathcal{A}_2$ at Decision 2. In our example, $\mathcal{A}_2 = \{\mathsf{M}_1, \mathsf{M}_2, \mathsf{S}_1, \mathsf{S}_2\}$. Note that not all options in $\mathcal{A}_2$ are feasible for all patients, as maintenance therapies are relevant only to patients who respond and salvage therapies are appropriate only for patients who do not. We return to this point shortly.

Here, with $K = 2$, let h_k denote the accrued patient information (history) at Decision k, $k = 1, 2$. Then $h_1 = x_1$ and, at Decision 2, $h_2 = \{x_1, a_1, x_2\}$, where a_1 is the treatment option that was administered at Decision 1. Thus, the accrued information at Decision 2 includes all that was known about the patient at Decision 1 plus additional information ascertained in the intervening period. With these definitions, we denote decision rules at each decision as

$$\begin{array}{lll} \text{Decision 1:} & d_1(h_1), & h_1 = x_1 \\ \text{Decision 2:} & d_2(h_2), & h_2 = (x_1, a_1, x_2). \end{array} \tag{13.1}$$

Here, d_1 is a function of the accrued information h_1 at Decision 1 and takes values in the set of treatment options $\mathcal{A}_1$; similarly, d_2 is a function of the accrued information h_2 at Decision 2, taking values in $\mathcal{A}_2$. We then denote a dynamic treatment regime d consisting of a collection of rules as in (13.1) by

$$d = \{d_1(h_1), d_2(h_2)\}. \tag{13.2}$$

All of the foregoing definitions can be extended in the obvious way to $K > 2$ decision points. If the focus is on a single decision point, $K = 1$, a regime d is defined by a single rule d_1 corresponding to that decision point, i.e., $d = \{d_1(h_1)\}$.

We now illustrate the notion of a decision rule by presenting examples of possible rules d_1 and d_2 corresponding to each decision point in our example. At Decision 1, the simplest type of rule is one that always selects a particular treatment option without taking into account any information on the patient; i.e., the rule "Give C_1" selects treatment C_1 regardless of the value of the information h_1 on the patient. We can express this rule as

$$d_1(h_1) = \mathsf{C}_1 \quad \text{for all } h_1, \tag{13.3}$$

and similarly for the alternative rule "Give C_2." Rules of this form obviously do not take into account any patient information and thus do not attempt to personalize treatment; accordingly, they can be described as being static or non-dynamic, as the treatment action recommended does not vary depending on patient information.

A more complex rule at Decision 1 is one that takes into account patient information. For example, if h_1 includes the variables age (years) and white blood cell count (WBC $\times 10^3/\mu$l), then a possible rule incorporating this information is "If $\mathsf{age} < 50$ and $\mathsf{WBC} < 10$, then give C_2; otherwise, give C_1." Coding $\{\mathsf{C}_1, \mathsf{C}_2\}$ as $\{0, 1\}$, as is commonplace with two treatment options, and defining as usual $I(\cdot)$ to be the indicator function such that $I(A) = 1$ if the event A is true and 0 otherwise, we can write this rule compactly as

$$d_1(h_1) = I(\mathsf{age} < 50 \text{ and } \mathsf{WBC} < 10). \tag{13.4}$$

The rule d_1 in (13.4) returns a 1 corresponding to C_2 if the event inside the indicator function is true and returns a 0 corresponding to C_1 otherwise. This rule is based on cutoff or threshold values for age and WBC. Clearly, other rules involving these variables are also possible; for example, "If $\mathsf{age} + 7.8 \log(\mathsf{WBC}) - 60 > 0$ give C_2; otherwise give C_1," which can be written formally as

$$d_1(h_1) = I\{\mathsf{age} - 7.8 \log(\mathsf{WBC}) - 60 > 0\}. \tag{13.5}$$

Here, instead of involving cutoff values, the rule d_1 in (13.5) is based on the value of a linear combination of variables.

The examples in (13.3)–(13.5) demonstrate that it is possible to conceive of an infinitude of possible rules; e.g., by simply changing the age cutoff in (13.4) from 50 to 51, say, a different rule is defined. With high-dimensional information $h_1 = x_1$ at Decision 1, quite complex rules can be conceived.

The situation is similar for Decision 2, with some modification. Here, as noted above, feasibility of the treatment options in $\mathcal{A}_2 = \{\mathsf{M}_1, \mathsf{M}_2, \mathsf{S}_1, \mathsf{S}_2\}$ for a given patient is dictated by the status of that patient's response to the induction therapy he or she received at Decision 1. Accordingly, any realistic Decision 2 rule must depend on the patient variable "response status," and thus all rules at Decision 2 are dynamic in the sense that the treatment action will vary according to response status. The simplest possible such rules depend only on response status; e.g., one such rule is "If patient is a responder, give maintenance therapy M_1; if patient is a nonresponder, give salvage therapy S_1." In our example there are four possible such simple rules corresponding to each combination of M_k and S_ℓ, $k, \ell = 1, 2$. Defining $r = 1$ if a patient responded to Decision 1 therapy and $r = 0$ otherwise, clearly r is contained in $x_2 \in h_2$, and such rules can be written formally for a particular choice $k, \ell = 1, 2$ as

$$\begin{aligned} d_2(h_2) &= \mathsf{M}_k \quad \text{if } r = 1, \\ &= \mathsf{S}_\ell \quad \text{if } r = 0. \end{aligned} \tag{13.6}$$

Assuming that x_1 includes the variables age, WBC, gender (= 1 if male), and percent CD56 expression (CD56, %), and x_2 includes an indicator of a grade 3 or higher hematologic adverse event (HAE), post-induction ECOG performance status (ECOG, 0–5 scale), and platelets (PLT $\times 10^3/\mu$l) in addition to response status, a hypothetical example of a more complex Decision 2 rule is

> "If patient is a responder, age < 60, WBC $< 12 \times 10^3/\mu$l, CD56 $> 20\%$, then give M_1, else give M_2; if patient is not a responder, age > 45, gender $= 1$, HAE, ECOG < 3, PLT $< 40 \times 10^3/\mu$l, then give S_1, else give S_2."

With appropriate notation for the components of x_1 and x_2, a mathematical statement $d_2(h_2)$ of this rule can be formulated. In rules like this and those in (13.4) and (13.5), patient variables like age, WBC, CD56, and so on that are important for making treatment decisions are sometimes referred to as *tailoring variables*, as they are implicated in "tailoring" treatment to the patient.

As in (13.2), a treatment regime d is then a collection of rules like those above, where rules can range from the very simple, making use of no (static) or only limited patient information, to more complex, involving many potential tailoring variables (dynamic). Regimes comprising rule(s) that incorporate extensive patient information may be closer to achieving personalized treatment and to mimicking clinical practice. We now discuss *classes* of regimes, distinguished by their complexity, that may be of interest in different practical situations.

13.2.2 Classes of Treatment Regimes

In cancer clinical research, as with that in most chronic diseases, and from a regulatory perspective, the conventional approach to thinking about and studying treatment is to focus on a single key decision point and compare treatment options at that point. This situation may be placed in the context of studying treatment regimes defined for $K = 1$ decision in a specified class. For definiteness, suppose interest focuses on Decision 1 of the example in Figure 13.1 and comparing the two induction chemotherapies C_1 and C_2. Ideally, the question of interest can be stated precisely as follows: "If all patients in the population were to be given C_2, would mean outcome (mean survival time here) be different from (larger than) that if all patients in the population were to be given C_1?" It should be apparent that this is a question about comparing the two simple regimes comprising a single rule d_1 corresponding to this single decision point of the form in (13.3). Thus, if we let $\mathcal{D}$ denote the class of regimes of interest,

$$\mathcal{D} = \{\text{“Give } \mathsf{C}_1\text{”}, \text{“ Give } \mathsf{C}_2\text{”}\}, \tag{13.7}$$

this question can be addressed by finding the regime in $\mathcal{D}$ such that, if all patients in the population were to receive treatment according to it, mean outcome would be largest among the regimes in $\mathcal{D}$. That is, the classical primary treatment comparison in a conventional clinical trial can be likened to finding the optimal treatment regime within a class $\mathcal{D}$ like that in (13.7), where optimal corresponds to achieving the largest mean outcome among the regimes in $\mathcal{D}$.

For situations like that in Figure 13.1, involving treatments administered sequentially, a common question of interest focuses on determining the "best" treatment sequence. In our example, with $K = 2$ decision points, it is apparent that a "treatment sequence" can be characterized by a statement of the form

$$\text{“Give } \mathsf{C}_j \text{ followed by } \mathsf{M}_k \text{ if response or } \mathsf{S}_\ell \text{ if no response,”} \tag{13.8}$$

for specified choices of $j, k, \ell = 1, 2$. Analogous to the classical treatment comparison at a single decision point, the "best" treatment sequence is reasonably defined as that leading to the largest mean outcome if all patients in the population were to follow it. It should be clear that such a treatment sequence can be characterized as a dynamic treatment regime with rules $d_1^{(j)}(h_1) = \mathsf{C}_j$ for all h_1, say, as in (13.3) at Decision 1 and, in obvious notation, $d_2^{(k\ell)}(h_2)$ as in (13.6) at Decision 2. There are eight possible treatment sequences associated with each possible combination of (j, k, ℓ), which correspond to eight possible treatment regimes of this form. With the rules defined in this way, write the regime corresponding to the (j, k, ℓ) combination as $d^{(jk\ell)} = \{d_1^{(j)}(h_1), d_2^{(k\ell)}(h_2)\}$, $j, k, \ell = 1, 2$. Letting $\mathcal{D}$ denote the class comprising these eight possible regimes, determining the best treatment sequence is equivalent to finding the optimal regime in $\mathcal{D}$, i.e., such that, if all patients in the population were to receive treatment according to its rules, the mean outcome achieved would be the largest. We discuss study designs and methods that can be used to address this question in Section 13.4.

These classes of regimes are simple, with finite numbers of elements. Clearly, it is possible to conceive of more complex classes of regimes that would be relevant in the context of personalized treatment. For instance, suppose that for Decision 1 in our example, interest focuses on regimes that involve a single decision rule ($K = 1$) based on age and WBC, which are ordinarily ascertained in clinical practice. Suppose further that rules like that in (13.4), involving cutoff values for each variable, are of interest, where C_1 and C_2 are coded as $\{0, 1\}$. Then the class of interest involves regimes with rules of the form

$$d_1(h_1) = I(\mathsf{age} < \eta_1 \text{ and } \mathsf{WBC} < \eta_2), \tag{13.9}$$

where η_1 and η_2 in (13.9) are real-valued cutoff values. This class is infinite, with regimes indexed by all possible pairs of values $\eta = (\eta_1, \eta_2)^T$, which we highlight by denoting the class by $\mathcal{D}_\eta$. Intuitively, an optimal regime within $\mathcal{D}_\eta$ is defined by $\eta^{opt} = (\eta_1^{opt}, \eta_2^{opt})$, say, such that, if all patients in the population were to be given induction therapy according to the rule (13.9) with η^{opt} substituted, the mean outcome achieved would be maximized across all possible rules of this form and thus over all possible η and regimes in $\mathcal{D}_\eta$. Similar considerations apply to defining classes of regimes for $K > 1$.

The preceding example involves a richer class of regimes than the previous two, albeit one whose form is restricted to rules of form (13.9) indexed by η. Such a class may be relevant when it is of interest to develop a personalized treatment strategy subject to considerations of interpretability of the decision rules involved and the cost, burden, and/or logistics of implementing them. Obviously, realizing the full promise of personalized medicine involves considering the class $\mathcal{D}$ consisting of *all* possible regimes, which for $K = 2$ are of the form in (13.2), where no restrictions are placed on the rules d_1 and d_2. Thus, rules in $\mathcal{D}$ can in principle involve the accrued information h_1 and h_2 in an infinitude of combinations and possibly complicated ways. An optimal regime in $\mathcal{D}$ is one that maximizes the mean outcome that would be achieved if all patients in the population were to follow it. In Section 13.6, we characterize formally the form of an optimal regime in terms of the statistical framework we discuss next, and we describe methods for estimating optimal regimes both in this class and restricted classes of regimes like $\mathcal{D}_\eta$.

13.3 Potential Outcomes Framework

We have seen that, given a class of regimes of interest, the optimal regime within the class corresponds to that leading to the largest mean outcome if all patients were to receive treatment according to it. Questions of interest may then be characterized as concerning finding the optimal regime within the class. This may be made precise by adopting the perspective of *causal inference* and appealing to the concept of *potential outcomes.*

13.3.1 Single Decision

We first discuss the situation where interest focuses on a single decision. In our example, consider Decision 1 and the classical comparison of the two induction therapies C_1 and C_2, coded again as $\{0, 1\}$. As before, this comparison can be cast as finding the optimal regime in the class (13.7).

Let $Y^{(1)}$ be a random variable representing the outcome that *would be achieved* if a randomly chosen patient from the population of interest were to receive treatment according to the regime "Give C_2"; that is, were to be given induction therapy C_2. Define $Y^{(0)}$ analogously. Conceptually, all patients in the population have such a potential outcome, so that $E\{Y^{(1)}\}$ corresponds to the mean outcome if all patients were to be treated according to the regime "Give C_2"; i.e., receive C_2. Similarly, $E\{Y^{(0)}\}$ corresponds to the mean outcome if all patients were to follow regime "Give C_1"; i.e., receive C_1. Thus, the classical question of which therapy leads to the largest mean outcome, which is analogous to finding the optimal regime in the class (13.7), can be represented as comparing $E\{Y^{(1)}\}$ and $E\{Y^{(0)}\}$.

Now consider an arbitrary, possibly infinite class of regimes $\mathcal{D}$ corresponding to a single decision ($K = 1$); for example, a class of regimes indexed by a parameter η, as in (13.9), or the class of all possible regimes discussed at the end of Section 13.2.2. If there are two treatment options coded as 0 and 1, so that the set of treatment options is $\mathcal{A}_1 = \{0, 1\}$, then we can again conceive of potential outcomes $Y^{(0)}$ and $Y^{(1)}$ corresponding to each option. A regime $d \in \mathcal{D}$ comprises a rule $d_1(h_1)$ that returns a 0 or 1, the option recommended depending on the value of h_1. Let X_1 be a vector of random variables representing the information available on a randomly chosen patient at Decision 1, and write $H_1 = X_1$ to denote the corresponding history. Then we can define the potential outcome that would be achieved if the patient were to receive treatment according to a regime $d \in \mathcal{D}$ as

$$\begin{aligned} Y^{(d)} &= Y^{(1)} I\{d_1(H_1) = 1\} + Y^{(0)} I\{d_1(H_1) = 0\} \\ &= Y^{(1)} d_1(H_1) + Y^{(0)}\{1 - d_1(H_1)\}. \end{aligned} \tag{13.10}$$

That is, intuitively, the outcome that would be achieved if a randomly chosen patient with information H_1 at Decision 1 were to receive treatment according to regime d is equal to the potential outcome he or she would achieve under the option dictated by d. Finding the optimal regime thus amounts to finding a regime in $\mathcal{D}$ that maximizes $E\{Y^{(d)}\}$; it is common to refer to $E\{Y^{(d)}\}$ for any regime d as the *value* of d. We refer to such a regime as d^{opt}; thus, d^{opt} maximizes the value over all regimes $d \in \mathcal{D}$. In principle, it is possible for more than one regime to achieve the maximum value of $E\{Y^{(d)}\}$, in which case there may be more than one optimal regime in $\mathcal{D}$. Thus, to be precise, we should refer to "an," rather than "the," optimal regime; for simplicity, we downplay this subtlety and use the latter terminology.

If the class $\mathcal{D}$ is that in (13.7) consisting of the two regimes "Give C_1" and "Give C_2," so that $d_1(h_1)$ returns 0 or 1 regardless of the value of h_1, respectively, then note trivially that $Y^{(d)} = Y^{(0)}$ or $Y^{(1)}$, and maximizing $E\{Y^{(d)}\}$ corresponds to finding the larger of $E\{Y^{(0)}\}$ or $E\{Y^{(1)}\}$, as above.

For a general, finite set $\mathcal{A}_1$ of two or more treatment options a_1, for any regime d, the rule $d_1(h_1)$ returns an option $a_1 \in \mathcal{A}_1$ depending on the value of h_1. Letting $Y^{(a_1)}$ denote the potential outcome a randomly chosen patient would achieve if given option a_1, it should be clear that, for such a patient with available information H_1 at Decision 1, (13.10) can be generalized as

$$Y^{(d)} = \sum_{a_1 \in \mathcal{A}_1} Y^{(a_1)} I\{d_1(H_1) = a_1\},$$

and the optimal regime d^{opt} maximizes the value $E\{Y^{(d)}\}$ so defined.

In all of the above, the optimal regime is expressed in terms of potential outcomes rather than outcomes that can actually be observed on patients; e.g., participants in a clinical trial or observational study. Although this characterizes an optimal regime precisely, if the optimal regime is to be studied based on data, it must be possible to represent it equivalently in terms of observable quantities. In Section 13.4.1, we discuss assumptions under which this is possible and demonstrate how to express quantities such as $E\{Y^{(0)}\}$, $E\{Y^{(1)}\}$, $E\{Y^{(d)}\}$ equivalently in terms of observable outcomes.

13.3.2 Multiple Decisions

First consider finding the optimal treatment sequence in our example, which corresponds to finding the optimal regime within the class of regimes of the form in (13.8). Define the random variable $Y^{(d^{(jk\ell)})}$ to be the outcome a randomly chosen patient in the population would achieve if he or she were to follow the regime $d^{(jk\ell)}$; i.e., "Give induction therapy j followed by maintenance k if response or salvage ℓ if no response." Then, for example, $Y^{(d^{(211)})}$ represents the potential outcome that would be achieved if a patient were to follow "Give C_2 followed by M_1 if response or S_1 if no response." By the same reasoning as in Section 13.3.1, finding the optimal regime among the eight possible in the class involves comparison of $E\{Y^{(d^{(jk\ell)})}\}$, $j, k, \ell = 1, 2$. Again, to determine how to do this based on data on observed outcomes for patients who have followed each of the eight regimes, it must be possible, under appropriate assumptions, to express these expectations in terms of observable outcomes. We demonstrate in detail for a related situation in Section 13.4.3.

For K decision points and an arbitrary, possibly infinite class of regimes $\mathcal{D}$, a general potential outcome framework may be formulated. For definiteness, take $K = 2$, and suppose there are finite sets of treatment options $\mathcal{A}_1$ and

$\mathcal{A}_2$ at each of Decisions 1 and 2, respectively. For any regime $d \in \mathcal{D}$, the rules $d_1(h_1)$ and $d_2(h_2)$ return options $a_1 \in \mathcal{A}_1$ and $a_2 \in \mathcal{A}_2$ depending h_1 and h_2. Let X_1 be a random variable representing the information available on a randomly chosen patient at Decision 1, and write $H_1 = X_1$. Intuitively, once such a patient receives his or her Decision 1 treatment according to d_1, all of his or her subsequent achieved information and outcome will be predicated on this and the rule d_2. To characterize this precisely, we define the intermediate information such a patient would achieve if he or she received option a_1 at Decision 1 to be $X_2^{(a_1)}$ and define the outcome he or she would then achieve after also receiving option a_2 at Decision 2 as $Y^{(a_1,a_2)}$.

We can then use these random variables to define the potential intermediate information and potential outcome a randomly chosen patient with initial information H_1 would achieve if he or she were to receive treatment at both decisions according to the rules in d as follows. If $H_1 = h_1 = x_1$ and the option dictated at Decision 1 is $a_1 = d_1(h_1)$, then define $X_2^{(d_1)} = X_2^{(a_1)}$ to be the intermediate information the patient would achieve after following rule d_1. If $X_2^{(d_1)} = x_2$, then $h_2 = (x_1, a_1, x_2)$. If the option thus dictated at Decision 2 is $a_2 = d_2(h_2)$, then define the potential outcome the patient would achieve after following both rules in d as $Y^{(d)} = Y^{(a_1,a_2)}$.

With the potential outcome $Y^{(d)}$ for any $d \in \mathcal{D}$ defined in this way, an optimal regime d^{opt} maximizes the value $E\{Y^{(d)}\}$ over all $d \in \mathcal{D}$. This formulation may be generalized to $K > 2$ decisions in the obvious way; see [50].

13.4 Sequential, Multiple Assignment, Randomized Trials

13.4.1 Data for Studying Dynamic Treatment Regimes

Having defined precisely the notion of a treatment regime and the optimal regime in a specified class within the potential outcome framework, we now consider the study of regimes based on observable data.

In our example and the simplest case of a single decision ($K = 1$) and the class of two (static) regimes of the form (13.3), i.e., "Give C_1" and "Give C_2," estimation and comparison of the mean outcomes if all patients in the population were to receive C_1 (0) or C_2 (1), respectively, correspond to estimation of $E\{Y^{(0)}\}$ and $E\{Y^{(1)}\}$ based on suitable data. Data from a randomized clinical trial in which patients are randomly assigned to the two regimes are the gold standard for addressing this classical treatment question. Alternatively, data from an observational study can be used. In either type of study, the data available on each subject are (X_1, A_1, Y), where X_1 is baseline information as discussed above; A_1 is the assigned treatment, coded as $\{0, 1\}$ here; and Y is the *observed* outcome of interest. We thus consider how $E\{Y^{(0)}\}$ and $E\{Y^{(1)}\}$ can be expressed in terms of these observed data.

Intuitively, the observed outcome can be represented as

$$Y = Y^{(1)}I(A_1 = 1) + Y^{(0)}I(A_1 = 0) = Y^{(1)}A_1 + Y^{(0)}(1 - A_1), \tag{13.11}$$

which says that the outcome observed on a subject is the potential outcome he or she would achieve under the treatment he or she actually received. This is usually referred to as the *consistency assumption*. In a clinical trial, randomization guarantees that treatment assignment is independent of how a patient would fare under either treatment, so that $(Y^{(0)}, Y^{(1)}) \perp\!\!\!\perp A_1$, where "$\perp\!\!\!\perp$" means "independent of." It follows that

$$E\{Y^{(1)}\} = E\{Y^{(1)}|A_1 = 1\} = E(Y|A_1 = 1), \tag{13.12}$$

where the first equality follows because $Y^{(1)} \perp\!\!\!\perp A_1$ and the second from (13.11); similarly, $E\{Y^{(0)}\} = E(Y|A = 0)$. Thus, under randomization, $E\{Y^{(0)}\}$ and $E\{Y^{(1)}\}$ can be expressed in terms of the observed data. Moreover, from (13.12), given independent and identically distributed (iid) data (X_{1i}, A_{1i}, Y_i), $i = 1, \ldots, n$, from n participants, $E\{Y^{(1)}\}$ can be estimated by

$$\left\{\sum_{i=1}^{n} A_{1i}\right\}^{-1} \sum_{i=1}^{n} Y_i A_{1i}, \tag{13.13}$$

the sample average of observed outcomes among subjects who received treatment 1, and similarly for $E\{Y^{(0)}\}$. Thus, the potential outcome framework makes explicit the role of randomization in achieving valid inferences on the comparison of mean outcomes were all patients in the population to receive each treatment. Note that the baseline information $H_1 = X_1$ is not required.

If the data are from an observational study, then subjects were not assigned at random to treatments. Thus, independence and (13.12) no longer hold, and confounding of treatment assignment and subject characteristics could render inference on, e.g., $E\{Y^{(1)}\}$ using (13.13), biased. A stronger assumption involving $H_1 = X_1$ is needed, namely, that of *no unmeasured confounders*,

$$(Y^{(0)}, Y^{(1)}) \perp\!\!\!\perp A_1 | H_1; \tag{13.14}$$

i.e., that the potential outcomes are independent of treatment assignment conditional on $H_1 = X_1$. This assumption is standard in the analysis of observational studies and is trivially true for a clinical trial. Assumption (13.14) says that all information that might have been used by clinicians and patients to make treatment decisions is contained in X_1, so that, once X_1 is taken into account, within the subpopulation of patients with a particular value of X_1, assignment to treatment 0 or 1 is essentially at random. The challenge in practice is that it is not possible to verify (13.14) based on the observed data. Moreover, X_1 thought to validate (13.14) must be recorded in the database and be available to the data analyst. Thus, the potential outcomes formulation emphasizes explicitly the well-known difficulties associated with inferences from observational data.

The key result is that, under (13.14),

$$\begin{aligned} E\{Y^{(1)}\} &= E[\,E\{Y^{(1)}|H_1\}\,] \\ &= E[\,E\{Y^{(1)}|H_1, A_1 = 1\} = E\{E(Y|H_1, A_1 = 1)\}, \quad (13.15) \end{aligned}$$

where the first equality in (13.15) follows from (13.14) and the second from (13.11); and similarly for $E\{Y^{(0)}\}$. Then, if (13.14) holds, it is possible to express $E\{Y^{(0)}\}$ and $E\{Y^{(1)}\}$ in terms of the observed data; namely, the regression $E(Y|H_1, A_1)$ of observed outcome on $H_1 = X_1$ and A_1. Thus, if a regression model $Q_1(h_1, a_1; \beta_1)$ is posited for $E(Y|H_1 = h_1, A_1 = a_1)$; e.g., a linear or logistic model for continuous or binary outcome, and β_1 estimated by $\widehat{\beta}_1$ (e.g., by least squares or maximum likelihood), (13.15) suggests that $E\{Y^{(1)}\}$ can be estimated by

$$n^{-1} \sum_{i=1}^{n} Q_1(H_{1i}, 1; \widehat{\beta}_1),$$

and similarly for $E\{Y^{(0)}\}$. Other approaches based on so-called propensity scores are also possible [12, 35, 49].

These developments show that, in the simplest case of a single decision and the class of regimes (13.7), the optimal regime among "Give C_1" and "Give C_2" can be be deduced from data from a clinical trial or, if (13.14) is assumed, from an observational study using routine methods. We discuss methods for estimating the optimal regime within richer, infinite classes of regimes such as $\mathcal{D}_\eta$ involving regimes (13.9) or the class of all possible regimes in Section 13.6.

We now consider data that would be required to study regimes involving $K > 1$ decision points. Consider finding the optimal treatment sequence in the class of regimes of form (13.8) for $K = 2$ in our example. As in the case of a single decision, basing this on data from randomized clinical trials would be ideal. One approach is to try to exploit data from a series of trials. Suppose that data are available from a trial comparing induction therapies C_1 and C_2, while in another, maintenance treatments M_1 and M_2 were compared in patients who responded to any induction therapy. In still another, S_1 and S_2 were compared in patients for whom induction therapy did not induce a response. Clearly, each trial would have involved different samples of patients. Given such data, it is tempting to conclude that the regime involving the "best" C therapy as determined from the first trial coupled with the "best" M and S treatments from the second and third trials should be optimal in the sense of leading to the "best" mean outcome.

Unfortunately, there are difficulties with this reasoning. A major challenge is that of *delayed effects* of treatments. For example, induction therapy C_1 may yield a higher proportion of responders than C_2, making it appear superior

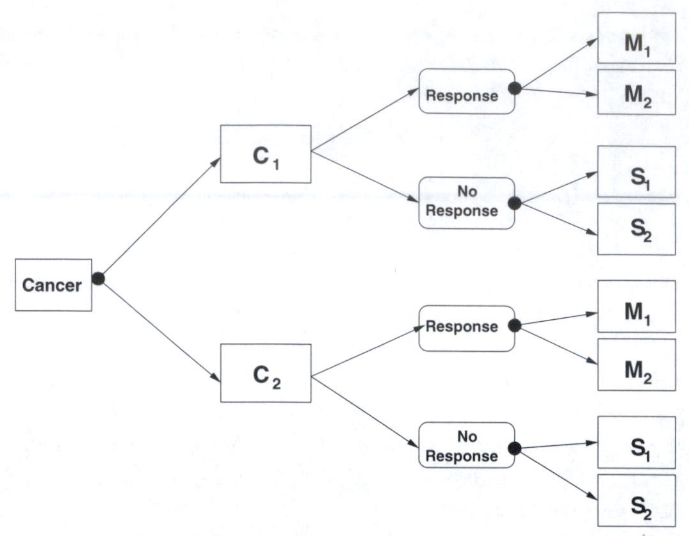

FIGURE 13.2: Schematic of a SMART embedding the eight possible regimes in the two-decision situation of Figure 13.1. Bullets represent points of randomization.

from a myopic point of view. However, C_1 may also have other effects that manifest only after some time has passed and render subsequent maintenance treatments less effective for survival. Such a delayed effect has obvious implications for determining the optimal treatment sequence. However, this would be impossible to elucidate from data from separate trials involving different samples of subjects. Accordingly, valid study of the optimal treatment sequence or, more generally, regimes in any class involving $K \geq 2$ decision points can only be carried out based on longitudinal data from the same subjects treated sequentially at each decision point.

These considerations underlie a clinical trial design that has been advocated for the purpose of studying dynamic treatment regimes, the sequential, multiple assignment, randomized trial, or SMART, which has been pioneered by Lavori and Dawson, Murphy, and others [14, 30, 31, 40]. In a SMART, the same subjects are randomized at each decision point to the available options. Intuitively, a SMART enjoys the advantages of randomization and provides a basis for taking possible delayed effects to be taken into account. In the next section, we discuss this and other issues surrounding the use of SMARTs.

13.4.2 Considerations for SMARTs

Consider Figure 13.2, which is a schematic representation of a SMART that could be undertaken to investigate treatment regimes involving the two decision points in our example in Figure 13.1. At the first decision point, patients present with cancer and are randomized to C_1 or C_2. When response status is ascertained, at the second decision point, responders are randomized to M_1 or M_2 and nonresponders to S_1 or S_2. Note that, at Decision 2, the randomization is restricted on the basis of responder status, in accordance with the fact that the maintenance (salvage) treatments are feasible only for subjects who responded (or not) to their assigned induction therapies.

The eight treatment sequence regimes of the form "Give C_j followed by M_k if response or S_ℓ if no response" in (13.8) are represented in the trial in the sense that there are "paths" through the schematic in Figure 13.2 corresponding to each regime. The regimes are thus said to be *embedded* in the SMART. Thus, a SMART yields data ideally suited to studying the embedded regimes; we describe methods for estimating mean outcomes associated with embedded regimes in the next section.

In addition to serving a natural framework for studying embedded regimes, a SMART can also provide data to inform the development of more complex, personalized (dynamic) regimes and estimation of the optimal regime in such a class. In particular, at baseline (Decision 1), rich patient information should be collected, and in the intervening periods between subsequent decision points, extensive longitudinal patient variables and characteristics should be recorded. The information collected should include all patient variables that potentially could be relevant tailoring variables. The resulting data set will be an ideal resource for this purpose, as we discuss below and in Section 13.6.

There is an extensive, evolving literature on design considerations for SMARTs [1, 3, 13, 14, 31–33, 40, 41, 43]. Clearly, design of a SMART is more complex than that of a conventional, single decision trial. Accordingly, a basic principle is to keep the design simple and straightforward. Pure randomization to all options at each decision point is preferred. If feasibility considerations require restricting randomization to subsets of options, this should be based on low-dimensional information; e.g., the single variable response status in our example in Figure 13.2. There is currently no consensus on criteria to be used for sample size determination. A common approach is to base sample size on a simple, primary hypothesis; e.g., comparison of the treatment options at Decision 1, which in our example can be interpreted as comparing sequences that start with C_1 with those starting with C_2. Other primary aims sometimes considered are to compare, for instance, the feasible options for responders at Decision 2, M_1 and M_2, or to compare embedded regimes; see the above references for discussion. When sample size is based on the latter, sample size calculators are available based on methods of the type we discuss in the next section. An overview of considerations for SMARTs in cancer research is given in [24].

A natural alternative to a SMART, in the context of our example, is an eight-arm trial in which subjects are randomized "up front" to follow each of the eight embedded regimes. That is, a patient randomized to, say, "Give C_1 followed by M_1 if response or S_1 if no response" would first receive C_1. If he responds, he would then receive M_1; if not, he would receive S_1, and similarly for the other seven embedded regimes. In principle, there is no real conceptual difference between a SMART and this design. In a SMART, there will be subjects whose realized treatment experiences under their sequentially randomized treatments are consistent with following each of the embedded regimes, so that, ultimately, all subjects may be viewed as being randomized to the eight regimes. One advantage of a SMART is the opportunity to randomize at decision points subsequent to the first based on factors such as response status that evolve during the study to achieve better balance in the numbers of subjects following each of the embedded regimes. There may be other advantages of a SMART in the context of securing patient consent; see the above references.

In the behavioral sciences, dynamic treatment regimes are referred to as *adaptive treatment strategies* [10], which has led to some confusion about the difference between a SMART and an adaptive clinical trial for classical, single decision treatment comparisons. An adaptive trial is one in which the accruing data from all participants are used to alter the design; e.g., to drop a treatment arm, change randomization probabilities, or modify the sample size. The design of a SMART does not change throughout its conduct, and it is focused on deducing strategies (regimes) for treating single patients, without regard to other subjects in a study.

The observed data on a subject in a SMART in which rich patient information is collected throughout can be written, for general K, as

$$(X_1, A_1, X_2, A_2, \ldots, X_K, A_K, Y), \tag{13.16}$$

where X_1 is baseline information as before; X_k, $k = 2, \ldots, K$, is observed patient information collected between decisions $k-1$ and k; A_k, $k = 1, \ldots, K$, is the treatment received at Decision k; and Y is the observed outcome. As in the single decision case, to study optimal, multiple decision regimes, it must be possible to express quantities involving potential patient information and outcomes in terms of the observed data (13.16).

For definiteness, take $K = 2$ and consider a situation with two treatment options at each decision, coded as 0 or 1 at each; i.e., $\mathcal{A}_1 = \{0, 1\}$ and $\mathcal{A}_2 = \{0, 1\}$. Then $X_2^{(0)}$ and $X_2^{(1)}$ are the potential intermediate information that a randomly chosen patient would achieve if he or she received option 0 or 1 at Decision 1, respectively. Likewise, $Y^{(0,0)}$ is the potential outcome that a patient would achieve if he or she received option 0 at Decision 1 and then option 0 at Decision 2, with $Y^{(0,1)}, Y^{(1,0)}$, and $Y^{(1,1)}$ defined similarly. Then

$$W = \{X_2^{(0)}, X_2^{(1)}, Y^{(0,0)}, Y^{(0,1)}, Y^{(1,0)}, Y^{(1,1)}\}$$

is the collection of all potential information and outcomes. A generalization of the consistency assumption discussed in the case of a single decision in Section 13.4.1 is that the observed intermediate information and outcome are those that potentially would be seen under the treatments received; i.e.,

$$X_2 = \sum_{a_1 \in \{0,1\}} X_2^{(a_1)} I(A_1 = a_1), \quad Y = \sum_{a_1, a_2 \in \{0,1\}} Y^{(a_1,a_2)} I(A_1 = a_1, A_2 = a_2).$$

In a SMART in which randomization at all decision points is unrestricted, as discussed above, by analogy to a classical clinical trial, this would guarantee $W \perp\!\!\!\perp A_1$ and $W \perp\!\!\!\perp A_2$. More generally, however, because at some decision points randomization is likely to be restricted depending on variables that are part of the accrued information, as in Figure 13.2, with $H_1 = X_1$ and $H_2 = (X_1, A_1, X_2)$, this may not hold. However, it is guaranteed that

$$W \perp\!\!\!\perp A_1 | H_1, \quad W \perp\!\!\!\perp A_2 | H_2. \tag{13.17}$$

For any regime d, it may be shown [50] that the consistency assumption and (13.17) allow $E\{Y^{(a_1,a_2)}\}$ for $a_1, a_2 = 0, 1$ and the value $E\{Y^{(d)}\}$ to be expressed in terms of the observed data. We demonstrate this in a particular case in the next section. These principles extend to general $K \geq 2$. This shows formally that data from a SMART are ideal for studying sequential treatment.

An alternative resource for studying regimes involving multiple decision points is data from a longitudinal observational study; e.g., a cohort study or registry. As with a single decision, there is the potential for confounding, but now at *each* decision point where treatment is given. In this case, it must be *assumed* that (13.17) holds to allow expression of quantities like $E\{Y^{(d)}\}$ in terms of the observed data. From this point of view, (13.17) is referred to as the *sequential randomization assumption* and can be thought of as a generalization of the no unmeasured confounders assumption (13.14) to $K > 1$ decision points and interpreted in an observational study as saying that treatment decisions depend only on a patient's accrued information and not on his or her prognosis. As above, the sequential randomization assumption holds by design for a SMART but is not verifiable from the data from an observational study. Indeed, (13.17) and its extensions to $K > 2$ may be suspect for a study that was not designed for the purpose of evaluating dynamic treatment regimes, as having confidence that the recorded, observed patient information $X_1, X_2, \ldots, X_K$ includes all variables used by clinicians and patients to make treatment decisions is difficult. Thus, the advantages of a SMART over an observational study for studying treatment regimes are considerable.

13.4.3 Inference on Embedded Regimes in a SMART

We demonstrate the foregoing principles in the context of cancer treatment by considering a certain type of SMART that has been conducted in cancer research, although not for the purpose of studying dynamic treatment regimes. Figure 13.3 depicts the design of Cancer and Leukemia Group B (CALGB) Protocol 8923 [51], which was a double-blind, placebo-controlled trial involving $n = 338$ elderly subjects with acute myelogenous leukemia (AML) and $K = 2$ decision points. At Decision 1, subjects were randomized to either standard induction chemotherapy C_1 or standard therapy augmented by granulocyte-macrophage colony-stimulating factor (GM-CSF) C_2. Subjects who responded to their assigned induction therapies were then randomized to one of two intensification treatments M_1 and M_2. In contrast to the trial in Figure 13.2,

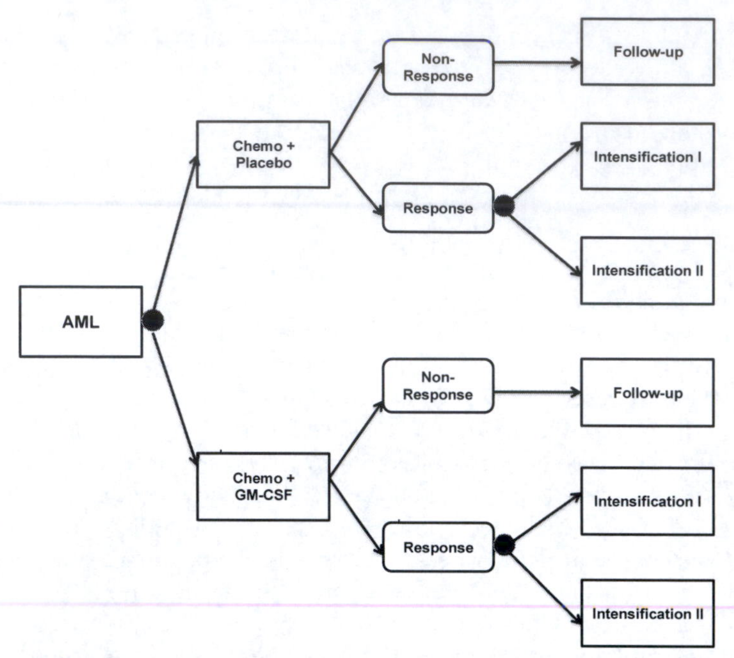

FIGURE 13.3: Schematic of the SMART design used in CALGB 8923. Bullets represent points of randomization.

there was only one option for subjects who did not respond, to follow up with the treating clinician. There was no protocol-specified treatment for patients who did not respond; thus, these subjects were not randomized, and many received other treatments according to best practices at the time at the clinician's discretion. All subjects were followed for a survival outcome.

Trials like CALGB 8923 are common in leukemia, and standard analyses include comparison of the response rates to Decision 1 induction therapies, comparison of survival outcomes between Decision 2 intensification treatments among responders, and comparison of survival between induction therapies regardless of response status. None of these analyses addresses questions regarding treatment sequences (treatment regimes). In CALGB 8923, there are four possible sequences, and thus four embedded regimes of the form

$$d^{(jk)} = \text{"Give } \mathsf{C}_j \text{ followed by } \mathsf{M}_k \text{ if response else follow up with clinician,"} \tag{13.18}$$

for $j, k = 1, 2$. Letting the class of regimes of interest $\mathcal{D}$ comprise the four regimes in (13.18), the relevant treatment sequence question is to find the regime in $\mathcal{D}$ such that, if all patients in the population were to receive treatment according to it, mean survival time would be the largest. That is, if we define $Y^{(d^{(jk)})}$ to be the potential survival outcome that a randomly chosen patient from the population would achieve if he or she were to receive treatment according regime $d^{(jk)}$, $j, k = 1, 2$, analogous to the development at the beginning of Section 13.3.2, we would like to estimate $E\{Y^{(d^{(jk)})}\}$, $j,k=1,2$, and deduce the largest. We focus on mean survival; by redefining the outcome to be $I\{Y^{(d^{(jk)})} > t\}$, survival probabilities can also be studied [36].

Before we discuss how to represent and estimate $E\{Y^{(d^{(jk)})}\}$ in terms of the observed data, we highlight some unique features of studying treatment sequences. Consider first two patients, each of whom receives treatment according to the regime in (13.18) with $j,k=1$. The first receives C_1, responds, and receives M_1. The second patient also receives C_1 but does not respond and follows up with his/her clinician. Note that these realized experiences are both consistent with having followed this regime. This demonstrates that individuals following the same regime can have different realized treatment experiences. Conversely, individuals who follow different regimes can have the same realized experience. For example, consider the experience of receiving C_1, not responding, and following up with the clinician. This experience could result from following the regimes of form (13.18) with $j=1$ and $k=1$ or 2.

These observations can be exploited to improve efficiency of inferences on $E\{Y^{(d^{(jk)})}\}$ for $j,k=1,2$. In particular, if a four-arm trial were conducted, with subjects randomized up front to follow one of the four regimes in (13.18), the conventional analysis would use only the data from subjects randomized to each arm to estimate the relevant mean outcomes. As we now demonstrate, it is possible to use data from all subjects whose realized experience is consistent with following each of the four embedded regimes. To emphasize the main ideas, we assume that there is no censoring, but see below.

Because we focus on the four embedded regimes, baseline information X_1 is not relevant, and of the intervening information X_2, only R, an indicator of response status, is relevant, where $R=1$ if a subject responds to his or her Decision 1 induction therapy, and $R=0$ otherwise. By convention, subjects who die before having a chance to respond are regarded as nonresponders.

To simplify notation, consider $j=1$ ($j=2$ is analogous) and a subject for whom $A_1=1$ (i.e., received C_1). Write the relevant remaining portion of the observed data as (R, A_2, Y), where Y is the observed survival outcome. Note that A_2 can take on possible values "follow up with clinician," M_1, or M_2, which we code as {0, 1, 2}, where the last two are feasible only if the subject is a responder to C_1. Suppose that responders are randomized to M_1 and M_2 with probabilities π and $1-\pi$, so that $\text{pr}(A_2=1|R=1)=\pi$; for nonresponders, $A_2=0$ by definition, so $\text{pr}(A_2=0|R=0)=1$.

The potential outcomes relevant when $A_1=1$ are $Y^{(d^{(11)})}$ and $Y^{(d^{(12)})}$; thus, we consider how to express their expectations in terms of these observed data. A subject who would not respond to C_1, so for whom $R=0$, would not go on to receive either of M_1 or M_2; rather, he or she would be treated at the clinician's discretion. Such a subject's experience, receiving C_1, not responding, and following up with the treating clinician, would be consistent with having followed either of the two regimes that assign M_1 or M_2 to responders. Thus, his or her potential outcomes under regimes $d^{(11)}$ or $d^{(12)}$ would be the same, as he or she would have this same experience following either of these regimes. Accordingly, when $R = 0$, $Y^{(d^{(11)})}$ and $Y^{(d^{(12)})}$ are the same, and a relevant consistency assumption is then

$$Y = (1 - R)Y^{(d^{(11)})} + RI(A_2 = 1)Y^{(d^{(11)})} + RI(A_2 = 2)Y^{(d^{(12)})}, \quad (13.19)$$

where $Y^{(d^{(11)})}$ in the first term could be replaced by $Y^{(d^{(12)})}$ because $Y^{(d^{(11)})} = Y^{(d^{(12)})}$ when $R = 0$ but are possibly different if $R = 1$.

Suppose that we have iid data (R_i, A_{2i}, Y_i), $i = 1, \ldots, n$. We deduce an estimator for $E\{Y^{(d^{(11)})}\}$ that is in the form of a weighted average of outcomes from all subjects i whose realized experience is consistent with following the regime (13.18) with $j = k = 1$; that for $E\{Y^{(d^{(12)})}\}$ can be deduced analogously. Take $\pi = 1/2$; then, ideally, half of the responders are assigned to M_1 in the SMART, and half to M_2. All nonresponders to C_1 are not randomized and follow up with their clinicians. Thus, all nonresponders represent themselves in the average, so receive a weight of 1. Each responder who is randomized to M_1 represents him/herself and another subject who was assigned by chance instead to M_2 but who could have received M_1; accordingly, he or she receives a weight of $2 = \pi^{-1}$. In general, these considerations suggest that the outcome for each subject who received C_1 at Decision 1 be weighted by

$$U = 1 - R + RI(A_2 = 1)\pi^{-1}. \quad (13.20)$$

It is straightforward to see that $U = 1$ if $R = 0$; $U = \pi^{-1}$ if $R = 1$ and $A_2 = 1$; and $U = 0$ if $R = 0$ and $A_2 = 2$, in which case the subject's realized experience is not consistent with having followed regime (13.18) with $j = k = 1$.

It can then be shown that $E\{Y^{(d^{(11)})}\} = E(UY)$, so can be expressed in terms of the observed Y and U. Substituting (13.19) and (13.20) and using $R(1 - R) = 0$, $I(A_2 = 1)I(A_2 = 2) = 0$, and so on yields

$$\begin{aligned} E(UY) = & \; E[Y^{(d^{(11)})}\{(1 - R) + RI(A_2 = 1)\pi^{-1}\}] \\ = & \; E[Y^{(d^{(11)})} \, E\{(1 - R) + RI(A_2 = 1)\pi^{-1}|R, Y^{(d^{(11)})}\}]. \quad (13.21) \end{aligned}$$

The inner expectation in (13.21) satisfies

$$\begin{aligned} & E\{(1 - R) + RI(A_2 = 1)\pi^{-1}|R, Y^{(d^{(11)})}\} \\ & \quad = E[(1 - R) + R\pi^{-1}E\{I(A_2 = 1)|R, Y^{(d^{(11)})}\}] = 1, \end{aligned}$$

which follows because, by randomization of responders at Decision 2, assignment to M_1 is independent of $Y^{(d^{(11)})}$, so that $E\{ I(A_2 = 1)|R = 1, Y^{(d^{(11)})}\} = \text{pr}(A_2 = 1|R = 1, Y^{(d^{(11)})}) = \text{pr}(A_2 = 1|R = 1) = \pi$. Substituting this in (13.21) yields $E\{Y^{(d^{(11)})}\} = E(UY)$, as desired and suggests estimating $E\{Y^{(d^{(11)})}\}$ by

$$n^{-1}\sum_{i=1}^{n} U_i Y_i \quad \text{or} \quad \left(\sum_{i=1}^{n} U_i\right)^{-1} \sum_{i=1}^{n} U_i Y_i \quad (13.22)$$

Estimators for $E\{Y^{(d^{(12)})}\}$, $E\{Y^{(d^{(21)})}\}$, and $E\{Y^{(d^{(22)})}\}$ analogous to those in (13.22) can be derived similarly. It follows from the derivations above that these estimators are consistent. Moreover, because the estimators for $E\{Y^{(d^{(j1)})}\}$ and $E\{Y^{(d^{(j2)})}\}$ for $j = 1$ or 2 both use data from all nonresponder subjects to C_j, they are correlated and are thus jointly asymptotically normal. These large sample results can be used to derive test statistics to compare $E\{Y^{(d^{(11)})}\}$, $j, k = 1, 2$, and deduce the optimal regime in the class; see [36].

These developments can be generalized to incorporate censoring by including an additional weight involving the censoring distribution and to arbitrary numbers of decisions K and options at each, and alternative estimators that improve on the efficiency of those in (13.22) are possible. See [16, 36, 40, 59, 60] for further developments for treatment regimes embedded in a SMART.

13.5 Thinking in Terms of Dynamic Treatment Regimes

In clinical research, complex questions arise that can not be addressed straightforwardly using conventional statistical models and methods. This is especially the case following completion of a clinical trial. As we now discuss, these questions can be cast as questions about appropriately defined dynamic treatment regimes. For example, in many cancer trials, assigned treatment is administered until disease progression; occurrence of a serious adverse event, at which point discontinuation of treatment is mandatory; or patient refusal to continue, and a question of interest may be how the study treatments compare if all subjects were to follow their assigned treatments. We present two examples that illustrate how this and related questions can be addressed by taking the perspective of treatment regimes. Although the examples are in the context of cardiovascular disease, they demonstrate the considerations involved, which may also be relevant to other challenges in cancer research.

As reported in [66], the SYNERGY trial randomized almost 10,000 subjects with acute coronary syndromes who were likely to undergo a cardiovascular procedure to the anticoagulant agents unfractionated heparin (UFH, control) and enoxaparin. An outcome of interest was time to death or myocardial infarction within one year. Because the routes of administration of UFH and enoxaparin are very different (bolus followed by infusion versus a series of subcutaneous injections at 12-hour intervals), the trial was not blinded. Per protocol, assigned drug was to be continued until the treating clinician deemed the subject to require no further anticoagulation, at which point the subject would be considered to have completed study treatment. The protocol also mandated immediate discontinuation of treatment if the subject experienced a serious adverse event or was to undergo surgery, as anticoagulation can be life-threatening under these conditions.

The primary, intent-to-treat analysis of the trial data did not show evidence of a difference, which was in contradiction to previous trials comparing these agents in other patient populations that concluded enoxaparin to be superior. The negative result could be attributed to the fact that the SYNERGY population was a sicker, more high risk group; alternatively, there was concern that it was a consequence of the considerable proportion of subjects in both treatment arms who switched from their assigned treatments to the other study drug or stopped altogether prior to completion. Such discontinuation of assigned treatment was differential by arm; because the trial was not blinded, treating clinicians easily were able to incorporate their preferences, resulting in more switching from enoxaparin to UFH than vice versa.

The investigators were thus interested in the treatment difference with respect to the outcome "had no subject discontinued his or her assigned treatment." Because in practice, as in the trial, both drugs would require immediate discontinuation in the case of an adverse event or procedure, the question as stated is not realistic. Thus, a careful definition of what is really meant by this question is required. This is facilitated by conceiving of two dynamic treatment regimes corresponding to each agent of the form

> "Take enoxaparin (UFH) until completion or discontinuation for mandatory reasons;"

here, the decision on whether or not to complete treatment is based on the binary variable indicating the occurrence of an event making discontinuation mandatory.

Thus, the question of interest can be addressed by comparing these two treatment regimes on the basis of the observed data. The data are observational with respect to this question, because, although some subjects did discontinue assigned treatment for mandatory reasons (and thus followed the associated treatment regime), others discontinued at the discretion of the treating clinician. Accordingly, such discretionary, or "optional," discontinuation may be confounded with patient characteristics, so that a valid approach to this problem requires a version of the sequential randomization assumption. As discussed in [66], common analyses that attempt to "adjust" for discontinuation do not distinguish between the two types of discontinuation, mandatory and optional, and consequently cannot yield valid inference on the comparison of the two regimes. In SYNERGY, completion and discontinuation times and reasons for discontinuation were recorded. In [66], a potential outcomes framework is established along with an appropriate sequential randomization assumption that allow derivation of valid estimators for mean potential outcome under each regime using these data, which are are similar in spirit to those discussed for embedded regimes in Section 13.4.3, involving weighting of observed outcomes. However, instead of involving randomization probabilities, the weighting is based on probabilities of continuing to receive assigned treatment without optionally discontinuing for discretionary reasons, which are modeled and estimated. The weighting thus takes into account confound-

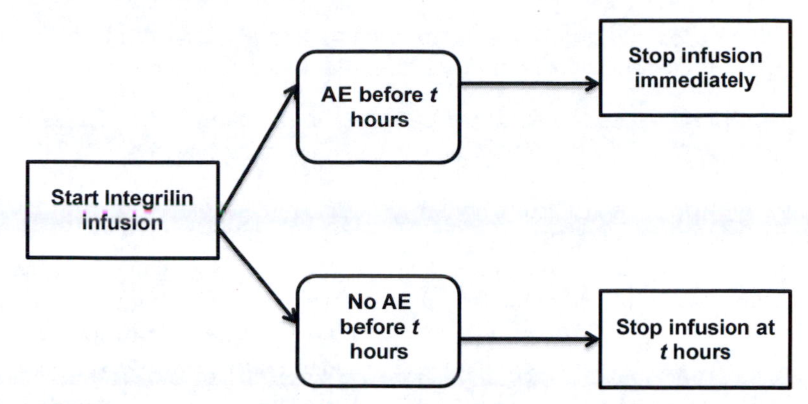

FIGURE 13.4: Schematic of a treatment duration regimes of duration t.

ing over time in a manner similar to that achieved by weighting by propensity scores; e.g., [35]. See [66] for details.

Our second example involves identifying an optimal duration of treatment; similar ideas could be relevant to questions regarding the optimal number of courses or dose of cancer therapies. Johnson and Tsiatis [21] discuss the ESPRIT trial, which randomized 2064 subjects with coronary artery disease who were scheduled to undergo percutaneous coronary intervention with stent implantation to two treatments: the anti-platelet therapy eptifibatide (Integrilin) or placebo. Integrilin and placebo were administered as a bolus injection followed by an infusion for 18–24 hours, where the protocol left the actual planned length of the infusion to the discretion of the treating clinician. The protocol also mandated that the infusion be stopped prior to completion if the subject experienced any one of a number of specified serious adverse events for which continued treatment with an anti-platelet therapy could be life-threatening. The outcome of interest was an indicator of whether or not a subject died or experienced a myocardial infarction or urgent target vessel revascularization within 30 days of treatment. The primary, intent-to-treat analysis based on this outcome suggested that Integrilin is superior to placebo.

Given the evidence favoring Integrilin, a natural follow-up question was to establish a recommended treatment duration (infusion length) for future patients. Clearly, in practice, as in the trial, it would be mandatory to terminate Integrilin therapy if a serious adverse event occurs. Accordingly, a realistic, precise definition of "recommended treatment duration" must acknowledge this. In particular, a recommended treatment duration of t hours necessarily must mean "Infuse for t hours or until an adverse event requiring discontinuation of treatment, whichever comes first." It should be evident that, for a given t, this can be interpreted as a dynamic treatment regime as in Figure 13.4. Here, realized length of the infusion, so whether or not the infusion lasts the full t hours or is curtailed, depends on the variable adverse event status. From this perspective, the question of recommended treatment duration can then be formulated as finding the optimal treatment regime in the class

$\mathcal{D}$ = { all regimes of the form "infuse for t hours or until an adverse event requiring discontinuation, whichever comes first" for $18 \leq t \leq 24$ };

that is, finding $t^{opt} \in [18, 24]$ leading to the largest mean outcome (probability of no event within 30 days).

Given this precise statement of the objective, the challenge is to use the data from the completed clinical trial to identify t^{opt}. Although subjects were randomized to receive Integrilin, the intended treatment durations were selected at the discretion of clinicians. Thus, the data are observational with respect to this question in that the chosen durations may be confounded with subject characteristics; e.g., clinicians may have selected shorter or longer intended durations based on the health status of the subjects. In [21], a potential outcomes framework and appropriate sequential randomization assumption are defined, and, taking the interval of possible t to be discrete, involving only integer values t_j, say, weighted estimators for the mean potential survival time corresponding to regimes in $\mathcal{D}$ for each t_j are developed. The weighting for each t_j is based on the probabilities of continuing to receive the infusion through time t_j as a function of accrued information, which are modeled and estimated. See [21, 22] for details.

In summary, these examples illustrate how thinking in terms of dynamic treatment regimes can clarify the statement of complex treatment questions. Through an associated potential outcomes formulation, this can lead to valid inferences addressing these questions.

13.6 Optimal Treatment Regimes for Personalized Medicine

13.6.1 Characterizing an Optimal Regime

We now consider data-based discovery of the optimal dynamic treatment regime in the class $\mathcal{D}$ of all possible regimes discussed at the end of Section 13.2.2, which has implications for personalized medicine. As the basis for estimators for the optimal regime d^{opt} in this class for both single and multiple decisions, discussed in the next two sections, we first characterize d^{opt}.

Consider first the case of a single decision discussed in Section 13.3.1, where, in the context of Decision 1 of our example, the two induction therapies C_1 and C_2 are coded as $\{0, 1\}$. Here, $\mathcal{D}$ is the class of all regimes d with a single rule $d_1(h_1)$ taking as input baseline information $h_1 = x_1$, where no restrictions are placed on the form of $d_1(h_1)$. With X_1 denoting as before observed baseline information for a randomly chosen patient in the population, recall from (13.10) that the potential outcome that would be achieved by such a patient if he or she received treatment according to d is can be written as $Y^{(d)} = Y^{(1)}d_1(H_1) + Y^{(0)}\{1 - d_1(H_1)\}$, where $H_1 = X_1$.

We now characterize d^{opt} maximizing the value $E\{Y^{(d)}\}$ in terms of both potential outcomes and observed data (X_1, A_1, Y) as in Section 13.4.1, where $Y = Y^{(1)}A_1 + Y^{(0)}(1 - A_1)$ by the consistency assumption. Assume that the data are from a clinical trial or an observational study in which it is reasonable to adopt the no unmeasured confounders assumption $(Y^{(0)}, Y^{(1)}) \perp\!\!\!\perp A_1|H_1$ in (13.14), which is, of course, trivially true for a clinical trial.

Under these conditions, it is straightforward that

$$E\{Y^{(d)}\} = E[\, E\{Y^{(d)}|H_1\}\,]$$
$$= E[E\{Y^{(1)}|H_1\}d_1(H_1) + E\{Y^{(0)}|H_1\}\{1 - d_1(H_1)\}] \tag{13.23}$$
$$= E[E(Y|H_1, A_1 = 1)d_1(H_1) + E(Y|H_1, A_1 = 0)\{1 - d_1(H_1)\}], \tag{13.24}$$

where (13.24) follows by the no unmeasured confounders assumption and calculations as in (13.15). Recalling that larger outcomes are preferred, from (13.23), it is immediate that the value $E\{Y^{(d)}\}$ will be maximized if the rule $d_1(h_1)$ is such that it selects treatment 1 if $E\{Y^{(1)}|H_1 = h_1\} > E\{Y^{(0)}|H_1 = h_1\}$ and 0 if $E\{Y^{(1)}|H_1 = h_1\} \leq E\{Y^{(0)}|H_1 = h_1\}$ for any h_1, which implies that the rule defining the optimal regime d^{opt} is

$$d_1^{opt}(h_1) = I[E\{Y^{(1)}|H_1 = h_1\} > E\{Y^{(0)}|H_1 = h_1\}]. \tag{13.25}$$

That is, the optimal decision is to select the treatment option that makes a patient's expected potential outcome given his or her baseline information as large as possible.

We highlight an important philosophical point: the difference between the *optimal treatment* and an *optimal decision* for a patient. There is a true, optimal treatment for each patient, that for which the corresponding potential outcome is largest. In our example, the true, optimal treatment is $I(Y^{(1)} > Y^{(0)})$. However, at the time treatment is selected, how a patient will fare on either treatment, and thus $Y^{(1)}$ and $Y^{(0)}$, is not known. Accordingly, we can not identify the optimal treatment for a patient. The best we can hope to do is to make an optimal decision, selecting the treatment option that leads to the largest expected outcome based on the information available.

Although (13.25) makes intuitively clear the form of the optimal regime, it is expressed in terms of potential outcomes. If we are to be able to estimate d^{opt}, it must be equivalently expressed in terms of the observed data. It follows from (13.24) that

$$d_1^{opt}(h_1) = I\{E(Y|H_1, A_1 = 1) > E(Y|H_1, A_1 = 0)\}. \tag{13.26}$$

Thus, the optimal rule may be represented in terms of the regression of outcome on $H_1 = X_1$ and A_1, suggesting that the optimal regime may be estimated using regression methods, as discussed in the next section. Note from

(13.24) that the value associated with any regime, including d^{opt}, can be expressed in terms of the observed data in a closed form.

Now consider the multiple decision case; we again focus on $K = 2$ and the situation in Section 13.4.2 with treatment options $\mathcal{A}_1 = \{0, 1\}$ and $\mathcal{A}_2 = \{0, 1\}$. Here, $\mathcal{D}$ is the class of all regimes d with rules $d_1(h_1)$ and $d_2(h_2)$ taking as input baseline information $h_1 = x_1$ and accrued information $h_2 = (x_1, a_1, x_2)$, with no restrictions on the form of either rule. In this case, $Y^{(d)}$ can be represented as in Section 13.3.2 in terms of potential information and outcome, and we again wish to characterize d^{opt} maximizing the value $E\{Y^{(d)}\}$.

It is possible to characterize d^{opt} in terms of the potential outcomes $W = \{X_2^{(0)}, X_2^{(1)}, Y^{(0,0)}, Y^{(0,1)}, Y^{(1,0)}, Y^{(1,1)}\}$ defined in Section 13.4.2; however, the formulation is somewhat complicated, so we do not present it here. It is shown in [50] that, as in the single decision case, it possible to express d^{opt} equivalently in terms of observed data (X_1, A_1, X_2, A_2, Y) from a SMART or observational study under the sequential randomization assumption in (13.17), which, of course, holds by design in a SMART. Both representations follow from the principle of *backward induction*, which underlies so-called reinforcement learning methods for sequential decision making developed in the computer science literature [53, 62]. With $H_1 = X_1$ and $H_2 = (X_1, A_1, X_2)$ as before, the characterization is as follows and works backward from the final decision.

Consider Decision 2. At this point, a patient has already accrued information h_2, so the best decision that can be made is to choose the treatment option in $\mathcal{A}_2$ that makes the patient's expected outcome as large as possible given this accrued information. In terms of the observed data, we thus have

$$d_2^{opt}(h_2) = I\{E(Y|H_2 = h_2, A_2 = 1) > E(Y|H_2 = h_2, A_2 = 0)\}. \quad (13.27)$$

Denote the maximized expected outcome under the option dictated by $d_2^{opt}(h_2)$ by

$$\widetilde{Y}_2(h_2) = \max\{E(Y|H_2 = h_2, A_2 = 1), E(Y|H_2 = h_2, A_2 = 0)\}. \quad (13.28)$$

At Decision 1, the best decision that can be made is to choose the treatment option in $\mathcal{A}_1$ that makes the patient's expected outcome as large as possible given the baseline information h_1 on the patient while also acknowledging that, at Decision 2 in the future, based on the accrued information at that point, the regime will choose the treatment option in $\mathcal{A}_2$ that maximizes expected outcome. This is the basis for the optimal rule

$$d_1^{opt}(h_1) = I[E\{\widetilde{Y}_2(H_2)|H_1 = h_1, A_1 = 1\} > E\{\widetilde{Y}_2(H_2)|H_1 = h_1, A_1 = 0\}]. \quad (13.29)$$

The optimal regime is then $d^{opt} = \{d_1^{opt}(h_1), d_2^{opt}(h_2)\}$. The maximized expected outcome under the options dictated by $d_1^{opt}(h_1)$ and $d_2^{opt}(h_2)$ in the future is then

$$\widetilde{Y}_1(h_1) = \max[E\{\widetilde{Y}_2(H_2)|H_1 = h_1, A_1 = 1\}, E\{\widetilde{Y}_2(H_2)|H_1 = h_1, A_1 = 0\}]. \tag{13.30}$$

It can be shown [50] that in fact the value of d^{opt} $E\{Y^{(d^{opt})}\} = E\{\widetilde{Y}_1(H_1)\}$. The expressions (13.28) and (13.30) are referred to as the *value functions.*

This formulation extends to arbitrary K and $\mathcal{A}_k$, $k = 1, \ldots, K$; see [50].

13.6.2 Regression-based Estimation of an Optimal Regime

From the results in the previous section, approaches to estimation of the optimal regime may be deduced. Consider first a single decision. Inspection of the form of (13.25) suggests immediately that the optimal rule $d_1^{opt}(h_1)$ comprising d^{opt} can be estimated by positing and fitting a regression model $Q_1(h_1, a_1; \beta_1)$ based on the observed data as at the end of Section 13.4.1 and substituting in (13.25), yielding the estimator

$$\widehat{d}_1^{opt}(h_1) = I\{Q_1(h_1, 1; \widehat{\beta}_1) > Q_1(h_1, 0; \widehat{\beta}_1)\}. \tag{13.31}$$

Using (13.24), it follows that the value $E\{Y^{(d^{opt})}\}$ can be estimated by

$$\widehat{V}(d^{opt}) = \sum_{i=1}^{n} \Big[Q_1(H_{1i}, 1; \widehat{\beta}_1)\widehat{d}_1^{opt}(H_{1i}) + Q_1(H_{1i}, 0; \widehat{\beta}_1)\{1 - \widehat{d}_1^{opt}(H_{1i})\}\Big].$$

Now consider the case of two decisions. The scheme to estimate d^{opt} follows from the backward induction argument and is referred to as *Q-learning* [42]. First, for Decision 2, posit and fit a suitable regression model $Q_2(h_2, a_2; \beta_2)$ for $E(Y|H_2 = h_2, A_2 = a_2)$, obtaining an estimator $\widehat{\beta}_2$. Then, from (13.27), the estimator for the optimal rule at Decision 2 is

$$\widehat{d}_2^{opt}(h_2) = I\{Q_2(h_2, 1; \widehat{\beta}_2) > Q_2(h_2, 0; \widehat{\beta}_2)\}. \tag{13.32}$$

Note that the optimal rule (13.29) at Decision 1 depends on the regression of the value function (13.28) on H_1 and A_1. Thus, for each subject i, form the "predicted value"

$$\widehat{\widetilde{Y}}_{2i} = \widetilde{Y}_{2i}(H_{2i}; \widehat{\beta}_2) = \max\{Q_2(H_{2i}, 0; \widehat{\beta}_2), Q_2(H_{2i}, 1; \widehat{\beta}_2)\}.$$

Then posit a model $Q_1(h_1, a_1; \beta_1)$ for the "regression" of $\widehat{\widetilde{Y}}_2$ on H_1 and A_1 and fit it to the "data" $(H_{1i}, A_{1i}, \widehat{\widetilde{Y}}_{2i})$ to obtain $\widehat{\beta}_1$. The estimator for the optimal rule at Decision 1 is then

$$\widehat{d}_1^{opt}(h_1) = I\{Q_1(h_1, 1; \widehat{\beta}_1) > Q_1(h_1, 0; \widehat{\beta}_1)\}. \tag{13.33}$$

From (13.32) and (13.33), the estimator for the optimal regime is then $\widehat{d}^{opt} = \{\widehat{d}_1^{opt}(h_1), \widehat{d}_2^{opt}(h_2)\}$. Forming for each subject i

$$\widehat{\widetilde{Y}}_{1i} = \widetilde{Y}_1(H_{1i}; \widehat{\beta}_1) = \max\{Q_1(H_{1i}, 0; \widehat{\beta}_1), Q_1(H_{1i}, 1; \widehat{\beta}_1)\},$$

the value $E\{Y^{(d^{opt})}\}$ is estimated by

$$\widehat{V}(d^{opt}) = n^{-1}\sum_{i=1}^{n} \widehat{\widetilde{Y}}_{1i}.$$

In this context, the required regressions and the models used to represent them are often referred to as the *Q-functions.* In the case of a single decision, the Q-learning estimator for d^{opt} reduces to (13.31). The Q-learning algorithm given here can be extended to $K > 2$ decisions; see [50].

In both the single and multiple decision cases, the form of the rules in the estimated optimal regime is dictated by the posited regression models. This raises concern over the effects of model misspecification on the quality of estimation of the optimal regime and has led to proposals to use more flexible, nonparametric modeling techniques [37, 67]. Model misspecification is a particular concern for multiple decisions because, except at the final decision (Decision 2 here), the modeling task is nonstandard, as one is developing a model for the maximum in (13.28). Thus, standard parametric models such as linear models are almost certainly misspecified; see [50] for an example.

An additional complication is that inference on the estimated optimal regime cannot be made by appealing to standard asymptotic theory. Because of the involvement of the nonsmooth max operator, usual large sample theory calculations are not valid. See [7, 9, 27, 28] for details.

13.6.3 Alternative Methods

A number of alternative approaches to estimation of optimal treatment regimes have been proposed [2, 20, 38, 39, 44, 46, 47]. Here, we describe briefly one class of techniques that is applicable when interest focuses on an infinite but restricted class of regimes as discussed in Section 13.2.2.

Consider a single decision, and suppose that interest focuses on a restricted class of regimes $\mathcal{D}_\eta$ indexed by a parameter η, as in (13.9). Denote regimes in $\mathcal{D}_\eta$ by $d_\eta = \{d_1(h_1;\eta)\}$, which emphasizes that the rule comprising a regime depends on η. Let d_η^{opt} denote the optimal regime within $\mathcal{D}_\eta$, that maximizes the value $E\{Y^{(d_\eta)}\}$ among all regimes $d_\eta \in \mathcal{D}_\eta$. The idea behind *value search* or *policy search* estimators is to develop directly an estimator for the value $E\{Y^{(d_\eta)}\}$ as a function of η and then maximize the estimator in η.

Zhang et al. [64] propose estimators for $E\{Y^{(d_\eta)}\}$ for fixed η based on inverse probability weighting similar to that discussed earlier. The simplest estimator is motivated by viewing whether or not a patient's actual treatment A_1 is consistent with having received treatment according to the rule $d_1(h_1;\eta)$ as a missing data problem. If it is, then the observed outcome Y for that patient is equal to the potential outcome $Y^{(d_\eta)}$ that he or she would achieve if following d_η; otherwise, Y does not reflect outcome under d_η, so the outcome that would be achieved under d_η is missing. Letting

$$C_\eta = A_1 d_1(H_1;\eta) + (1 - A_1)\{1 - d_1(H_1,\eta)\},$$

it is clear that $C_\eta = 1$ if the patient's actual treatment is consistent with d_η and $C_\eta = 0$ otherwise. Let

$$\pi(h_1) = \text{pr}(A_1 = 1|H_1 = h_1)$$

be the propensity score for treatment; in a clinical trial, $\pi(h_1)$ is known and likely constant, but in an observational study is not known and must be modeled and estimated. It may be shown that

$$\pi_C(H_1;\eta) = \text{pr}(C_\eta = 1|H_1) = \pi(H_1)d_1(H_1;\eta) + \{1 - \pi(H_1)\}\{1 - d_1(H_1,\eta)\}.$$

Semiparametric theory for missing data problems [48, 58] then suggests an estimator for the value $E\{Y^{(d_\eta)}\}$ for fixed η given by

$$\widehat{V}(d_\eta) = n^{-1}\sum_{i=1}^{n} \frac{C_{\eta,i}Y_i}{\pi_C(H_{1i};\eta)}. \tag{13.34}$$

Under the consistency (13.11) and no unmeasured confounders (13.14) assumptions, it can be shown that $\widehat{V}(d_\eta)$ is a consistent estimator for the value $E\{Y^{(d_\eta)}\}$ for fixed η. More efficient estimators can be constructed by "augmenting" (13.34) by another mean zero term that also serves to make the estimator *doubly robust*; see [64].

The estimator for d_η^{opt} is found by maximizing (13.34) in η. This is a nonstandard optimization problem because $\widehat{V}(d_\eta)$ is a nonsmooth function of η. This can be appreciated by inspection of (13.9), which incorporates η inside the nonsmooth indicator function. Accordingly, specialized optimization methods are required, the challenges of which are discussed in [64]. This approach can be extended to multiple decisions [65], although it becomes unwieldy for $K > 3$ decision points.

Related methods are based on calculations that show that maximization of the value can be likened to a weighted classification problem [63, 70], with the regime playing the role of a classifier. The restricted class of regimes is induced by the family of classifiers chosen by the analyst, for example, classification and regression trees [6] or support vector machines [11].

See [68] for an overview of estimation of optimal treatment regimes.

13.7 Discussion

Cancer is a chronic, progressing disease for which sequential treatment decisions must be made. Much of cancer clinical research has focused on study of treatment at single decision points in isolation. Placing the study of cancer treatment in the context of dynamic treatment regimes provides a principled approach to comparing sequential treatment strategies. In addition, the dynamic treatment regime paradigm offers a conceptual and methodological framework for developing optimal, evidenced-based personalized cancer medicine.

SMARTs are an ideal study design for achieving these objectives. Clinical trials with two or more sequential randomizations have been conducted in cancer research [45, 51], although not with the goal of investigating dynamic treatment regimes. However, this demonstrates that such trials are logistically feasible with existing infrastructure. See [4, 54, 55, 57, 61, 67, 71] for accounts of the use of sequential randomization toward the goal of studying optimal treatment sequences and strategies in the cancer context. In particular, Thall et al. [54] describe a sequentially randomized trial in prostate cancer for the purpose of generating hypotheses regarding optimal sequences of treatment, and [61] present analyses focused on the embedded regimes. SMARTs have seen broad acceptance in the study of behavioral and mental health disorders [15, 23, 52]. See `http://methodology.psu.edu/ra/smart/projects` for a list of ongoing SMARTs in this area.

There are several challenges relevant to cancer clinical research for which further methodological development is required. Although some progress has been made on methods for estimation of optimal treatment regimes based on a censored survival outcome [69], extensions of methods such as Q-learning and value search estimators for optimal treatment regimes based on, for example, a proportional hazards formulation are required. A key consideration in cancer treatment is balancing competing outcomes, such as efficacy and toxicity, cost, or burden. A popular approach to competing outcomes is to develop a composite outcome; however, patient and clinician preference may be heterogeneous or evolve over time, making formulation of meaningful composites with which to define an optimal treatment regime problematic. Moreover, estimated optimal regimes based on different composite outcomes can differ substantially [3]. Thus, this problem requires alternative frameworks in which a suitable notion of optimality can be defined; this may entail developing regimes that are "nearly optimal" with respect to efficacy to take into account competing unfavorable outcomes. There has been some methodology along these lines [26, 56], but more development is needed. One approach might be to develop methods to maximize expected outcome for efficacy subject to a constraint on toxicity or cost.

A broad, unresolved issue for discovery of dynamic treatment regimes is methods for variable selection for building of relevant statistical models. Existing methods for variable selection in regression focus on minimizing prediction error, while the goal of variable selection in the treatment regime context is identification of tailoring variables important for decision making. Some work along these lines has taken place [5, 17–19, 34], and more is required.

Design considerations for SMARTs need further development. Of particular interest are methods applicable when a goal is to estimate an optimal treatment regime for personalized medicine; see [29].

Software implementing several of the methods for estimating an optimal regime discussed in this chapter and for design of SMARTs is available or under development. User-contributed R packages for comparison of the regimes embedded in a SMART (`DTR`) and for estimation of an optimal regime via Q-learning for two decisions points (`iqLearn`, `qLearn`) are available on the Comprehensive R Archive Network (CRAN), `http://cran.r-project.org/`. SAS and R implementations and sample size calculators are available at `http://methodology.psu.edu`. A comprehensive R package implementing both value search and Q-learning approaches for single and multiple decisions, `DynTxRegime`, is available on CRAN.

Recent books [8, 25] offer comprehensive overviews of concepts and methodology for dynamic treatment regimes.

Bibliography

[1] D. Almirall, S. N. Compton, M. Gunlicks-Stoessel, N. Duan, and S. A. Murphy. Designing a pilot sequential multiple assignment randomized trial for developing an adaptive treatment strategy. *Statistics in Medicine*, 31:1887–1902, 2012.

[2] D. Almirall, T. Ten Have, and S. A. Murphy. Structural nested mean models for assessing time-varying effect moderation. *Biometrics*, 66:131–139, 2010.

[3] D. Almirall, D. Lizotte, and S. A. Murphy. SMART design issues and the consideration of opposing outcomes, *Discussion of "Evaluation of Viable Dynamic Treatment Regimes in a Sequentially Randomized Trial of Advanced Prostate Cancer" by Wang et al. Journal of the American Statistical Association*, 107:509–512, 2012.

[4] S. F. Auyeung, Q. Long, E. B. Royster, S. Murthy, M. D. McNutt, D. Lawson, A. Miller, A. Manatunga, and D. L. Musselman. Sequential multiple-assignment randomized trial design of neurobehavioral treatment for patients with metastatic malignant melanoma undergoing high-dose interferon-alpha therapy. *Clinical Trials*, 6:480–490, 2009.

[5] P. Biernot and E. E. M. Moodie. A comparison of variable selection approaches for dynamic treatment regimes. *International Journal of Biostatistics*, 6, 2010.

[6] L. Breiman, J. H. Freidman, R. A. Olshen, and C. J. Stone. *Classification and Regression Trees.* Wadsworth, Belmont, CA, 1984.

[7] B. Chakraborty, E. B. Laber, and Y. Zhao. Inference for optimal dynamic treatment regimes using an adaptive m-out-of-n bootstrap scheme. *Biometrics*, 69:714–723, 2014.

[8] B. Chakraborty and E. E. M. Moodie. *Statistical Methods for Dynamic Treatment Regimes: Reinforcement Learning, Causal Inference, and Personalized Medicine.* Springer-Verlang, New York, NY, 2013.

[9] B. Chakraborty, S. A. Murphy, and V. Strecher. Inference for non-regular parameters in optimal dynamic treatment regimes. *Statistical Methods in Medical Research*, 19:317–343, 2010.

[10] L. M. Collins, S. A. Murphy, and K. Bierman. A conceptual framework for adaptive preventive interventions. *Prevention Science*, 5:185–196, 2004.

[11] C. Cortes and V. Vapnik. Support-vector networks. *Machine Learning*, 20:273–297, 1995.

[12] R. B. D'Agostino, Jr. Tutorial in biostatistics: Propensity score methods for bias reduction in the comparison of a treatment to a non-randomized control group. *Statistics in Medicine*, 17:2265–2281, 1998.

[13] R. Dawson and P. W. Lavori. Sample size calculations for evaluating treatment policies in multi-stage designs. *Clinical Trials*, 7:643–652, 2010.

[14] R. Dawson and P. W. Lavori. Efficient design and inference for multi-stage randomized trials of individualized treatment policies. *Biostatistics*, 13:142–152, 2012.

[15] M. Fava, A. J. Rush, M. H. Trivedi, A. A. Nierenberg, M. E. Thase, H. A. Sackeim, F. M. Quitkin, S. Wisniewski, P. W. Lavori, J. F. Rosenbaum, and D. J. Kupfer. Background and rationale for the Sequenced Treatment Alternatives to Relieve Depression (STAR*D) study. *Psychiatric Clinics of North America*, 26:457–494, 2003.

[16] W. Feng and A. S. Wahed. Sample size for two-stage studies with maintenance therapy. *Statistics in Medicine*, 28:2028–2041, 2009.

[17] L. Gunter, J. Zhu, and S. A. Murphy. Variable selection for optimal decision making. In *Proceedings of the 11th Conference on Artificial Intelligence in Medicine*, 2007.

[18] L. Gunter, J. Zhu, and S. A. Murphy. Variable selection for qualitative interactions. *Statistical Methodology*, 8:42–55, 2011.

[19] L. Gunter, J. Zhu, and S. A. Murphy. Variable selection for qualitative interactions in personalized medicine while controlling the family-wise error rate. *Journal of Biopharmaceutical Statistics*, 21:1063–1078, 2011.

[20] R. Henderson, P. Ansell, and D. Alshibani. Regret-regression for optimal dynamic treatment regimes. *Biometrics*, 66:1192–1201, 2010.

[21] B. A. Johnson and A. A. Tsiatis. Estimating mean response as a function of treatment duration in an observational study, where duration may be informatively censored. *Biometrics*, 60:315–323, 2004.

[22] B. A. Johnson and A. A. Tsiatis. Semiparametric inference in observational duration-response studies, with duration possibly right-censored. *Biometrika*, 92:605–618, 2005.

[23] C. Kasari, A. Kaiser, K. Goods, J. Nietfeld, P. Mathy, R. Landa, and D. Almirall. Communication interventions for minimally verbal children with autism: A sequential multiple assignment randomized trial. *Journal of the American Academy of Child and Adolescent Psychiatry*, 53:635–646, 2014.

[24] K. M. Kidwell. Smart designs in cancer research: learning from the past, current limitations and looking toward the future. *Clinical Trials*, 11:445–456, 2014.

[25] M. R. Kosorok and E. M. M. Moodie. *Dynamic Treatment Regimes in Practice: Planning Trials and Analyzing Data for Personalized Medicine.* SIAM, Philadelphia, PA, 2015.

[26] E. B. Laber, D. J. Lizotte, and B. Ferguson. Set-valued dynamic treatment regimes for competing outcomes. *Biometrics*, 70:53–61, 2014.

[27] E. B. Laber, D. J. Lizotte, M. Qian, W. E. Pelham, and S. A. Murphy. Dynamic treatment regimes: technical challenges and applications. *Electronic Journal of Statistics*, 8:1225–1271, 2014.

[28] E. B. Laber and S. A. Murphy. Adaptive confidence intervals for the test error in classification. *Journal of the American Statistical Association*, 106:904–913, 2011.

[29] E. B. Laber, Y. Zhao, T. Regh, M. Davidian, A. A. Tsiatis, J. Stanford, D. Zeng, R. Song, and M. R. Kosorok. Using pilot data to size a two-arm randomized trial to find a nearly optimal personalized treatment strategy. *Statistics in Medicine*, 2015 (in press).

[30] P. W. Lavori and R. Dawson. A design for testing clinical strategies: biased adaptive within-subject randomization. *Journal of the Royal Statistical Society: Series A*, 163:29–38, 2000.

[31] P. W. Lavori and R. Dawson. Dynamic treatment regimes: practical design considerations. *Clinical Trials*, 1:9–20, 2004.

[32] P. W. Lavori and R. Dawson. Sample size calculations for evaluating treatment policies in multi-stage designs. *Clinical Trials*, 7:643–652, 2010.

[33] Z. Li and S. A. Murphy. Sample size formulae for two-stage randomized trials with survival outcomes. *Biometrika*, 98:503–518, 2011.

[34] W. Lu, H. H. Zhang, and D. Zeng. Variable selection for optimal treatment decision. *Statistical Methods in Medical Research*, 22:493–504, 2013.

[35] J. K. Lunceford and M. Davidian. Stratification and weighting via the propensity score in estimation of causal treatment effects: A comparative study. *Statistics in Medicine*, 23:2937–2960, 2004.

[36] J. K. Lunceford, M. Davidian, and A. A. Tsiatis. Estimation of survival distributions of treatment policies in two-stage randomization designs in clinical trials. *Biometrics*, 58:48–57, 2002.

[37] E. E. M. Moodie, N. Dean, and Y. R. Sun. Q-learning: flexible learning about useful utilities. *Statistics in Biosciences*, 6(2):223–243, 2014.

[38] E. E. M. Moodie, T. S. Richardson, and D. A. Stephens. Demystifying optimal dynamic treatment regimes. *Biometrics*, 63:447–455, 2007.

[39] S. A. Murphy. Optimal dynamic treatment regimes (with discussions). *Journal of the Royal Statistical Society: Series B*, 65:331–366, 2003.

[40] S. A. Murphy. An experimental design for the development of adaptive treatment strategies. *Statistics in Medicine*, 24:1455–1481, 2005.

[41] I. Nahum-Shani, M. Qian, D. Almiral, W. Pelham, B. Gnagy, G. Fabiano, J. Waxmonsky, J. Yu, and S. A. Murphy. Experimental design and primary data analysis methods for comparing adaptive interventions. *Psychological Methods*, 17:457–477, 2012.

[42] I. Nahum-Shani, M. Qian, D. Almiral, W.. Pelham, B. Gnagy, G. Fabiano, J. Waxmonsky, J. Yu, and S. A. Murphy. Q-learning: a data analysis method for constructing adaptive interventions. *Psychological Methods*, 17:478–494, 2012.

[43] A. I. Oetting, J. A. Levy, R. D. Weiss, and S. A. Murphy. Statistical methodology for a smart design in the development of adaptive treatment strategies. In P.E. Shrout, K.M. Keyes, and K. Ornstein, editors, *Causality and Psychopathology: Finding the Determinants of Disorders and their Cures*, pages 179–205, Arlington, VA, 2011. American Psychiatric Publishing, Inc.

[44] L. Orellana, A. Rotnitzky, and J. M. Robins. Dynamic regime marginal structural mean models for estimation of optimal dynamic treatment regimes, Part I: Main Content. *International Journal of Biostatistics*, 6, 2010.

[45] B. L. Powell, B. Moser, W. Stock, R. E. Gallegher, C. L. Willman at R. M. Stone, J. M. Rowe, S. Coutre, J. H. Feusner, et al. Arsenic trioxide improves event-free and overall survival for adults with acute promyelocytic leukemia: North American Leukemia Intergroup Study C9710. *Blood*, 116:3751–3757, 2010.

[46] J. M. Robins. Optimal structural nested models for optimal sequential decisions. In D. Y. Lin and P. Heagerty, editors, *Proceedings of the Second Seattle Symposium on Biostatistics*, pages 189–326, New York, 2004. Springer.

[47] J. M. Robins, L. Orellana, and A. Rotnitzky. Estimation and extrapolation of optimal treatment and testing strategies. *Statistics in Medicine*, 27:4678–4721, 2008.

[48] J. M. Robins, A. Rotnitzky, and L. P. Zhao. Estimation of regression coefficients when some regressors are not always observed. *Journal of the American Statistical Association*, 89:846–866, 1994.

[49] P. R. Rosenbaum and D. B. Rubin. The central role of the propensity score in observational studies for causal effects. *Biometrika*, 70:41–55, 1983.

[50] P. J. Schulte, A. A. Tsiatis, E. B. Laber, and M. Davidian. Robust estimation of optimal dynamic treatment regimes for sequential treatment decisions. *Statistical Science*, 129:640–661, 2014.

[51] R. M. Stone, D. T. Berg, S. L. George, R. K. Dodge, P. A. Paciucci, P. Schulman, E. J. Lee, J. O. Moore, B. L. Powell, and C. A. Schiffer. Granulocyte macrophage colony-stimulating factor after initial chemotherapy for elderly patients with primary acute myelogenous leukemia. *New England Journal of Medicine*, 332:1671–1677, 1995.

[52] T. S. Stroup, J. P. McEvoy, M. S. Swartz, M. J. Byerly, I. D. Glick, J. M. Canive, M. McGee, G. M. Simpson, M. D. Stevens, and J. A. Lieberman. The National Institute of Mental Health clinical antipschotic trials of intervention effectiveness (CATIE) project: schizophrenia trial design and protocol deveplopment. *Schizophrenia Bulletin*, 29:15–31, 2003.

[53] R. S. Sutton and A. G. Barto. *Reinforcement Learning: An Introduction.* MIT Press, Cambridge, 1998.

[54] P. F. Thall, C. Logothetis, Lance C. Pagliaro, S. Wen, M. A. Brown, D. Williams, and R. E. Millikan. Adaptive therapy for androgen-independent prostate cancer: a randomized selection trial of four regimens. *Journal of the National Cancer Institute*, 99:1613–1622, 2007.

[55] P. F. Thall, R. E. Millikan, and H. G. Sung. Evaluating multiple treatment courses in clinical trials. *Statistics in Medicine*, 30:1011–1128, 2000.

[56] P. F. Thall, H. G. Sung, and E. H. Estey. Selecting therapeutic strategies based on efficacy and death in multicourse clinical trials. *Journal of the American Statistical Association*, 97:29–39, 2002.

[57] P. F. Thall, L. H. Wooten, C. J. Logothetis, R. E. Millikan, and N. M. Tannir. Bayesian and frequentist two-stage treatment strategies based on sequential failure times subject to interval censoring. *Statistics in Medicine*, 26:4687–4702, 2007.

[58] A. A. Tsiatis. *Semiparametric Theory and Missing Data*. Springer, New York, 2006.

[59] A. S. Wahed and A. A. Tsiatis. Optimal estimator for the survival distribution and related quantities for treatment policies in two-stage randomized designs in clinical trials. *Biometrics*, 60:124–133, 2004.

[60] A. S. Wahed and A. A. Tsiatis. Semiparametric efficient estimation of survival distributions in two-stage randomisation designs in clinical trials with censored data. *Biometrika*, 93:163–177, 2006.

[61] L. Wang, A. Rotnitzky, X. Lin, R. E. Millikan, and P. F. Thall. Evaluation of viable dynamic treatment regimes in a sequentially randomized trial of advanced prostate cancer. *Journal of the American Statistical Association*, 107:493–508, 2012.

[62] C. J. C. H. Watkins and P. Dayan. Q-learning. *Machine Learning*, 8:279–292, 1992.

[63] B. Zhang, A. A. Tsiatis, M. Davidian, M. Zhang, and E. B. Laber. Estimating optimal treatment regimes from a classification perspective. *Stat*, 1:103–114, 2012.

[64] B. Zhang, A. A. Tsiatis, E. B. Laber, and M. Davidian. A robust method for estimating optimal treatment regimes. *Biometrics*, 68:1010–1018, 2012.

[65] B. Zhang, A. A. Tsiatis, E. B. Laber, and M. Davidian. Robust estimation of optimal dynamic treatment regimes for sequential treatment decisions. *Biometrika*, 100:681–694, 2013.

[66] M. Zhang, A. A. Tsiatis, M. Davidian, K. S. Pieper, and K. W. Mahaffey. Inference on treatment effects from a clinical trial in the presence of premature treatment discontinuation: the SYNERGY trial. *Biostatistics*, 12:258–269, 2011.

[67] Y. Zhao, M. R. Kosorok, and D. Zeng. Reinforcement learning design for cancer clinical trials. *Statistics in Medicine*, 28:3294–3315, 2009.

[68] Y. Zhao and E. B. Laber. Estimation of optimal dynamic treatment regimes. *Clinical Trials*, 11:400–4077, 2014.

[69] Y. Zhao, D. Zeng, E. B. Laber, R. Song, M. Yuan, and M. R. Kosorok. Doubly robust learning for estimating individualized treatment with censored data. *Biometrika*, 102:151–168, 2015.

[70] Y. Zhao, D. Zeng, A. J. Rush, and M. R. Kosorok. Estimating individual treatment rules using outcome weighted learning. *Journal of the American Statistical Association*, 107:1106–1118, 2012.

[71] Y. Zhao, D. Zeng, M. A. Socinski, and M. R. Kosorok. Reinforcement learning strategies for clinical trials in nonsmall cell lung cancer. *Biometrics*, 67:1422–1433, 2011.

Index